Cancer Nursing

A Holistic Multidisciplinary Approach

Second Edition

nursing outline series

Ardelina A. Baldonado,
B.S.N., R.N., M.S., Ph.D.

Dulcelina Albano Stahl,
R.N., B.A., M.A., M.S., Ph.D., C.N.A.A.

 Medical Examination Publishing Co., Inc.
an Excerpta Medica company

Baldonado, Ardelina A.
   Cancer nursing.

   (Nursing outline series)
   Bibliography: p.
   Includes index.
   1. Cancer--Nursing. I. Stahl, Dulcelina
Albano. II. Title. III. Series: [DNLM:
1. Neoplasms--Nursing. 2. Holistic health--
Nursing texts.   WY 156 B178c]
RC266.B34   1982   610.73'698   82-2183
ISBN 0-87488-374-1   AACR2

Contents

Part V   COMMON MALIGNANCIES:
         DIAGNOSIS AND MANAGEMENT

Part VI   CANCER METASTASES AND MANAGEMENT

Part VII   APPLICATION OF A MULTIDISCIPLINARY
           APPROACH TO CARE OF THE CANCER PATIENT

About the Authors

ARDELINA A. BALDONADO, B.S.N., R.N., M.S., Ph.D.
Assistant Professor, Loyola University of Chicago, Chicago,
Illinois; Formerly Instructor, Medical-Surgical Nursing, Uni-
versity of Illinois, Chicago, Illinois; Acting Chairman, Second
Level Faculty and Instructional Program, St. Francis Hospital
School of Nursing, Evanston, Illinois; Nursing Instructor,
Passavant Memorial Hospital School of Nursing and Alexian
Brothers Hospital School of Nursing, Chicago, Illinois.

DULCELINA ALBANO STAHL, R.N., B.A., M.A., M.S.,
Ph.D., C.N.A.A.
Assistant Hospital Administrator for Clinical Services and
Director of Nursing Services, Olympia Fields Osteopathic
Medical Center Hospital, Olympia Fields, Illinois; Faculty,
Elmhurst College of Business Administration, Elmhurst,
Illinois; Formerly Adjunct Professor of Nursing, Rush Univer-
sity College of Nursing, Chicago, Illinois; Director of Nursing,
Bethany Hospital, Chicago, Illinois; Assistant Director of
Nursing, University of Illinois Hospital, Chicago, Illinois;
Vice-Chairperson, Faculty Organization and Chairperson Third
Level Faculty, South Chicago Community Hospital School of
Nursing, and Nursing Instructor, Michael Reese Hospital and
Medical Center School of Nursing, Chicago, Illinois.

Acknowledgment

We wish to thank the American Cancer
Society for providing us with invaluable
reference materials.

Preface

Cancer nursing is unique in the magnitude, complexity, and depth of its challenges and rewards. This book is designed to enhance the effectiveness of a holistic care of the cancer patient through:

inclusion of universal concepts such as: pain, sexuality, death and dying, hospice and home-care services, nutrition and cancer, rehabilitation oncology, and cancer and aging;

update of current methods of prevention, detection, diagnosis, treatment, and control of malignant diseases;

provision of models, schemes/paradigms to summarize the relevant factors, concepts, and theories as bases of care;

use of review questions to facilitate the learning and sharing of knowledge; and

presentation of case studies demonstrating the holistic-multidisciplinary approach to cancer nursing from the pre-diagnostic to the bereavement phase of patient-family care.

For the sake of clarity and consistency the authors have referred to "the nurse" as "she" and "the patient" as "he," with no slight intended toward male nurses or female patients.

To the health care providers and clients; to our beloved parents, Jovita and Rosalino; and to

Al, Rozelda Fredelyn, Bradshaw Mark, and Erika-Gina

- Ardel

Wendelin, Astania, Bryan, and Vivian Larraine

- Dulce

notice

The authors and the publisher of this book have made every effort to ensure that all therapeutic modalities that are recommended are in accordance with accepted standards at the time of publication.

The drugs specified within this book may not have specific approval from the Food and Drug Administration in regard to the indications and dosages that are recommended by the authors. The manufacturer's package insert is the best source of current prescribing information.

PART I
Introduction

CHAPTER 1
Perspectives

Oncology, the study of neoplastic disease generally referred to as cancer, involves the investigation of a large variety (approximately 270 identified neoplasms) of malignant growths with potentially lethal sequelae. Although clinical research has made our knowledge and understanding of cancer much deeper and broader, the effective management of this complex disease remains a tremendous challenge to the medical, nursing, and allied health professions.[1,2,4]

There continues to be a staggering number of new cases of cancer each year, with an estimated 785,000 cases in 1980.[5] The 1980 American Cancer Society Cancer Facts and Figures reveals the following new cases in the major sites of cancer:

Major Site	Number of Cases
Colorectal	114,000
Lung	117,000
Breast	109,000
Prostate	66,000
Uterus (including carcinoma, in situ)	99,000
Urinary	52,000

The Department of Health, Education and Welfare report of 1979 indicates that the direct cost of treating neoplasms (mostly cancers) in 1975 was $5.3 billion and indirect cost estimates ranged from $13.7 billion to $22.7 billion.[4]

The etiology of cancer continues to be the subject of investigation among scientists and clinicians. Some researchers have postulated the oncogenic theory. Others have found evidence of the causative role of a virus in certain animal cancer, although none has been definitely established for human cancer. Some immunologists have suggested that there is a correlation between immunologic factors and cancer. Most recently, there is growing evidence that certain substances called carcinogens - tobacco tars, for example - can cause body cells to multiply wildly.[4,6]

The great advances made in clinical research have aided in the control of the disease and have prolonged the survival of the cancer patient. In the 1930s only one in five cancer patients could expect to survive for five years or more. Today one in three have a better chance of living longer than five years. This marked increase in survival rate has been achieved through a combination of the three major cancer treatment modalities: chemotherapy, surgery, and radiotherapy. Experimental procedures have also been carried out in cancer management, such as tumor transplant, bone marrow transplant, and immunotherapy. Positive results have been derived from plasmapheresis (replacement of platelets) and leukopheresis (replacement of leukocytes) when there is a dangerously low level of platelets and leukocytes, respectively. In an effort to combat infection, which is the major cause of morbidity and mortality in a number of cancer patients, the laminar airflow room has been developed. This device is a semiportable horizontal airflow isolator that is placed in a standard two-bed patient room which provides for a "germ free" living space for the patient. The almost sterile environment of the patient reduces his exposure to pathogenic organisms, thereby minimizing the risk of infection. Although these available therapeutic methods have enhanced the curative management of cancer, it is known that higher cure rates and better prognoses will ensue if tumors are detected and treated in their early stages. As the American Cancer Society has long advocated, the early recognition of the following seven warning signs of cancer would influence the course of the disease:[1]

1. Change in bowel or bladder habits
2. A sore that does not heal
3. Unusual bleeding or discharge
4. A thickening lump in the breast or elsewhere
5. Indigestion or difficulty in swallowing
6. Change in wart or mole
7. Nagging cough or hoarseness.

In cancer nursing, the challenge lies in the ability of the nurse to meet the individual patient's physical, psychosocial, and spiritual needs. A holistic patient care approach and a multidisciplinary health care system provide avenues for the nurse to meet this challenge.

The role of the nurse in the management of a cancer patient is unique in that it is in caring for this kind of patient that her technical, psychosocial, and communication skills are exercised with deep sensitivity to the patient's needs. However, before the nurse can be in this unique position, she must cope with her own feelings and attitudes towards cancer. Cancer is usually associated with grim feelings of death and dying which not only affect the patient and his relatives but also the nurse. We suggest that an existentialist viewpoint be adopted in dealing with the cancer patient. In this regard, the existential "here and now" becomes the focus of nursing care. The patient during this moment of crisis, at the realization of his terminal illness, and during the course of his disease, need not be treated in the traditional manner of a dying patient, but as a patient whose "here and now" necessitates support in making him achieve satisfactory adaption to his maximum level of functioning. The patient is in the "process of living right now first and dying second."* Jose Ortega y Gasset, the Spanish philosopher has said: "I am myself and my circumstance, if I do not save it, I do not save myself." The "circumstance" of the cancer patient is his living present - his relationships with others, including those who care for him. Thus the nurse can make the patient's circumstance be more meaningful through a positive attitude and a conscious effort to facilitate his adjustment to his illness and the effects of his disease.

REVIEW QUESTIONS

1. Define oncology.
2. Identify the major sites of human cancer.
3. What is the current survival rate of cancer patients?
4. What are the three major methods of cancer treatment?
5. Define plasmapheresis and leukopheresis.
6. List the seven warning signs of cancer.
7. Describe the role of the nurse in the management of a cancer patient.

REFERENCES

1. Essentials of Cancer Nursing. American Cancer Society, pp. 1-6, 1963.
2. Isler, C., The Cancer Nurses. RN Magazine, pp. 4-13, (February, 1972).
3. Marino, L.B., Cancer Patients: Your Special Role. Nursing 76, pp. 26-29, (September, 1976).
4. The Challenge of Cancer Nursing, U.S. Department of Health, Education, and Welfare, DHEW Publ. No. (NIH) 76-760.
5. American Cancer Society Cancer Facts and Figures, 1980. American Cancer Society, p. 8, 1980.
6. Pollack, E.S., Trends in Cancer Incidence and Mortality in the United States, 1969-76. J. N. Cancer Inst. 64(5):1091-1103 (May, 1980).

---

* Lisa Begg Marino, Cancer Patients: Your Special Role. Nursing '76, p. 29, September 1976

CHAPTER 2
Pathogenesis of Cancer

The origin and development (pathogenesis) of cancer have been attributed to certain mutations of a previously normal cell or group of cells. In the neoplastic process, the normal cellular growth-controlling mechanisms are impaired as a result of ever changing internal and external environmental factors and the susceptibility of the host to oncogens (carcinogens). In effect, the resultant neoplastic cell proliferates independently in a rapid, uncontrolled, and disordered fashion and spreads from the original local focus (primary site) to the surrounding tissues. These proliferated cancer cells are usually larger than normal cells, have bigger nuclei, and are of varying sizes (angiocytosis) and abnormal shapes (poikilocytosis). Thus, cancer cells are found in varying degrees of maturity.[2,4]

Unlike normal cells which effect precise and highly specialized functions that are homeostatically and harmoniously congruent with other body cells, cancer cells do not serve any useful physiologic function. Hence, cancer cells may lay dormant for a prolonged period of time without any observed effects. In fact, it is known that hyperplasia and dysplasia often precede the neoplastic process by months and years.[1,3,5]

A malignant cell can arise from any tissue at any age and may develop following a variety of stimuli such as physical or chemical agents, viruses, radiant energy, enzymes, and hormones. The biologic behavior of some malignant cells may be modified by the immune system, hormones, chemotherapy, or radiotherapy. If the neoplastic process is uninterrupted, a mass of tissue (growths or tumor) is formed. The tumor mass essentially has two parts: the parenchyma (major part) and the stroma, which is composed of connective tissue and blood vessels that support and provide structure for the parenchymal tumor cells. This tumor may continue to grow and invade other local tissues by direct extension (expansion or infiltration) or by permeation of the lumina of blood vessels (expecially veins) and of the lymphatic system. Circulatory neoplastic cells may

4

be trapped in the microcirculation of tissues and/or organs and with a suitable environment metastatic growths develop.[5]

Malignant neoplasms have been classified according to the parent tissue as shown in Table 1.[1,2,5]

Table 1: Classification of Malignant Neoplasms

Parent Tissue (Embryonic Origin)	Malignant Neoplasm
Epithelium	Melanoma Squamous cell carcinoma
Skin and mucous membranes	Epidermoid carcinoma Basal cell carcinoma
Transitional epithelium Glandular epithelium	Transitional cell carcinoma Adenocarcinoma
Endothelium	Endothelioma Hemangioendothelioma
Blood vessels	Angiosarcoma
Lymph vessels	Lymphangiosarcoma Lymphangioendothelioma
Bone marrow	Multiple myeloma Ewing's sarcoma Leukemia
Lymphoid	Malignant lymphoma Lymphosarcoma Reticulum cell sarcoma Lymphatic leukemia
Connective Tissue	
Embryonic fibrous tissue Fibrous tissue	Myxosarcoma Fibrosarcoma

Table 1 (cont'd)

Parent Tissue (Embryonic Origin)	Malignant Neoplasm
Adipose Tissue	Liposarcoma
Cartilage	
	Chondrosarcoma
Bone	Osteogenic sarcoma
Synovial membrane	Synovial sarcoma
Muscle Tissue	
Smooth muscle	Leiomyosarcoma
Striated muscle	Rhabdomyosarcoma
Nerve Tissue	
Nerve fibers and sheath	Neurogenic sarcoma
	Neurofibrosarcoma
Ganglion cells	Neuroblastoma
Glia cells	Glioblastoma
	Spongioblastoma
Pigmented Neoplasm	
Melanoblasts	Malignant melanoma
	Melanocarcinoma
Miscellaneous	
Placenta	Choriocarcinoma
	(Chorionepithelioma)
Gonads	Embryonal carcinoma
	Embryonal sarcoma
	Teratocarcinoma

REVIEW QUESTIONS

1. Define pathogenesis.
2. What is meant by anisocytosis and poikilocytosis ?
3. Differentiate between a normal cell and cancer cell.
4. What factors can affect the development and growth of cancer cells?
5. Enumerate some of the malignant neoplasms according to embryonic origin.

REFERENCES

1. Essentials of Cancer Nursing. American Cancer Society, pp. 19-25 (1963).
2. Bouchard, R., Nursing Care of the Cancer Patient. C.V. Mosby Co., St. Louis (1976).
3. Luckmann, J. and Sorensen, K.C., Medical-Surgical Nurssing. W.B. Saunders Co., Philadelphia (1974).
4. Richards, V., Cancer: The Wayward Cell. University of California Press, Los Angeles , 1972).
5. Broder, S. and Waldmann, T.A., The Suppressor-Cell Network in Cancer. N. Eng. J. Med. : 1335-1341 (December 1978).

CHAPTER 3
Etiology of Cancer

The exact etiology of neoplastic disease is unknown. Current research is focused on investigation of the neoplastic process as a disease of the cell, as a disease of the organism, and as a disease of organized tissue.

The transformation of a normal cell into a neoplastic cell remains a highly complex problem of medical science. To date there are more than 270 types of neoplasms which have been identified. In the light of the ever-changing histologic characteristics of neoplastic cells, there is reason to believe that there are as many neoplastic diseases as there are patients.

In general, the causation of neoplastic disease has been attributed to:

1. Genetic and chromosome factors
2. Hormones and enzymes
3. Chemical agents
4. Physical agents
5. Viruses
6. Immunological factors.

GENETIC AND CHROMOSOMAL FACTORS

The somatic mutation in cancer pathogenesis has been attributed to either genetic or chromosomal factors. Included in the genetic theory is the transmission of cancer and/or cancer susceptibility from parents to offspring. One rare form of human cancer, retinoblastoma, a cancer of the eye that usually occurs in childhood, has been established as hereditary.

It has also been found that embryonal structures may undergo malignant changes producing such neoplastic diseases like Wilms' tumor, melanoma, medulloblastomas, glioblastoma, and neurofibromatosis. It is believed that certain changes occur in

8

the DNA molecule producing an oncogene (cancer-producing substance). Some autosomal dominant neoplasms have also been identified. Certain chromosomes have been found to play a role in some types of cancer. The Ph-type chromosome 21 is associated with chronic myeloid leukemia.[24]

In view of the documented types of cancer which are hereditary in nature as well as of familial tendency, early detection of cancer through genetic counseling has been advocated.[26]

HORMONES AND ENZYMES

Animal experiments have demonstrated that there is a relationship between hormonal secretion and function and tumor growth. Excess hormones, particularly estrogens, produce cancer when given to animals. Recent studies have revealed that mothers treated with estrogen diethylstilbestrol (DES) tend to develop vaginal cancer. It has been found that changes in the hormone balance in man can either stimulate or retard cancer development, particularly in hormone-dependent tissues such as the prostate gland or the breast. Steroid hormones have a chemical structure similar to that of carcinogenic hydrocarbons. The significance of this similarity is not fully comprehended, but the occurrence of neoplastic disease due to hormonal factors cannot be overlooked.

The role of enzymes in neoplastic cell formation has been demonstrated in the increased enzyme activity of malignant cells. These enzymes are hyaluronidase, hexokinase, glucose-6-phosphodehydrogenase, proteases, and amino peptidases.

CHEMICAL AGENTS

Some scientists believe that chemical carcinogens are the major culprit in the causation of human cancer. Biologically the effects of chemical carcinogens are dose-dependent and genetically linked.

The major classification and types of carcinogenic chemicals affecting man are shown in Table 2.

Other chemical compounds considered carcinogenic include: asphalt, cobalt, aniline dyes, certain plastics, and air pollutants (i.e., crude paraffin oil, fuel oils, arsenicals, beryllium, lactones, aminostilbenes, agricultural insecticides, herbicides, fertilizers, and some preservatives).[1,3,20]

Table 2: Chemical Carcinogens

Major Classification	Chemical Compounds
Polycyclic aromatic hydrocarbons	Soots, tars, and cigarette smoke
Aromatic amines	Benzedine, 4-aminobiphenyl, 2-naphthylamine, N, N-bis (2-chloroethyl), 2-naphthylamine
Alkylating agents	Mustard gas Nitrogen mustard and derivatives
Nitrosamines and other nitroso compounds	4-Nitrobiphenyl
Drugs	Diethylstilbestrol (DES) Nitrogen mustard
Industrial carcinogens	Chloromethyl methyl ether Vinyl chloride
Naturally occurring products	Aflatoxin B Betel nut
Metals	Asbestos (calcium-magnesium silicate fibers) Cadmium compounds Chromium compounds Nickel compounds

Source: Ryser, 1974.

PHYSICAL AGENTS

Various agents and chronic trauma causing tissue irritation and injury are considered carcinogenic. Examples include: ionizing radiation, sunlight, and ultraviolet radiation. Pipe smoking is believed to be a predisposing factor to lip cancer and a multi-parous woman is more prone to develop cancer of the cervix. It is also known that lung cancer and cancers of the oral cavity are closely related to heavy, long-term cigarette smoking.[2,3]

VIRUSES

A variety of malignant tumors and leukemias in several animal species have been found to be caused by filterable viruses. In men, indirect evidence strongly suggests the theory that certain types of cancer are caused by viruses. Data on the viral etiology of human cancer have been accumulated by monitoring the ability of a virus to transform cells in culture. Evidence of oncogenic transformation includes alteration of surface properties of the cell, loss of contact inhibition, capability to grow indefinitely, and frequently the capacity to induce tumor growths.

Several studies on a number of human viruses that can transform cells in vitro suggest oncogenic potential. In addition, seroepidemiological surveys of human populations are correlating the presence of antivirus antibody, indicative of previous viral exposure, with tumor incidence. The result of these studies indicated the association or role of Epstein-Barr herpes virus (EBV) with Burkitt's lymphoma and herpes simplex virus type 2 with cervical cancer. Thus far, there are three general types of viruses implicated in adult patients with cancer:

1. Type C viruses: certain sarcomas and leukemias
2. Type B viruses: breast cancer
3. Epstein-Barr viruses (EBV): carcinomas of the cervix, lymphoma, nasopharyngeal carcinoma (a rare epithelial tumor prevalent in Chinese).

Although there appears to be tremendous evidence linking RNA and DNA containing viruses in human cancer, there is not a single human cancer with a proven viral etiology.[2,4,5]

IMMUNOLOGICAL FACTORS

Cancer research during the past decade documented the role played by the immune system in the occurrence of and therapy of neoplastic diseases. The relationship of immunocompetence and prognosis has been established and the presence of tumor-specific and tumor-associated antigens and the immune response to them has been recognized.[6] In general, immunologic deficiency or incompetence leads to:

1. Poor response to therapy and poor prognosis
2. Shortened survival time
3. Uncontrolled spread of the disease.

A competent immune system affords the individual the ability to maintain functional integrity and physiological survival through the interaction of complex processes in warding off, fighting, or killing and/or modifying the effects of disease-producing microorganisms (viral or bacterial), foreign tumor cells, or antigens which may be of extrinsic or intrinsic origin.

The biology and development of the immune system can be best understood by reviewing the equivalent immune system of the chicken. The chicken has two distinct lymphoid organs: the thymus and the bursa of Fabricius. The thymus is responsible for converting stem cells from the bone marrow into T lymphocytes (thymus-dependent cells). Similarly, the bursa of Fabricius converts stem cells to B lymphocytes (bursa-dependent cells also referred to as thymus-independent cells).[7]

The human immune system consists of stem cells from the bone marrow which will become differentiated into either the T lymphocytes (T cells) or B lymphocytes (B cells). With the presence of T-cell precursors, the stem cells mature in the thymus gland and then become transformed into T cells (small and large T lymphocytes). Similarly, the B-cell precursors transform the stem cells in a bursa-equivalent site into B cells (small and large B lymphocytes). The T lymphocytes are mainly responsible for cellular immunity while the B lymphocytes are for humoral immunity. Other stem cells in the bone marrow develop into blood monocytes (immature macrophages) and mature into tissue macrophages.[8]

The thymus gland apparently influences the development of lymphocytes by promoting differentiation of stem cells in the bone marrow and by secreting a humoral factor which influences the development of lymphocytes elsewhere in the body. The lymphocytes migrate into lymphoid tissues in the lymph nodes, liver, spleen, gastrointestinal tract, and bone marrow.

In summary, immunological competence, i.e., the ability to detect and respond to foreign materials (antigens), depends on the thymus gland which transforms stem cells into T lymphocytes and prevents the release into the circulation of any immunocytes that can destroy the body itself. Another function of the immune system is the production of the bursa-dependent lymphocytes (B lymphocytes). This process occurs in unidentified sites, possibly the tonsilar, and gut-associated lymphoid tissue. Together, the T and B lymphocytes contribute to antibody production, cellular immunity, and immunologic memory.[12]

There are various theories regarding the cellular-mediated and humoral-mediated immunity. As previously mentioned, the cellular-mediated immunity involves the T lymphocytes. This immune response is initiated when a T cell becomes sensitized with a specific antigen. The T cells (T lymphocytes) release chemicals called lymphokines which act on target cells (antigens). The humoral-mediated immunity involves the presence of antibodies (produced by plasma cells as a result of the interaction of B lymphocytes and an antigen) and the "complement system." The serum complement systems consist of various proteins and enzyme precursors which, in the presence of antigen-antibody reaction, stimulate the enzymes necessary for the occurrence of complement fixation, which will cause the death of a viable antigen. It is the complement system that bridges the cellular and humoral immune responses.[7]

The characteristics of cellular and humoral immunity are summarized in Table 3. The relationship of an immune response to the life course of a tumor cell is shown in Figure 1.

Most tumors invoke an immune response in the host.[9,10] If the immune system becomes weak, improperly functions, becomes totally incompetent or becomes overwhelmed by massive invasion, then the manifestations and sequelae of disease processes become obvious.[8] For the host to react immunologically against a neoplastic cell, his immune system must recognize the "foreign cell" as a different or as a non-self cell (recognition factor). It is believed by most scientists that neoplastic cells are constantly being developed but the immune system seems to confer a natural immunity against cancer.[8,11,12] It is also believed that the immune response against cancer is relative rather than absolute. In other words, the immune system can handle only limited numbers of tumor cells, up to 10 million. When there is growth to more than 100 million cells, the immune response is usually no longer capable of preventing further proliferation.[11,12] In conjunction to the relative response to cancer, the immune system may become depressed or rendered incompetent by:

1. Genetic causes such as absence of thymus gland or stem cells (the precursors of T and B lymphocytes, agammaglobulinemia (absence of gamma globulins), or intrinsic deficiencies of the lymphoid tissues.
2. Blocking factors that cover the tumor cells with substances which prevent its destruction by immune response.
3. Malnutrition syndromes due to poor intake or absorption of essential nutrients, thereby decreasing the ability to form circulating antibodies.

Table 3:   Cellular and Humoral Immunity:
Summary of Characteristics

Cellular Immunity	Humoral Immunity
Immunity depends on the presence of intracellular antibodies that remain in the cell.	Acquired immunity conferred primarily by circulating antibodies.
T lymphocytes become sensitized by contact with specific antigen.	Highly differentiated plasma cells formed by interaction of B lymphocytes and an antigen.
T lymphocytes release numerous chemical factors (lymphokines):	Plasma cells release antibodies (immunoglobulins):
Chemotactic factor promotes migration of macrophages and sensitized lymphocytes to the area of the antigens.	Immunoglobulin G (Ig G): constitutes the majority of antibody in the secondary response to subsequent contact with the same antigen; activates the complement system and is frequently involved in opsonization.
Migration-inhibiting factor (MIF): prevents further migration of the T cells and macrophages.	IgA (serum IgA) and secretory IgA (sIgA) antiviral activity: production of IgA and sIgA are stimulated by oral vaccines and aerosol immunizations. The sIgA is the predominant class of immunoglobulin in saliva, tears, colostrum, milk, and secretions of the respiratory, urogenital, and gastrointestinal tracts.
Macrophage activation factor (MAF): transforms local macrophages into highly phagocytic state.	IgM: major component of the primary antibody response destroys foreign invaders during the initial exposure to the antigen. It also activates the complement system much more so than IgG.

Table 3 (cont.)

Cellular Immunity	Humoral Immunity
Transfer factor (TF): transforms nonsensitized T lymphocytes into sensitized lymphocytes.	IgE (or reagenic antibody): implicated in the etiology of atopy or allergy. Concentration in the serum is normally lower than any of the immunoglobulins. Increasing levels occur in persons with allergic diseases such as extrinsic asthma, hay fever, atopic dermatitis, urticaria, and anaphylactic shock.
Blastogenic factor: initiates rapid mitosis of sensitized T lymphocytes.	IgD: function is still unknown; serum concentration is very low.
Response can become very intense.	Each type of immunoglobulin serves a specific function as described above.
Produces a delayed-type hypersensitivity reaction.	Immunity remains active for months.
Cannot be transferred from one person to another by cell-free plasma and is dependent, therefore, on the presence of immune cells.[2,7]	Antibodies (immunoglobulins) in general act by aiding phagocytosis through opsinization, activating or causing complement fixation, serving as antitoxins, and causing agglutination and neutralization of bacteria.
	Produces an immediate hypersensitivity reaction.[2,7]

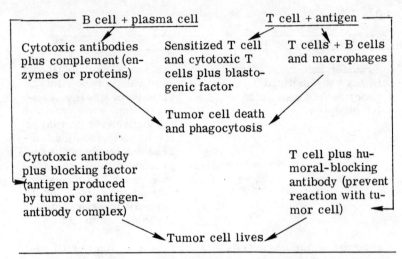

Figure 1: Life Course of a Tumor Cell

4. Age as a factor: people at extremes of the life span are more apt to develop immunologic depression. Premature infants have temporary passive immunity conferred by maternal antibodies. Eventually they will develop their own immune systems.

5. Diseases such as burns and treatment of diseases with immunosuppressants contribute to the development of cancer. Neoplastic disease itself is also an immunosuppressant. A large tumor can produce a steady leak into the blood which subsequently combines with circulatory antibodies and prevents them from attacking the tumor. Together, antigens and carcinogens can lead to immunosuppression.

6. Iatrogenic conditions: radiation and certain drugs such as chloramphenicol (Chloromycetin), azathioprine (Imuran), mechlorethamine (Mustargen) corticosteroids, chlorpromazine (Thorazine), heroin, and alcoholism can cause immunosuppression.

7. Overwhelming systemic infection depresses the immune system.

8. Cumulative effects of treatments, infections, and stress cause immunosuppression. [1,8,26,27,28]

SOME RESULTS OF STUDIES SHOWING
RELATIONSHIPS OF THE IMMUNE
SYSTEM AND NEOPLASTIC PROCESSES

1. Antigens which are specific to cancer, tumor-specific antigens (TSA), are not found in normal tissues.
2. Unexplained spontaneous cancer regression will sometimes occur.
3. There is an increased incidence of malignancy in immunoincompetent patients due to congenital or acquired deficiencies.
4. Patients receiving a battery of immunosuppressive drugs develop cancer at a rate at least 80 times greater than does the general population.
5. Reactions to skin testing indicate that most healthy persons can be sensitized to known antigens. Anergy (the inability to develop delayed cutaneous hypersensitivity to the antigen used) found in cancer patients almost uniformly indicates rapidly growing tumors and poor prognosis.[11]
6. Blastogenic response studies show that antigens and mitogens induce blastogenic transformation and proliferation of lymphocytes. Lymphocytes of patients with poor prognosis showed less than normal blastogenic response.[6]
7. Release of the immunosuppressive factor by tumor cells appears to be related to polypeptides in the alpha-2-macroglobulin fraction of the serum. They often disappear after surgical extirpation of the neoplastic growth.[6]
8. The presence of tumor antigens has been found in the surface or within the malignant cells.[6]
9. Tumor cell growth inhibition by lymphocytes has been noted, indicating cell-mediated response.
10. The occurrence of tumor-specific and tumor-associated (TSTA) antigens has been demonstrated in neoplastic processes such as malignant melanoma, Burkitt's lymphoma, osteosarcoma, choriocarcinoma and others.[13,14]

In summary, the characteristics of malignant cells may be described as:

1. Cancer cells are derived from normal cells but their structural and physiologic potential do not serve a useful function.
2. Cancer cells are atypical, live longer, and divide in a disorganized pattern and more often than normal cells.
3. Malignancy correlates to the degree of inflexibility of the biochemical enzymes pattern which determines the cell response to therapeutic cellular manipulation, e.g., chemoradiotherapy or immunotherapy.[16]

4. Cancer cells have a hyperchromatin nucleus with some in-
   clusions, as well as a larger amount of DNA molecules.
5. Some malignant cells produce a plasminogen activator which
   results in fibrinolysis, thus enhancing the process of invasion of other tissues.
6. The concept of "progression" indicate worsening of the biologic potential of the disease.[16] This progression is a
   stepwise process of loss of tissue characteristic and therefore becomes more anaplastic.
7. The higher the percentage of undifferentiated (anaplastic)
   cells, the greater the malignancy.[16]
8. Some variant cancer cells produce a paraendocrine syndrome, e.g., bronchial cancer producing insulin.[16]
9. Some cancer cells are hormone-dependent, therefore hormonal manipulation is possible and cycle related.
10. The production of hyaluronidase and other enzymes by ma-
    lignant cells facilitates invasion through tissue substance.
11. Cancer cells penetrate neighboring cells and metastasize
    by direct invasion and permeation through the blood, lymph,
    and serous fluid of the body.
12. Predilection for certain sites of metastatic is anatomical
    dependent.[16]

A conceptual scheme on the etiologic and causal factors related
to cancer is depicted in Figure 2.

The multiplicity theory of cancer causation is depicted by the
interrelatedness of specific theories, e.g., carcinogenesis/on-
cogenesis, genetic, viral, hormonal, and evolutionary reversion
theory.[15,17,19,20]

The space/time/developmental continuum reflects individual
growth and sex-stage-related crises within one's spatial-temporal space. The greater the intensity and length of absolute
and relative exposure in a contained, stress-filled environment,
the greater is the chance to develop cancer.

REVIEW QUESTIONS

1. Enumerate the factors believed to play a role in the origin
   and development of neoplastic disease.
2. What are some malignant conditions arising from embryonal
   structures?
3. List some of the chemical carcinogenic agents.
4. What physical agents can be carcinogenic?
5. What are the three types of viruses associated with human
   cancer development?

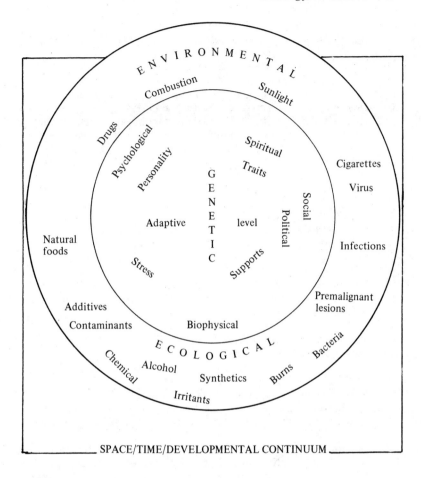

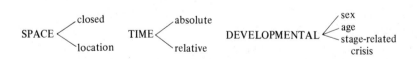

Figure 2. Multiplicity theory of cancer causation.

6. What is a competent immune system?
7. Which gland of the body determines to a large extent immunological competence?
8. Differentiate between cellular immunity and humoral immunity.
9. Enumerate factors which depress the immune system.
10. Describe the life course of a tumor cell.
11. Discuss the results of studies concerning the relationship
    between the immune system and the neoplastic process.
12. Describe the multiplicity theory of cancer causation.
13. Enumerate at least eight characteristics of malignant cells.

REFERENCES

1. Ryser, H., Special Report: Chemical Carcinogenesis.
   CA. 24(6):353 (November/December, 1974).
2. Luckman, J. and Sorensen, K., Medical Surgical Nursing:
   A Psychophysiologic Approach. W.B. Saunders Co., Philadelphia, p. 170 (1974).
3. Smith, D. and Germain, C., Care of the Adult Patient:
   Medical-Surgical Nursing. J.B. Lippincott Co., Philadelphia (1975).
4. Gross, L., The Role of Viruses in the Etiology of Cancer
   and Leukemia. JAMA, pp. 1029-1032 (November 18, 1974).
5. Rapp, F. and Westmoreland, D., Do Viruses Cause Cancer in Man? CA. 25(4):215-299 (July/August, 1975).
6. Hersh, et al., Immunology: Where Do We Go From Here?
   Med. World News, 4(4):33-37, (April, 1975).
7. Nysather, J.O., et al., The Immune System: Its Development and Functions. Am. J. Nurs. pp. 1614-1616 (October, 1976).
8. Bochow, A.J., Cancer Immunotherapy: What Promise
   Does it Hold? Nursing 76, pp. 50-56 (October, 1976).
9. Isler, C., Cancer Immunotherapy. R.N. pp. 35-38 (April,
   1976).
10. Isler, C., Cancer Immunotherapy. R.N. pp. 29-31 (May,
    1976).
11. Silverstein, M. and Morton, D., Cancer Immunotherapy.
    Am. J. Nurs. pp. 1178-1181 (July, 1973).
12. Donley, D., The Immune System - Nursing the Patient Who
    Is Immunosuppressed. Am. J. Nurs. pp. 1619-1625 (Oc-
    tober, 1976).
13. American Cancer Society, Clinical Oncology for Medical
    Students and Physicians: A Multidisciplinary Approach,
    P. Rubin and R. Bakemeier, eds. (1974).
14. McKhan, C., Tumor Immunology. CA. 25(4):187-197
    (July/August, 1975).

15. Burkhalter, P.K. and Donley, D.L. Dynamics of Oncology Nursing, McGraw-Hill Book Co., New York (1978).
16. Kruse, L., et al., Cancer Pathophysiology, Etiology and Management - Collected Readings, The C.V. Mosby Co., St. Louis (1979).
17. Castro, B. and Di Paolo, J., Prog. Med. Virol. pp. 1-47 (1973).
18. Comings, D.E., A General Theory of Carcinogenesis, Proc. Nat. Acad. Sci. pp. 3324-3328 (December, 1973).
19. Epstein, S.S., Environmental Determinants of Human Cancer. Cancer Res. pp. 2425-2435 (October, 1974).
20. Magee, P.N., Carcinogens in the Environment. Proc. R. Soc. Med. pp. 741-743 (August, 1974).
21. McAllister, R.M., Viruses in Human Carcinogenesis. Prog. Med. Virol. pp. 48-85 (1973).
22. Meek, E., Viruses as Possible Factors in Human Cancer. J. Iowa Med. Soc. pp. 535-538 (October, 1972).
23. Nastac, R., Results in the Study of Virus - Tumor Relationships Obtained in the Stefan S. Nicolau Institute of Virology. Virologie 30(4):307-318 (October-December, 1979).
24. Knudson, A.G., Genetics and Cancer. Am. J. Med. 69(1): 1-3 (July, 1980).
25. Zahradnik, J.M., et al., Adenovirus Infection in the Immunocompromised Patient. Am. J. Med. 68(5):725-732 (May, 1980).
26. Doll, R.S., The Epidemiology of Cancer. Cancer 45(10): 2475-2485 (May, 1980).
27. Klein, G., Immune and Non-Immune Control of Neoplastic Development: Contrasting Effects of Host and Tumor Evolution. Cancer 45(10):2486-2499 (May, 1980).
28. Monkman, G., Orwall, G., and Ivins, J., Trauma and Oncogenesis. Mayo Clin. Proc. pp. 157-163 (March, 1974).

CHAPTER 4
General Aspects of Cancer Detection and
Diagnostic Procedures

The key to possible cancer cure is early detection. Unfortunately, because of the fear associated with cancer, by the time an individual seeks medical attention the lesion is usually already widespread. In view of this dilemma, the nurse by virtue of her daily interactions with her patients can be in a vital position to make her patients cognizant of the value of cancer prevention and control. Through patient education, the nurse can share with her patients the most current trends in oncology and instill a feeling of hope and confidence in the possible beneficial effects of the various modalities of treatment now available in cancer therapy. [9,10,15]

CANCER CONTROL MEASURES

There are several measures that should be undertaken to promote early cancer detection.

1. Patient education
   a. The fact that pain and weight loss are not early signs of cancer, but the persistence of any of the seven danger signs of cancer as previously mentioned in Chapter 1, Part I, these should be reported immediately to the patient's physician.
   b. The most common sites of cancer in women are the breast, cervix of the uterus, the skin, and the gastrointestinal tract. Among men, the most common sites are the skin, lungs, gastrointestinal tract, and prostate gland. [1]
   c. Breast self-examination should be done monthly on the third day postmenstrual period or on a regular day designated on a monthly basis for menopausal women.
   d. Any abnormal bleeding per vagina postmenopause must be reported to the patient's physician.
   e. The relationship between cigarette smoking and cancer should be understood.

  f. Protective measures should be taken against skin can-
      cer.
  g. The relationship between individual hazards and cancer
      should be comprehended.

2. Patients should comply with the protocol for the early de-
    tection of cancer in asymptomatic persons as specified in
    Table 4. It should be noted that as a result of an 18-month
    study of the American Cancer Society expert committees and
    task forces, the previous recommendation of annual chest
    x-ray has been deemed unnecessary due to a lack of strong
    scientific and medical evidence that the test or procedure
    is medically effective in reduction of morbidity, that the
    medical benefits outweigh any possible risks, that the costs
    are reasonable in relation to expected benefits.

3. Nurses should recognize their responsibility for and con-
    tribution to early cancer detection by:
    a. Being a role model and having an annual physical exam-
        ination
    b. Assessment of the patient's complaints and symptoms
    c. Encouragement of persons with suspected symptoms to
        seek medical attention promptly
    d. Explanation of diagnostic procedures to persons with
        suspected symptoms.

SPECIFIC PROCEDURES FOR CANCER DETECTION AND DIAGNOSIS

Bone Marrow Aspiration

The skin area over the sternum or iliac crest is cleansed with
providone-iodine (Betadine) solution as for any minor surgery.
Then a small area is anesthetized through the skin, subcutaneous tissue, and to the periosteum of the bone. The bone marrow needle with a stylet is introduced into the marrow cavity,
and when the stylet is removed a syringe is attached and a small
volume (0.5 cc) of blood and marrow is aspirated. If a bone
marrow biopsy is to be done, then a small skin incision of 3 to
4 mm is made with a surgical blade (No. 9 or 11). In this case,
only the iliac bone is used for this procedure since the sternum
is too thin.

Table 4: Cancer Detection Protocol Recommended by the American Cancer Society, 1980

Test or Procedure	Sex	Recommended Frequency	Age
Pap test	F	At least once every 3 years after two negative examinations of 1 year apart; more frequently in high-risk women (i.e., first intercourse at early age, multiple sex partners)	20-65; under 20 if sexually active
Digital rectal exam	M & F	Annual	Over 40
Stool guaiac slide test	M & F	Annual	Over 50
Sigmoidoscopy	M & F	Every 3-5 years; after 2 negative examinations of 1 year apart	Over 50
Pelvic exam	F	Every 3 years Annual	20-40
Mammography	F	Baseline Consult private physician Every year	35-40 Under 50 Over 50
Health counseling and cancer checkup*	M & F M & F	Every 3 years Annual	Over 20 Over 40
Chest x-ray		No longer recommended	
Sputum cytology		No longer recommended	

* - Note: This includes examination for cancers of the lymph nodes, oral region, skin thyroid, testicles, ovaries, and the prostate.

Nursing Management

1. Most patients need no special preparation except adequate and simple explanation of the procedure. If the patient is very anxious, however, a minor tranquilizer such as diazepam (Valium) and meperidine (Demerol) may be given as prescribed by the physician. These drugs are given intramuscularly one hour before the test.
2. Warn the patient that he may experience brief discomfort in the actual aspiration of the marrow.
3. Apply pressure to the aspiration or needle biopsy site for five to ten minutes after the procedure to prevent bleeding, since some patients tend to have thrombocytopenia.

Needle Aspiration

Cleanse the skin with providone-iodine (Betadine) solution before the area is anesthetized. A #18 needle is inserted by the physician into the tissue to be sampled. Using a syringe, tissue is drawn into the syringe by suction and the material obtained is put on a glass slide and stained before it is sent to the laboratory for examination.

Biopsy

This entails an excision of a piece of tissue from a suspicious growth. This tissue is then examined under a microscope by the pathologist as a frozen section (rapid) or a paraffin section (permanent). The former enables the pathologist to quickly examine and report his findings on the nature of the cells. The latter takes longer for the results but the sliced tissue can be kept for a period of time and offers a clearer view of the cells.

Nursing Management

1. Consent for surgery must be signed after a simple explanation of the procedure by the physician. Ascertain how much the patient has comprehended and reinforce the physician's explanations.
2. The type of anesthesia to be used is discussed with the patient by the anesthesiologist or Certified Registered Nurse Anesthetist during a preanesthetic visit, preferably the day before. The nurse should reassure patient about the fact that general anesthesia is relatively safe.
3. The patient is kept N.P.O. (nothing by mouth) after 12 midnight if general anesthesia will be used.
4. On the day of surgery, the nurse should insure that the physical preparation of the patient is completed, i.e., enemas the night prior, any shaving as indicated, the patient has had a bath, and the patient's bladder has been emptied.

5. Before administration of the preoperative medication ordered to allay the patient's anxiety and to sedate the patient, the vital signs should be taken and charted.
6. Provide emotional support.
7. If general anesthesia is administered, maintain on N.P.O until gag or coughing reflex returns, after which time sips of fluid may be given.
8. The biopsy site should be observed for any bleeding. If it occurs, apply pressure dressings and notify the physician.
9. Check the patient's vital signs every 15 minutes in the immediate postoperative period until stable and then every hour for the first eight hours and every four hours thereafter.

Cytology

An examination of the cells from a vaginal or cervical smear and the sputum may reveal the presence or absence of cancer cells.

Transillumination

This is performed by using a powerful cold light in a completely darkened room. A mass that transilluminates is probably cystic (benign) unless it is lipomatous or filled with opaque material.

Radiologic Tests

1. Thermography: An infrared scanner is used to measure heat emissions. The patient is placed in a room under 70°F for 20 to 30 minutes. Abnormal variations in an area due to increased vascularization may indicate the presence of a neoplasm.

2. Mammography: This is a roentgenography of the breast without the injection of a contrast medium. Although this may detect breast cancer before any signs and symptoms are manifested, many carcinomas noted on clinical examination are not detected by a mammogram.

3. Xerography: In this test, a selenium-coated plate is subjected to an electric charge, the x-ray exposure is made, and the plate is then developed by a special process under careful observation. The outcome is a xerogram in which all tissues of the breast, including the skin, are portrayed in a bas-relief effect. It is useful for early cancer detection. However, this has not been established as routine procedure.

4. Tomography: A sharp focus is made on the structure in question by blurring out the shadows of surrounding areas. Also, by simultaneously moving both the x-ray source and the roentgenographic films, "slices" of a particular site can be studied at different depths. This is useful in demarcation of the extension of a soft-tissue tumor in the bones, brain, or lungs.[6]

5. Computerized Transverse Axial Tomography and EMI Scanner: This combines the transmission of x-ray protons with tomographic techniques and computerized information resulting in an accurate indication of the location and nature of a lesion. The machine scans at different angles by a narrow x-ray beam, then the differential absorption by tissues in contiguous slices is calculated by a computer in the machine. This information is later displayed as a printout of numerical values and an oscilloscopic visualization in shades of gray which correspond to the density of the tissue. Malignant lesions can be precisely defined and localized. The lesion's specific volume and surrounding edema are visualized by their respective densities on polaroid pictures. The accuracy of the machine is even greater when combined with nuclear medicine scanning. (As many as 98% of lesions are diagnosed by this procedure accurately.) In about 20 to 30 minutes, the procedure is usually completed. With the EMI (Electric and Musical Instruments) scanner, the readouts cannot display or pick up scalp lesions and bone metastases. These are picked up only by nuclear medicine scans.[11,12]

Nursing Management

1. To prepare a patient for the EMI scanner of the brain, the hair is shampooed before the test so there will be no hair spray to cause artifacts; no hair pins or bobby pins should be worn.
2. Reassure the patient that the amount of radiation obtained from the scan is similar to the simple x-ray examination and therefore virtually harmless.
3. Instruct the patient on remaining immobile during the test.
4. Inform the patient that he will lay supine on a table in front of the scanner while his head is placed in a semispherical cap.

Automated Computerized Transverse Axial (ACTA) Scanner

This can take cross sections in color, not only of the brain as the EMI scanner does, but of any site in the body. In the EMI scanner machine, the x-ray beam is fed into a computer which assembles the information and presents a black and white picture. In the ACTA scanner the picture is re-read by a second computer that analyzes the various tones of gray and produces a color picture. The color picture makes it easier to see anatomical structures and lesions. The visualized color picture does not correspond to the actual color of the tissue x-rayed but rather to the density of the tissues as indicated by their resistance to the passage of the x-ray beam. In 4.5 minutes a picture of any lesion can be taken and in another two minutes a printout of information is obtained regarding the extent and precise location of the lesion.[11]

Nursing Management

1. Except in brain scans, there is no special preparation of the patient for any of the radiologic tests discussed above.
2. Psychologically, however, assist the patient in coping with anxiety and fear of radiation by encouraging verbalization of fears and concerns and by providing reassurance.

Ultrasound

This test uses a machine that sends high-frequency sound vibrations to the structure being investigated. The structure will return the echoes derived from the ultrasound. Motions of the echoes are traced on an oscilloscope and recorded on film. If there is a solid tumor, there will be increased echoes and the motions of the echoes recorded will show an irregular outline.[16]

Intravenous Pyelogram (IVP)

Radio-opaque dye is injected into the patient's vein and then x-ray films are taken. Filling defects may indicate a space-occupying lesion or displacement of normal structures.

Nursing Management

1. Inform patient of the procedure to be done.
2. A laxative may be given the night prior to testing.
3. A light evening meal is given the evening prior to testing.
4. No food or fluids are allowed after midnight.

5. Check any history of allergy such as allergy to fish or to iodine.
6. Inform patient that he may experience feelings of warmth, flushing of the face, and a salty taste in the mouth while the dye is being injected into the vein. These sensations will disappear in a few minutes.
7. After the I.V.P. watch for any allergic reactions to the dye such as respiratory difficulty, diaphoresis, clamminess, urticaria, numbness, and tingling of extremities. Notify the physician if any of these occur. Have available antihistamine drugs, epinephrine, steroids, and oxygen to combat allergic reaction.

Arteriography

Contrast medium is injected into specific arteries to demonstrate stenosis, obstruction, thrombi, neoplastic vasculature, or the extent of a tumor.[8]

Endoscopic Procedures

The use of fiberoptic scopes in direct inspection and observation of the respiratory tree and the gastrointestinal system has proved very effective in tumor detection and diagnosis. The fiberscope has a shaft made of rubber or plastic that allows for greater flexibility and permits greater visualization. Incorporated into the shaft of the instrument are glass fibers which transmit light from the mucosa and the image is transmitted back to the examiner's view. Cameras may be attached to the instrument to take pictures of abnormalities. The most common endoscopic procedures done for cancer detection and diagnosis follow.

Nursing Management

1. Bronchoscopy: The direct inspection and observation of the larynx, trachea, and bronchi is performed through a fiberoptic bronchoscope passed through the trachea. This would show the location and the extent of the tumor.[4]
   a. A signed consent for bronchoscopy is obtained.
   b. The procedure is explained in simple and understandable language by the physician and then reinforced by the nurse.
   c. No food or fluids are allowed for at least six hours before the procedure. The nurse should explain the importance of this and the reason why it is necessary.
   d. Before administering atropine IM, inform the patient of a possible experience of dryness of the mouth after receiving the drug.

e. An intramuscular analgesic such as meperidine to decrease anxiety and promote sedation should be given at least 45 minutes before the test so that its maximum effect will not be worn out by the time the patient is taken for the procedure. After administration of the drug, instruct the patient to remain in bed as it can cause drowsiness and he may fall. Raise the bed siderails if the patient is left unattended.

f. Contact lenses, dentures, and other prostheses are removed before the patient goes to the operating room.

g. After the test, ascertain what type of anesthesia was used. If it was local, an anesthetic spray would have been applied to the pharynx and some drug would have been instilled on the epiglottis or vocal cords. Hence, the patient should be kept NPO until the cough or gag reflex returns.

h. After the return of the gag or cough reflex, crushed ice is given and then sips of fluids, as tolerated. In a few hours, a regular diet may be given.

2. Esophagoscopy: Direct viewing of the interior of the esophagus is performed through a tube with a light source (esophagoscope). The nursing management is similar to bronchoscopy.

3. Gastroscopy: Direct examination of the gastric mucosa using a gastroscope.

4. Gastroduodenoscopy: Direct examination of the esophagus, stomach, and colon is performed with a fiberoptic instrument called a gastroduodenoscope. This instrument is passed through the patient's oropharynx, into the esophagus, and then into the stomach which is then examined through the sideview of the fiberscope. The tip of the scope is then advanced gently through the pyloric ring into the duodenal bulb and the descending duodenum.

5. Ampullary cannulation: This uses the same basic setup as in gastroduodenoscopy with the addition of a side view fiberduodenoscope which enables the radiologist to visualize the pancreatic and biliary ducts. [3,5,14]

Nursing Management of Patient Undergoing
Gastrointestinal Endoscopic Examination

a. Explain the procedure in simple, nontechnical terms and what will be expected during the procedure, i.e., to keep immobile while the scope is being introduced and passed through the esophagus.

b. Foods and fluids are withheld for at least six to eight hours before the examination to prevent regurgitation.

c. Dentures, glasses, and other prostheses must be removed.

d. Signed consent of the patient must be obtained.

e. The patient should be sedated to allay his anxiety. Reassurance is most effective in allaying fear of the procedure.

f. Instruct the patient on the need to hold his breath when the physician sprays the posterior pharynx with local anesthetic such as tetracaine hydrochloride (Pontocaine). This would prevent aspiration of the medication.

g. After the examination, instruct the patient not to eat or drink for at least four hours or until the gag reflex has returned in order to prevent aspiration.

h. Inform the patient of the possibility of experiencing discomfort and hoarseness of voice after the test, but that these will be temporary and last only a few days. Saline gargles may be given to help relieve discomfort.

i. Provide adequate rest after the procedure because it is very exhausting.

j. Have available for the physician's use atropine or glucagon which may be administered intravenously to produce a quiet, atonic duodenum and relaxed ampullary sphincter.

k. After a gastroduodenoscopy and ampulla cannulation, observe for any rise in temperature, chills, and abdominal pain. The patient may also experience a transient elevation of serum amylase, mild clinical pancreatitis, or an ascending cholangitis. Hence, serum amylase levels are checked after the examination.

6. Anoscopy, proctoscopy, and sigmoidoscopy: These are tubular instruments used to examine the lower bowel. The anal canal is viewed directly by an anoscope, the anus and the rectum with a proctoscope, and the sigmoid colon and the rectum are examined through a sigmoidoscope. [17,18]

Nursing Management

a. Give the patient a clear liquid diet the day before the examination.

b. A cathartic is given the evening prior to testing.

c. A warm tap water enema is administered on the morning of the examination.

The objective of preparing the patient for the procedure is to insure that the lower bowel be clean for better visualization.

7. Colonoscopy: This is perhaps the most significant advance in the diagnosis of colon and rectal cancer. The colonoscope is an instrument consisting of a flexible 4-mm glass bundle containing some 250,000 glass fibers with a lens at either end to focus and magnify the image. Light from an external source is transmitted by a fiberoptic bundle to the tip of the colonoscope. This light is for visualization and photography of the bowel. There are two types of colonoscopes available. One measuring about 105 cm in length is used for the left side of the colon; the other varies from 165 to 186 cm and can visualize the entire colon. There is a newer version of the colonoscope with two open channels which can be used for both polypectomy and diagnostic procedures.12,13,18
   a. Indications for colonoscopy
      (1) Any unexplained colonic sign or symptom
      (2) Lower gastrointestinal bleeding
      (3) Assessment of inflammatory bowel disease
      (4) Any abnormality on barium enema examination or sigmoidoscopy
      (5) Postoperative evaluation of the colon
   b. Contraindications for colonoscopy
      (1) Severe fulminant ulcerative or granulomatous colitis
      (2) Acute diverticulitis

Nursing Management

1. The patient is put on a clear liquid diet 48 hours prior to procedure.
2. The night before, give patient 10 ounces of citrate of magnesia, P.O.
3. Three hours before procedure, tap water or saline enemas are given until clear, allowing time for the colon to empty.
4. Premedicate as ordered to produce sedation, making colonoscopy more tolerable.
5. Anticipate the necessity for further analgesics, since pain can occur despite initial sedation.

It is felt that most, if not all, colon and rectal cancers originate in polyps. Generally, the larger the polyp the more likely it is to be malignant. It is also known that the incidence of cancer is higher in villous adenomas, although the more common pedunculated variety can also become malignant. Patient teaching on the importance of colonoscopy as a procedure to detect any polyps, since these may be precancerous, is essential.

8. Hysteroscopy: The cervix is dilated to 6 mm and the uterine cavity is distended with carbon dioxide gas or 5% dextrose, or 32% dextran-70 (preferred). Visualization of the endocervix and endometrial cavity is made and biopsy can be taken as indicated. This is of value in the diagnosis of endometrial carcinoma. The criticism leveled at this procedure is the possibility of tumor spread due to the instillation of fluid into the uterus. To counteract this, irrigation of the endometrial cavity should be done after the procedure. [7]

9. Laparoscopy: Visualization of the nature of an adnexal mass and/or any abnormality suspected of the internal reproductive system is performed via a laparoscope. [1]

10. Colposcopy: This is an examination of the fornix of the vagina and the cervix uteri. It is useful in identifying the abnormal area in the cervix which can be sampled through a biopsy.

Nursing Management

a. A signed consent obtained from the patient.
b. NPO for at least six hours before the procedure.
c. If done under general anesthesia, fear of anesthesia and the unknown should be discussed with the patient. A preanesthetic visit by the anesthesiologist would be beneficial. This visit can be arranged by the nurse if there is no protocol requiring it to be done.

REVIEW QUESTIONS

1. To promote early cancer detection, what measures should be undertaken by the nurse?
2. What should an annual physical examination for women consist of? What should the examination be for men over 40 years?
3. Identify the most common sites of cancer in women and in men.
4. What is bone marrow aspiration?
5. Describe the preparation of a patient for: (a) biopsy, (b) bronchoscopy, (c) sigmoidoscopy, (d) gastroduodenoscopy.
6. Define transillumination, thermography, xerography, mammography, tomography.
7. What is an EMI scanner? What is its diagnostic value?
8. What is the advantage of an Automated Computerized Transverse Axial (ACTA) Scanner over the EMI scanner?

9. Describe the diagnostic technique called ultrasound.
10. List the allergic reactions that may occur following an injection of a contrast medium (dye) into the veins or arteries.
11. Describe a fiberscope.
12. Identify the nursing management of a patient who has had endoscopy and radiologic examination.

REFERENCES

1. Berlin, N., Research Strategy in Cancer: Screening Diagnosis, Prognosis. Hosp. Practice 10(1):83-91 (June 1975).
2. Berlin, N., How to Color a Brain Tumor Blue. Med. World News, p. 41 (November 2, 1973).
3. Belinsky, I., Fiberoptic Advances: Visualizing the Pancreatic and Biliary Ducts. Am. J. Nurs., pp. 936-939, (June, 1976).
4. Marsh, B.R., Flexible Fiberoptic Bronchoscopy - Its Place in the Search for Lung Cancer. Ann. Otol. Rhinol. Laryngol., 82:757 (1973).
5. McCune, W.S., et al., Endoscopic Cannulation of the Ampulla of Vater: A Preliminary Report. Ann. Surg. 167: 752-756 (May, 1968).
6. New, P.F.S., Computed Tomography: A Major Diagnostic Advance. Hosp. Practice, 10(2):55-64 (February, 1973).
7. Nelson, J., et al., Detection, Diagnostic Evaluation, and Treatment of Dysplasia and Early Carcinoma of the Cervix. CA, 25(3):134 (May/June, 1975).
8. Osborne, R., The Differential Radiologic Diagnosis of Bone Tumors. American Cancer Society (1975).
9. Shafer, K., et al. Medical-Surgical Nursing. C.V. Mosby Co., St. Louis (1971).
10. Brunner, L.S. and Suddarth, D.S., Textbook of Medical-Surgical Nursing. J.B. Lippincott Co., New York (1975).
11. Pohutsky, L. and Pohutsky, K., Computerized Axial Tomography of the Brain: A New Diagnostic Tool. Am. J. Nurs., pp. 1341-1342 (August, 1975).
12. Overholt, B., Colonoscopy. CA, 25(2):74-81 (March/April, 1975).
13. Williams, C. and Muto, T., Examination of the Whole Colon with the Fiberoptic Colonoscope. Br. Med. J., 3:278 (1972).
14. Vennes, J.A. and Silvis, S.E., Endoscopic Visualization of the Bile and Pancreatic Ducts. Gastrointest. Endosc., 18:149-152 (May, 1972).

15. Russell, W., The Pathologic Diagnosis of Cancer - A
    Crescendo of Importance in Current and Future Therapies.
    Am. J. Clin. Pathol., 73(1):3-11 (January, 1980).
16. Samuels, B.I. and Silver, T.M., Diagnostic Ultrasound
    in the Evaluation of Patients with Gynecologic Cancer.
    Surg. Clin. North Am., 58(1):3-18 (February, 1978).
17. Leffall, L.D., Jr., Early Diagnosis of Colorectal Can-
    cer. CA, pp. 152-159 (1974).
18. Wolff, W.E. and Shinya, H., A New Approach to Colonic
    Polyps. Ann. Surg., pp. 367-378 (1973).

CHAPTER 5
Immunodiagnosis: Tumor Markers of Malignancy

The presence of antigenic substances in the circulation has been demonstrated through immunoassay of the blood or urine. Some of the identified tumor markers include:[1,2,3,4]

1. Carcinoembryonic antigen (CEA), a protein polysaccharide complex normally found in fetal gut which has been implicated in cancer of the colon, pancreas, liver, bronchus, cervix, endometrium, breast, ovary prostate, bladder, kidney, neuroblastoma, leukemia, and lymphoma. CEA assay is most valuable in monitoring metastases. Rising values of CEA are related to poor prognosis and positive levels posttreatment (i.e., surgery) may indicate metastases.
2. Carcinoplacental phosphatase (Regan and non-Regan isoenzyme) is a nonspecific tumor marker found in some patients with pancreatic, ovarian, and testicular cancer.
3. α-2-H fetoprotein (alpha-2-HFP), an antigen migrating with the α-globulins is found in patients with primary liver cancer, colorectal, testicular, pancreatic, gastric, bronchogenic, and embryonal carcinoma.
4. β-S fetoprotein (beta-SFP) found in liver cancer.
5. γ-fetoprotein (gamma-FP), found in serum of some patients with cancer.
6. γ-fetoprotein is found in a variety of human tumors and in fetal serum.
7. Fetal sulfoglycoprotein antigen (FSA) is found in some patients with gastric carcinoma.
8. Oncofetal antigen is a tumor-associated antigen found in some patients with carcinoma of the pancreas.

The identification of certain tumor markers is of particular significance in that it paves the way for further research on the etiology of cancer cells. Moreover, the value of immunoassay as a diagnostic tool is thereby reaffirmed.

REVIEW QUESTIONS

1. Define immunoassay.
2. List some of the tumor markers found in various types of cancer.
3. What is the significance of rising levels of CEA?
4. What would be the value of immunoassay in the detection and diagnosis of cancer?

REFERENCES

1. Bakemeier, R., Basic Principles of Tumor Immunology and Immunotherapy, in Clinical Oncology for Medical Students and Physicians: A Multidisciplinary Approach. (Rubin, P. and Bakemeier, R., eds.) University of Rochester School of Medicine and Dentistry, and American Cancer Society, New York, pp. 566-577 (1974).
2. Di Luzio, N., Globulin May be a Cancer Tipoff. Med. World News, p. 22 (September 28, 1973).
3. Keating, M., et al., Acute Leukemia in Adults. CA, pp. 2-3 (January/February, 1977).
4. Zamcheck, N. and Pusztaszeri, G., CEA, AFP and Other Potential Tumor Markers. CA, pp. 204-213 (July/August, 1975).

CHAPTER 6
The Role of Radioisotopes in Cancer Diagnosis

Several radioisotopes have been used in cancer diagnosis. When endoscopic and radiologic techniques fail to establish a diagnosis of cancer, radioisotope scanning is done since lesions that cannot be picked up by radiologic methods can be picked up by radioisotope. Among the commonly used radioisotopes for cancer diagnosis are:

1. Iodine-131 (sodium iodide, ^{131}I): This type of radioisotope has a physical half-life of 8.1 days. It is used in screening thyroid nodules and scanning the neck and body after thyroidectomy for diagnosis of metastases.
2. Radioiodinated serum albumin (RISA): This is human serum albumin with a physical half-life of 8.1 days. It is used in brain tumor diagnosis through scintillation scanning at 6 to 48 hours. There is increased concentration by malignant cells.
3. Phosphorus-32 (sodium phosphate, ^{32}P): Its physical half-life is 14.3 days and it is used for eye tumor, other head and neck tumors, and lung tumor in a limited way. This is done by using the Geiger-Müller counter. There is increased phosphorus uptake of malignant tumors.
4. Colloidal gold-198 (colloidal gold, ^{198}Au): This has a physical half-life of 2.7 days and is used in the diagnosis of liver tumors which are greater than 2 cm in diameter. This is done through scintillation scanning at 30 minutes to 5 hours. Space-occupying lesions do not concentrate this isotope.
5. Rose bengal-I-131 (rose bengal, ^{131}I): This has a half-life of 8.1 days and is done through scintillation scanning at 20 to 30 minutes for the diagnosis of liver tumors. The malignant tumors do not concentrate this isotope.
6. Selenomethionine-75 (selenomethionine, ^{75}Se): This has 127 days physical half-life and is done through scintillation scanning at 30 minutes to an hour, and is used in pancreatic tumor diagnosis. Benign and malignant tumors do not concentrate this.

7. Mercury-203-neohydrin (chlormerodin, ^{203}Hg): This has a physical half-life of 47.9 days and is used in renal scanning and in the diagnosis of squamous cell carcinomas of the skin and nasopharynx, and in bone, bowel, and lung tumors.
8. Strontium-85 (strontium chloride, ^{85}Sr): This has a physical half-life of 65 days; scintillation scanning at 24 to 48 hours is done for diagnosis of primary and metastatic bone tumors.
9. Calcium-47 (calcium chloride, ^{47}Ca): This has a physical half-life of 4.9 days, is done by scintillation scanning at one to two days and is useful in the diagnosis of primary and metastatic bone tumors. However, it is difficult to differentiate benign from malignant tumors since this compound, like strontium-85, localizes mainly in actively metabolizing bone tumors.

It should be noted that the amount of radiation received by the patient during the diagnostic procedure is minimal and therefore there is no need to exercise radiation precautions in caring for the patient after the test.[4]

Scanning in diagnostic terminology refers to the use of radionuclides and instrumentation to produce patterns of radioactivity for interpretation. Among the commonly done scanning tests are brain scan, thyroid scan, lung scan, and liver scan. In the case of a brain scan, only a few of the many radioactive tracers are used. Among those used are ^{99m}Tc technetium pertechnetate, ^{203}Hg and ^{197}Hg chlormerodin and RISA. Radioiodinated human serum albumin is mostly given intravenously in brain scanning procedures and the scan is done when the radioisotope uptake has reached a peak. Through external detection, the patterns of abnormal radioactive isotope uptake in the brain are transmitted to photographic films (scan) or an imaging screen (image). The physiologic rationale of a brain scan is centered upon the presence of the blood-brain barrier. Under normal conditions, the brain does not permit the passage of the radioisotope from the plasma to the brain tissue. Under abnormal conditions, this selective permeability is no longer effective; hence, the isotope passes to the site of the lesion. This phenomenon is attributed to breakdown of the blood barrier, increased vascularity, and metabolic factors.[1,3,5,6]

The preparation of a patient for a brain scan depends upon the type of isotope that will be used. For instance, in radioiodinated human serum albumin, 10 drops of Lugol solution is given three times a day for three days prior to the test. The purpose of this is to inhibit the uptake by the thyroid. The nurse should inform the patient that there is no pain and no need for enemas or withholding of fluids or food prior to the test. The patient is also instructed not to cough or move so that the picture will not be a false image. If ^{99m}Tc is used, the patient is instructed to keep hands away from the eyes, tears, face, and saliva because the radioactivity of the injected compound persists for a few hours, although there are no after effects. [2]

In thyroid scan, selenomethionine, ^{75}Se, an analog of methionine in which sulfur has been replaced by the gamma emitter isotope ^{75}Se, has been found to be useful in differentiating cystic and benign lesions from neoplastic ones. Both cystic and neoplastic thyroid lesions show cold areas of little or no concentration of radiotracer when scanned with pertechnetate ^{99m}Tc. With the use of selenomethionine ^{75}Se, however, cystic areas show cold areas on the scan whereas neoplastic lesions show "hot" areas of high uptake of the radiotracer.

REVIEW QUESTIONS

1. Identify the commonly used radioisotopes in the diagnosis of cancer.
2. Define scanning.
3. What is meant by physical half-life?
4. List the respective physical half-lives of the following radioisotopes:
   a. Iodine-131 (^{131}I)
   b. RISA
   c. Rose bengal
   d. Phosphorus-32 (^{32}P)
   e. Strontium-85 (^{85}Sr)
5. What is the preparation of a patient for a brain scan with RISA?
6. What is the advantage of ^{75}Se over ^{99m}Tc in thyroid scan?

REFERENCES

1. Peterson, B.H. and Kellog, C.J., Current Practice in Oncologic Nursing. C.V. Mosby Co., St. Louis (1976).
2. Mandrillo, M., Brain Scanning. Nurs. Clinics N. Am., 9(4):633-669 (December, 1974).
3. Ackermann, N.B., Use of Radioisotopic Agents in the Diagnosis of Cancer. CA, 15:257-269 (1965).
4. Posner, J., Diagnosis and Treatment of Metastases to the Brain. Nurs. Digest, 3(6):58-59 (November/December, 1975).

5. Walker, M., Malignant Brain Tumor - A Synopsis. CA, 25(3):116 (May/June, 1975).
6. Loken, M. and Frick, M., Scanning the Brain: Radionuclide Scintigraphy. Mod. Med., pp. 50-55 (May 1, 1976).

PART III
Treatment Modalities and Nursing Care Principles

CHAPTER 7
Chemotherapy

The recent advances in knowledge of the pharmacologic effects of old and new antineoplastic drugs and how best to use them greatly enhanced a safer and more efficacious treatment modality for cancer. Today, certain chemotherapeutic agents can help produce permanent arrest in some cases of malignancy, relieve symptoms, and prolong life.

ACTION OF ANTINEOPLASTIC
DRUGS ON THE CELL LIFE CYCLE

The life cycle of a normal cell or malignant cell is directed towards replication. This cycle consists of several distinct phases as follows:

1. Resting phase (G_0): The cell remains dormant until a stimulus triggers the onset of the replication process.
2. RNA and protein synthesis (G^1): Commences after the stimulus for replication is triggered and continues until the DNA synthesis begins.
3. DNA synthesis (S): This follows the RNA and protein synthesis.
4. Small amounts of RNA synthesis: These take place while the cell enters a quiet period (G).
5. Mitosis phase (M): The cell divides into two daughter cells which enter either a resting phase or, if the stimulus still exists, continue through the life cycle.

The cell life cycle duration can either be short or long. Cells that proliferate rapidly have a short life cycle, whereas those that proliferate slowly have a long life cycle. It is this life cycle that is interrupted specifically or nonspecifically by antineoplastic drugs.

Drugs that affect the cell during only one phase of the cell's life cycle are called cell-specific drugs. For instance, antimetabolite drugs interfere with the DNA synthesis. Plant alkaloids inhibit mitosis. Those drugs that affect more than one phase of the cell's life cycle are cell-cycle nonspecific drugs. Alkylating agents, for example, destroy completed DNA by settling within the nucleus of the cell and altering the DNA molecules. Antibiotics such as actinomycin-D destroy completed DNA and inhibit the transcription of RNA. Hormones alter cell metabolism by creating an unfavorable environment for cell growth and reproduction.

MODE OF ACTION OF ANTINEOPLASTIC DRUGS

1. Antimetabolites interfere with the metabolic pathways normally used in synthesizing certain chemicals (metabolites) essential to the normal cell. They are similar in structure to vitamins, coenzymes, or normal intermediary metabolic products. They act by affecting cell nucleic acid synthesis. They may affect the biosynthesis of DNA or RNA by interfering with the rates of synthesis of the purines or pyrimidines. They may also substitute abnormal components for those essential to biosynthesis.

2. Polyfunctional alkylating agents are known as antimitotic drugs because they settle within the nucleus of the cell and alter the deoxyribonucleic acid (DNA) molecules so that cell growth and division are inhibited. These include cyclophosphamide (Cytoxan), melphalan (Alkeran), chlorambucil and busulfan.

3. Hormones change the chemical environment of the cancer cells by providing a hormonal imbalance that may interfere with the growth of the hormone-dependent tumors. These hormones include prednisone, the progestins, estrogens, and androgens.

4. Enzymes (L-asparaginase) work in this manner: Cells make use of an amino acid called asparagine. While normal cells make their own, leukemic cells cannot. Thus, when L-asparaginase is administered to a leukemic patient, it breaks down the asparagine available in the body fluids, thereby causing starvation of the leukemic cells and consequently a remission of the disease ensues.

5. Natural products are not clear how their major action works but these drugs are believed to inhibit mitosis by interfering with the metabolic pathways. These include antibiotics like actinomycin-D, urethane, and the vinca alkaloids, which

are extracted from the periwinkle plant and include vincristine and vinblastine.

6. Antifolics block the conversion of folic acid to tetrahydrafolic acid, a substance needed for DNA synthesis and mitosis. An example is methotrexate.

7. Antipurines inhibit purines, which are proteins needed for DNA synthesis. Purine antagonists include mercaptopurine (6-MP).

8. Antipyramidines inhibit pyramidines which are also proteins needed for DNA synthesis. Examples of pyramidine antagonists are fluorouracil (5-FU) and cytosine arabinoside (Cytosar or ara-C).

9. Miscellaneous drugs comprise a variety of investigational drugs which are effective against malignant cells. Some of these drugs have been proven to be efficacious in certain specific cases of cancer while others are still in the process of further investigation. Exact mechanisms of action of these drugs are still not totally known. For example, mitotane (O, p-DDD or Lysodren) is chemically similar to DDT and has been found to be effective in treating adrenocortical tumors, although its mechanism of action is unknown. Recently interferon, a protein substance produced by a virus-infected animal cell, has been shown to shrink tumors in animals and has already helped some humans. Hydroxyurea (Hydrea) inhibits DNA synthesis, while procarbazine (Matulane) inhibits DNA, RNA, and protein synthesis.

The various types of anticancer drugs, the specific dosage, method of administration, toxic effects and side effects, indications for use, and the subsequent nursing management of the patient's reactions can best be understood through Table 5.

Table 5: Cancer Chemotherapy and Principles of Nursing Intervention

Agents	Indications for Use	Method of Administration	Side Effects/ Toxic Effects	Nursing Intervention
Polyfunctional Alkylating Agents				
Methylbis (B-Chloroethyl) Amine HCL (HN₂, Mustargen) Mechlorethamine nitrogen mustard	Chronic leukemias, Cancers of the lung, breast, ovary, Hodgkin's disease, lymphosarcoma, reticulum cell sarcoma	IV	Nausea, vomiting, local phlebitis, marrow depression alopecia, jaundice, vertigo, tinnitus, decreased hearing, weakness, diarrhea, decreased sperm, skin eruptions, convulsions	Provide an emesis basin at bedside and empty after each use. Allay anxiety and stay with patient. Instruct patient to take deep breaths while nauseated. Give antiemetic drug as ordered, bland diet. Give mouth care to make patient feel refreshed. Note color, amount of vomitus and record. Avoid spillage on skin or infiltration since it can cause severe damage, use sodium thiosulfate to decrease reactions. Kaopectate, antispasmodics or Lomotil may be given for diarrhea. Wear gloves.
Busulfan (Myeleran)	Chronic granulocytic leukemia, polycythemia vera, primary thrombocytosis	PO	Pulmonary fibrosis, marrow depression, gynecomastia, hyperpigmentation of skin, amenorrhea, nausea, vomiting, testicular atrophy, bone marrow depression, systemic infection can occur, pseudomonas, candidiasis	Check results of lab tests, report abnormalities of CBC platelets. Initiate reverse isolation

Table 5 (Cont'd)

Agents	Indications for Use	Method of Administration	Side Effects/ Toxic Effects	Nursing Intervention
Chlorambucil (Leukeran)	Lymphosarcoma, Hodgkin's disease, cancers of breast, testis and ovary, chronic lymphocytic leukemia, lymphoma	PO	Nausea, vomiting, moderate depression of peripheral blood count, marrow depression, hepatic toxicity, bleeding, megaloblastic anemia	SAME AS ABOVE plus observe any bleeding. Check color of urine
Cyclophosphamide Endoxan, Cytoxan CTX	Acute lymphocytic leukemia, chronic lymphocytic leukemia, cancer of the breast, ovary, lung, colon; Burkitt's sarcoma; Ewing's sarcoma, lymphosarcoma, Hodgkin's disease, multiple myeloma, neuroblastoma, reticulum cell sarcoma, Wilms' tumor; rhabdomyosarcoma	IV	SAME AS ABOVE, alopecia, hemorrhagic cystitis, anaphylactic reaction, liver dysfunction, stomatitis, mucositis, delayed wound healing, loss of virility, amenorrhea, dermatitis, darkened skin pigments	SAME AS ABOVE plus allow patient to verbalize feelings about self-image. Suggest use of wig or hair piece. Provide physical comfort and emotional support. Ensure adequate hydration to prevent irritation of kidneys and bladder that cause hemorrhagic cystitis. For stomatitis give mouth care using lemon swabs rather than toothbrushes. Give soft, bland foods; do not give commercially prepared mouthwashes since they only irritate; instead give H_2O and H_2O_2 (1:1 proportion) then rinse with water; in case of severe pain, Xylocaine or Chloroseptic mouthwash may be given before meals.

Drug	Route	Side Effects	Nursing Measures
Melphalan (Alkeran Compound CB 3025, L-Sarcolysin) L-PAM, L-Phenylalanine mustard)	PO	Nausea, vomiting, marrow depression, stomatitis	Stay with patient. Allay anxiety. Provide emesis basin and clean after each use. Give antiemetic as ordered. Note amount, color of vomitus and record. Check lab work and report findings if abnormal. Give after meals to prevent nausea.
Triethylenethiophosphoramide (ThioTEPA, TSPA)	IV, PO	Marrow depression, local pain, nausea, vomiting, dizziness, headache, anemia, GI perforation, potential allergic reaction	Check lab work. Report abnormal findings. Initiate reverse isolation. Protect patient from infection; use with caution if kidneys are impaired.
Triethylene melamine (TEM)	PO	Severe marrow depression, anorexia	Same measures as above. In addition, give sodium bicarb to promote absorption and activity of drug. Give before meals, acids inactivate the drug.

Table 5 (Cont'd)

Agents	Indications for Use	Method of Adminis-tration	Side Effects/ Toxic Effects	Nursing Intervention
ANTIMETABOLITES				
Methotrexate (Amethopterin) MTX	Acute lymphocytic leukemia; breast cancer; choriocarcinoma; head and neck cancer; and testicular cancer; CNS leukemia; osteogenic sarcoma	PO, IV intra-thecal	Impaired kidney function, chills, fever, nausea, vomiting, pruritus, urticaria, drowsiness, visual blurring, headaches, photosensitivity, gastrointestinal ulceration; stomatitis; bone marrow depression; diarrhea; alopecia; fibrosis of lung, cystitis, diabetes, liver atrophy and necrosis	Provide mouth care. Protect from infection. Check vital signs at least q.i.d. Give adequate fluids, watch for bleeding. Since drug is excreted through the kidneys, it should not be given in the presence of impaired renal function; keep antidote for drug on hand, i.e., leukovorin (folinic acid). Caution: not given to those with liver dysfunction; check liver function test results. Note: effect of MTX is decreased by salicylates, sulfonamides, and aminobenzoic acid; do not give with tetracyclines, vitamins, vaccines or chloramphenicol, dilantin)
Cytosine arabinoside (Ara-C, Cytarabine, Cytosar)	Lymphocytic and acute granulocytic leukemia	IV	Marrow depression; megaloblastosis; leukopenia; thrombocytopenia, nausea, vomiting; hepatic toxicity; esophagitis, thrombophlebitis	Check vital signs; report any rise in temperature. Care for nausea and vomiting as previously stated. Reduce exposure to infection; reverse isolation; drug crosses blood-brain barrier

5-Fluorouracil (5-FU),	Bladder cancer, ovarian cancer, breast cancer, cancer of stomach and colon, lung cancer, cancer of uterus, liver, skin, oropharynx and prostate	IV	Stomatitis, GI injury, marrow depression; nausea, diarrhea, alopecia, dermatitis, nail changes; cerebellar dysfunction	Meticulous mouth care. Avoid foods that cause curds. Give plenty of fluids. Check lab work and vital signs. Give Kaopectate as ordered; stomatitis indicates impending bone marrow depression
6-Mercaptopurine (6-MP, Purinethol)	Acute granulocytic and lymphocytic leukemia, chronic granulocytic leukemia, and choriocarcinoma	PO	Marrow depression, nausea, vomiting (rare), hepatic toxicity, stomatitis, mouth ulcers	Check lab work and report abnormalities. Encourage verbalization of feelings.
6-Thioguanine (6-TG, Thioguan)	Acute myelogenous leukemia, chronic granulocytic leukemia		Photosensitivity, bone marrow depression, hepatic dysfunction, nausea, vomiting, skin rash, stomatitis, jaundice	SAME AS ABOVE. Avoid alcohol. Observe for rash and jaundice and report immediately to doctor.
Floxuridine (FUDR, Fluorodeuxyuridine)	Cancer of colon; gallbladder, bile duct; liver metastasis	IV	Nausea, vomiting, diarrhea, stomatitis, alopecia, bone marrow depression	Give antiemetics; mouth care as previously stated, note any loose, watery stools and report; check WBC levels

Table 5 (Cont'd)

Agents	Indications for Use	Method of Administration	Side Effects/ Toxic Effects	Nursing Intervention
ANTIBIOTICS				
Actinomycin D (Dactinomycin) Cosmegen, Meractinomycin)	Choriocarcinoma, rhabdomyosarcoma, Ewing's sarcoma, Wilms' tumor, testicular cancer, oat cell cancer of lung	IV	Stomatitis, GI disturbances, alopecia, marrow depression, local phlebitis, tissue necrosis, nausea, vomiting, diarrhea, dermatitis, acne, abdominal pain, fatigue, malaise, lethargy, proctitis	Avoid skin infiltration (very toxic) Note: Not given if child has chicken pox since it would cause CNS chicken pox and resultant death. If given post-radiotherapy, it may reactivate radiation site.
Adriamycin (ADRIA, Doxorubicin	Ewing's sarcoma, acute granulocytic and lymphocytic leukemia, cancer of breast, bladder, thyroid; lung; Hodgkin's disease; multiple myeloma, neuroblastoma, osteogenic sarcoma, reticulum cell sarcoma	IV	Alopecia, GI disturbances, bone marrow depression, cardiac toxicity at cumulative doses over 600 mg/m^2 can cause congestive heart failure, immediate toxicity: abdominal pain, nausea and vomiting within 4-6 hrs; mouth ulcers; thrombophlebitis at injection site	SAME AS ABOVE, check any irregular and increased pulse rate and abnormal rhythm. Observe for signs of cardiac decompensation (edema of legs, dyspnea, weakness). Dose is limited to 550 mg/m^2. Drug is red and causes red urine, thus <u>not</u> hematuria.

Drug	Route	Uses	Side Effects/Toxicity	Nursing Considerations
Bleomycin (Blenoxane)	IV	Head and neck cancer, lymphosarcoma, reticulum cell sarcoma, testicular cancer, Hodgkin's disease, epidermoid cancer lymphoma, urinary tract cancer, soft tissue sarcoma	Phlebitis, fever, chills, pneumonia, mucocutaneous ulcerations, alopecia, pulmonary fibrosis, rarely stomatitis and myelosuppression, may have pain and hemorrhage from tumor site due to rapid destruction of tumor tissue	Check vital signs q 4 hrs. Report any fever, chills. Give antipyretic drugs as ordered. Maintain proper room temperature and humidity. Avoid exposure to those with respiratory symptoms. Give mouth care. Note any difficult breathing. Dose limit is 400 mg total. Test dose is given before first dose.
Daunomycin (Rubidomycin, Daunorubicin)	IV	Acute granulocytic and lymphocytic leukemia, neuroblastoma	Nausea, vomiting, phlebitis, necrosis, marrow depression, alopecia, stomatitis, cardiac toxicity at cumulative doses over 25 mg/kg, mouth ulcer; diarrhea; fever with skin rash; CHF; PVC's; ST changes	Protect from infection. Check vital signs. Note pulse rhythm and rate. Drug is red and causes red color of urine. Dose is limited to 600 mg/m.
Mithramycin (Mithracin)	IV	Testicular cancer, malignant hypercalcemia, trophoblastic tumors	Anorexia, nausea, drowsiness, azotemia, thrombocytopenia, marrow depression, hypocalcemia, hepatic toxicity, hypokalemia, epistaxis, hematemesis, vomiting, diarrhea, stomatitis, change in renal and liver function with increased BUN and SGOT, headache	Note any complaint of tingling of extremities and muscle spasms. Serve foods attractively. Give nutritive fluids. Watch any bleeding and report immediately to physician, toxic to skin if infiltrated. Instruct patient not to drive or operate heavy machinery after dose

Table 5 (Cont'd)

Agents	Indications for Use	Method of Administration	Side Effects/ Toxic Effects	Nursing Intervention
Mitomycin C (Mutamycin)	Cancer of colon, pancreas, cervix, breast, lung, head and neck cancers; gastric carcinoma, malignant melanoma	IV	Bone marrow depression nausea, vomiting, severe skin reaction if given subcutaneously, stomatitis, severe malaise, fever, alopecia, pruritus, renal damage, paresthesias	Have vitamin B6 on hand to counteract severe skin reaction to be given stat after extravasation
STEROID HORMONES				
Androgen Testosterone propionate (Oreton) Halotestin, Teslac, Delatestryl, Drolban, Methosarb Cupusterone	Breast cancer postmenopausal or postcastration	PO IM	Fluid retention; masculinization, hirsutism, dyspepsia, increase libido, deepening of voice, hot flashes	Watch for edema. Weigh daily. Monitor blood pressure.
Estrogens Diethylstilbestrol (DES, Stilbestrol)	Breast cancer (palliative only) prostatic cancer (palliative therapy for advanced disease)	PO	Diarrhea, breast tenderness, headache, rash, paresthesias, anxiety, insomnia, changes in libido, changes in calcium and phosphorus metabolism, muscle weakness, polyuria, polydypsia	Note: urinary output; push fluids, limit calcium intake in milk, cheese, etc. Encourage ambulation to keep calcium in bones.
Estradiol cypionate (Depo-Estradiol)	Prostatic cancer	IM		
Chlorotrianesene (TACE)	Prostatic cancer	PO		
Estradiol valerate (Delestrogen)	Prostatic cancer	IM		

Estrone (Theelin)	Prostatic cancer	IM	Possible nausea, vomiting, sodium retention	Assess for occurrence of possible side-effects.
Polyestradiol phosphate (Estradurin)	Prostatic cancer	IM		
Estrogenic substances, conjugated (Premarin), esterified (Evex, Amnestrogen, Menest)	Breast and prostatic carcinomas	PO		
Progestin	Renal and breast cancer		When used with estrogens may cause nausea and vomiting, anorexia, abdominal cramps, thromboembolitic disorders, depression, backache, breast tenderness, hypercalcemia, fluid retention, libido changes	
Megestrol acetate (Megace)	Endometrial cancer	PO		
Prednisone (Deltasone, Merticorten, Orasone, Paracort, Deltra-Dome, Servisone)	Acute leukemia (as combination chemotherapy; COAP)	PO	Stomatitis, gastric ulcers, alopecia, increased pigmentation, acne, urticaria, nail changes	Give with antacids and continue for at least 1 week after discontinuation of drug

Table 5 (Cont'd)

Agents	Indications for Use	Method of Adminis-tration	Side Effects/ Toxic Effects	Nursing Intervention
Hydrocortisone sodium succinate (Solu-cortef)	Acute and chronic lymphocytic leukemia, breast cancer, lymphosarcoma	IV	Potassium loss, sodium and fluid retention, gastric bleeding	Give foods high in potassium such as bananas, oranges, prunes, dates. Monitor blood pressure, weight and electrolytes
Dexamethasone (Decadron)	Same as above	PO	Immunosuppression, fluid retention, hypertension, diabetes	Protect from infection. Watch for edema. Weigh daily. Check BP q 4 hrs. Clinitest and Acetest urine after each voiding.
Methylprednisolone sodium succinate (Solu-Medrol)	Acute and chronic lymphocytic leukemia, breast cancer, miscellaneous tumors	IM IV	Depression, headache, hypertension, increased intraocular pressure, ulcer, menstrual abnormalities, atrophy at IM injection, muscle weakness, withdrawal symptoms, hypotension, dyspnea, fatigue, fever, hypokalemia, hypernatremia	Avoid sudden withdrawal of drug. Check BP, weight, serum electrolytes. Teach patient signs of early adrenal insufficiency: fatigue, muscular weakness, joint pain, fever, anorexia. Watch for depression or psychotic episodes.

MISCELLANEOUS DRUGS

Drug	Uses	Route	Side Effects	Nursing Considerations
BCNU (1.3-bis (B-Chloroethyl)-1-nitrosurea, Carmustine	Brain tumor, breast cancer, cancer of the lung and colon, myeloma, melanoma, lymphomas, gastric cancer, renal cancer	IV	Facial flushing, nausea, vomiting 6 hrs after dose, renal toxicity, burning pain along vein, marrow depression, diarrhea, mild hepatotoxicity, anorexia	Observe amount and color of urine. Maintain I&O. Protect from infection. Give analgesics as prescribed. Crosses the blood-brain barrier, avoid skin contact (causes brown spots).
Hydroxyurea (Hydrea)	Brain tumor, chronic granulocytic leukemia, melanoma	PO	Marrow depression; anorexia, diarrhea, megaloblastic anemia, nausea, vomiting, skin rash, rarely alopecia, oral and GI ulceration	Protect from infection. Note any complaints of feeling tired and report to physician. Watch for pallor. Serve frequent, small feedings that are attractively set up. Note amount and frequency of defecation. Synergistic action with radiotherapy and may cause erythema. Note: Give with caution if liver or kidney are impaired. Crosses blood-brain barrier.
Mitotane (O, p'DDD, lysodren, Ortho-para-DDD)	Adenocortical cancer after excision	PO	Nausea, vomiting, anorexia, GI toxicity, diarrhea, CNS depression, dizziness, altered steroid metabolism, tremors, bone marrow depression	Instruct patient to be careful if concentration and coordination is needed. Steroid replacement may be necessary.

Table 5 (Cont'd)

Agents	Indications for Use	Method of Administration	Side Effects/ Toxic Effects	Nursing Intervention
Streptozotocin (probably acts by alkylation)	Pancreatic insulinoma, carcinoid tumor, Hodgkin's disease, lung	IV	Nausea, vomiting, renal tubule defects, abdominal cramps, stomatitis, may cause hypoglycemia, nephrotoxicity, diabetogenic	Inform patient of burning sensation on administration. Test urine for glycosuria (urinalysis)
Neocarzinostatin antibiotic (Investigational Drug)	Advanced bladder cancer, carcinoma of pancreas, stomach, ovaries, uterus, liver and kidneys, malignant melanoma, acute leukemia	IV	Nausea and vomiting, anorexia, diarrhea, anaphylactic reaction, elevation of liver enzymes, acute renal failure, skin rash, stomatitis, headache, chills	Give antiemetics as ordered, watch urinary output and report any oliguria. Mouth care as previously mentioned. Avoid sudden changes in room temperature. Report any chills or signs of anaphylaxis.
CCNU (1-(2-chloroethyl) 3-cyclohexyl-1-nitrosourea; Lomustine) Investigational Drug (Alkylating agent)	Hodgkin's disease, primary/secondary CNS tumors, gastric, renal, bronchogenic carcinomas	PO	Nausea and vomiting, gastric irritation, hepatotoxicity, bone marrow depression	Give antiemetics. Take fluids on empty stomach. Crosses blood-brain barrier. NPO for 4-6° post drug intake.

Drug	Use	Route	Side Effects	Nursing Considerations
Methyl-CCNU (1-2-chloroethyl)-3(4-methylcyclohexyl)-1-nitrosoureal); MeCCNU; Semustine, Lomustine) <u>Investigational Drug</u> (More useful than BCNU in cancer of gastrointestinal tract)	Primary/secondary CNS tumors; cancer of stomach, colon, lung, pancreas; squamous cell carcinoma; malignant melanoma	PO	Nausea and vomiting, gastric irritation, anorexia, bone marrow depression, leukopenia, thrombocytopenia, renal and hepatotoxicity	Give on empty stomach 4 hrs. after meal. Give antiemetics and fluids. Avoid sources of infection.
Hexamethylmelamine (probably acts as an antimetabolite) <u>Investigational Drug</u>	Cancer of lung and ovary	PO	Nausea, vomiting, diarrhea, peripheral neuropathy after repeated doses, bone marrow depression, alopecia, motor weakness, incoordination	Give antiemetics. Note: record and report watery stools. Drug may have to be stopped. Infection/bleeding caution.
Imidazole carboxamide dimethyltriazino (DIC, DTIC, BIC, Imidazole Carboxamide, TIC Mustard, Imidazole Mustard) <u>Investigational Drug</u>	Hodgkin's disease, malignant melanoma	IV	Nausea, vomiting 1-2 hrs after IV dose, improves with further doses, flu-like syndrome with myalgia, headache and malaise up to 10 days, mild hepatotoxicity, rare bone marrow depression	Protect from light. Inform patient of possible burning sensation on injection, metallic taste, give antiemetics.
Cycloleucine (1-amino cyclopentane carbosylicacid) <u>Investigational Drug</u>	Sarcomas	IV push or scalp vein needle	Nausea, vomiting, mild bone marrow depression, CNS toxicity, vertigo, slurred speech, ataxia, weakness, diplopia, disorientation, immunosuppression	Give antiemetics. Protect from infection. Observe for early signs of CNS toxicity (drug may need to be stopped).

Table 5 (Cont'd)

Agents	Indications for Use	Method of Administration	Side Effects/ Toxic Effects	Nursing Intervention
Procarbazine (Matulane, Natulane, methylhydrazine, ibenzmethyzin)	Hodgkin's disease, myeloma, ovarian and oat cell cancer, non-Hodgkin's lymphomas	PO IV	Sedative effect, nausea, vomiting, bone marrow depression, myalgia, CNS irritability, rare psychosis, orthostatic hypotension, inhibition of monoamine oxidase, mental depression, convulsion	Synergistic action with phenothiazine and barbiturates, narcotic intolerance to alcohol. Note any facial edema. Instruct patient to avoid eating cheese, yogurt, bananas; do not drink chianti wine; avoid antihistamines, narcotics, sedatives, and alcohol. Drug crosses the blood-brain barrier. Watch for evidence of infection or bleeding and report stat
BCG (Bacille Calmette-Guerin) substrains: 1. Pasteur 2. Connaught 3. Tice 4. Glaxo nonspecific immunostimulant	Acute and chronic leukemia, lymphoma, malignant melanoma lung cancer	Intralesional, intradermal, IV, heaf gun, scarification, multipuncture	After injection, local inflammation occurs (red papule in 7-10 days), then necrosis, eschar, and healing unless secondary infection sets in; flu-like syndrome with fever, myalgia, nausea, vomiting, lymphadenopathy near tumor sites, anaphylactic reaction	Avoid autoinnoculation, keep site clean, dry, and exposed to air; give aspirin for flu-like syndrome; give antiemetics
cis-Platinum (II) diammine dichloride Inorganic metallic salt	Testicular and ovarian cancers, epidermoid tumors, head and neck cancer	IV	Nausea, vomiting, renal toxicity, deafness, diarrhea, bone marrow depression	Give anti-emetics. Observe urinary output. Safeguard against infection.

PLANT EXTRACTS

Drug	Route	Indications	Side Effects	Nursing Considerations
Vinblastine (Velban)	IV	Breast cancer, choriocarcinoma, Hodgkin's disease, lymphosarcoma, reticulum cell sarcoma, testicular cancer	Stomatitis, marrow depression, paresthesia, headache, vomiting, alopecia, constipation, diarrhea, abdominal pain, depression, loss of deep tendon reflexes, vesiculation of mouth, ileus, pain in tumor site, urinary retention	Apply previously mentioned principles on care of nausea, vomiting, alopecia and marrow depression. Reassure patient when anxious about paresthesia. Avoid infiltration (very toxic.) Caution: if splashed in the eye it can cause corneal ulceration, thus be careful in handling drug and wash hands after use; drug has cumulative toxicity.
Vincristine sulfate (Oncovin)	IV	Acute lymphatic leukemia, breast cancer, Ewing's sarcoma, Hodgkin's disease, lymphosarcoma, reticulum cell sarcoma, Wilms' tumor; rhabdomyosarcoma, testicular cancer, choriocarcinoma	Paresthesias, areflexia, muscular weakness, hoarseness, paralytic ileus, mental depression, constipation, mild marrow depression, impotence, visual disturbances, seizures, loss of deep tendon reflexes, upper colon impaction	Reassure patient. Assist in self-care. Watch for abdominal distention. Show interest in patient. Encourage involvement in some activities. Give plenty of fluids and fruits. Check lab results. Prophylactic stool softeners should be given; dosage limited by neurotoxicity; prevent skin infiltration - very toxic. Note: Use with caution in patients with pre-existing neuropathies.

Table 5 (Cont'd)

Agents	Indications for Use	Method of Administration	Side Effects/ Toxic Effects	Nursing Intervention
ENZYME				
L-Asparaginase (Elspar)	Acute lymphocytic leukemia	IV	Fever, allergic reactions, hyperglycemia, hepatic toxicity, nausea, vomiting, renal toxicity, reversible encephalopathy, hypoalbuminemia, blood dyscrasias, malaise, hyper/hypo-lipidemia, decreased clotting factor, pancreatitis	Check vital signs. Give anti-pyretics as ordered. Check lab work. Report any abnormalities. Note urinary output, amount, and color of urine. Test urine for glucose at least once a day. Avoid shaking vial - it harms enzymes.

Note: Due to the continued aggressive search for additional agents that can be used therapeutically in the treatment of cancer, this table cannot be completely exhaustive of everything that is being subjected to research and investigation.

RESISTANCE TO CHEMOTHERAPY

The effectiveness of chemotherapy can be curtailed by the kind of resistance exhibited by the neoplasm. There are three types of resistance to chemotherapy that have been identified:

1. Type I resistance: Permanently resistant tumor cells cannot be affected by the drug at all. For example, one in a million to 10 million tumor cells become resistant to a specific drug or class of drug. When this occurs, another type of combined chemotherapy should be used.
2. Type II resistance: Temporarily resistant tumor cells can be affected if a combined modality of treatment is used such as surgery, chemotherapy, and irradiation.
3. Type III resistance: Tumor cells that receive less than average drug exposure due to anatomic site or architecture, e.g., those that cannot be reached by drugs that do not have the capacity of crossing the brain barrier. In this case, intrathecal administration of a specific drug is advocated.

PERFUSION AND INTRA-ARTERIAL INFUSION CHEMOTHERAPY

In cancer chemotherapy, it is sometimes necessary to give large doses of extremely toxic drugs to an isolated extremity, organ, or region of the patient's body. In such a case, perfusion technique is used. This technique involves the use of a pump oxygenator so that the patient's blood is circulated in a closed system for the involved part of the body. The chemotherapeutic drug is injected in concentrated doses. The duration of the perfusion depends on the drug and the extent and location of the tumors. During the procedure, efforts are made by tourniquets and/or ligatures to prevent seepage of the drug into the systemic circulation. The vessels perfused for a lesion in the lower extremity are the iliac, femoral, and popliteal arteries and veins. For the upper extremity the axillary artery and vein are used, and for pelvic perfusion the abdominal aorta and the vena cava are used.

Intra-arterial infusion is the introduction of a catheter into a major artery with the aid of a fluoroscope. This has the advantage of not requiring surgery and it can be repeated at intervals. Routes used are the brachial, axillary, carotid, and femoral arteries, depending on the location of the cancer.

To prepare a patient for perfusion, he should be weighed, as the weight would determine the amount of chemotherapeutic drugs to be given. Moreover, heparin is calculated on the basis of the patient's weight. Blood, urine, and x-ray studies as ordered by the physician should be done and the results made available prior to perfusion.

Nursing Management

The nursing care of the patient following perfusion and intra-arterial infusion is as follows:

1. Blood tests are done to check any bone marrow depression.
2. Check tissue around area of perfusion for any reaction such as erythema, mild edema, blistering, and petechiae.
3. Pain is usually not a problem but if it occurs and is severe, it may indicate injury to the tissues. It is very important for the nurse to note any complaints of soreness at the injection site.
4. Observe for signs of malaise, nausea, vomiting, rise in temperature, and signs of hypotension in patients who had aortic perfusion.
5. Fluids and electrolytes are maintained for the first 48 hours after therapy to prevent adverse reactions.
6. Keep an accurate intake and output record of the patient's daily fluid intake and elimination.
7. Provide emotional support to the patient.

DETERMINATION OF
APPROPRIATE CHEMOTHERAPY

The Goals of Chemotherapy

1. Effect cure, and/or remission induction. Therefore, the specific objective is to give the right drug in the right amount at the proper time.
2. Prolong the disease-free interval and maintain remission.
3. Shrink tumor masses.
4. Palliate symptoms and minimize immunosuppression.
5. Improve patient's well-being.
6. Reossify lytic bone lesions.
7. Relieve pressure on lymphatic, nerve, and vascular elements.

Factors considered in the selection of appropriate drugs and/or regimen (to achieve one or more of the goals of chemotherapy as mentioned above) include the following:

1. Cell type: Certain drugs are cell-type-specific. For example, bleomycin is most effective against tumors of squamous cell origin whereas 5-fluorouracil is most effective

against adenocarcinoma, a glandular tissue tumor.

2. Tumor location: Brain tumor cannot be affected by 5-fluorouracil because this drug does not cross the blood-brain barrier.

3. Rate of drug absorption: In isolated organ tumors such as liver cancer, an intra-arterial infusion drug is necessary but for some cases oral drugs are preferred. As a general rule, localized tumors are treated with localized (instillation) drugs and systemic tumors are treated with systemic drugs.

4. Patient's eligibility for chemotherapy: Some patients may not be good candidates for certain drugs due to more harmful than desirable side effects.

5. Status of bone marrow functioning: Evidence of adequate hemoglobin, white blood cell count, platelet count, and lymphocytic count are essential before drug treatment, especially if the drug to be given can cause myelosuppression.

6. Histologic proof of cancer diagnosis: To prevent administration of drugs for a nonmalignant tumor and to determine recurrence of disease or metastases, histologic proof should be obtained.

7. Weight of patient: If the patient is underweight, drug dosage is based on actual weight, but if he is underweight and edematous, dosage is based on estimated dry weight. If the patient is overweight or edematous, drug dosage is based on the ideal weight for the patient's height and age.

8. Nutritional status and state of hydration: Some drugs may cause decreased absorption of vitamins, nutrients, and water in the gastrointestinal mucosa. On the other hand, nutrition is important in promoting efficacy of chemotherapy. Cells must be well nourished to be maximally affected by antineoplastic agents. For example, the sensitivity of DNA during synthesis can be blocked by a lack of essential amino acids or uracil. [12]

9. Expectation of longevity: If the patient is moribund and is not likely to live longer than four weeks, a drug may only hasten death rather than prolong life as well as cause misery on the patient due to the toxic effects of the drug. Therefore, prior to chemotherapy the possible positive and negative outcomes should be carefully weighed and a decision made based upon the most desirable benefits for the patient.

10. Presence of liver and/or renal disease: Since the majority of these drugs are detoxified by the liver and then excreted by the kidneys, impairment of these organs can cause drug overdose or increased toxicity.

11. History of chemotherapy: Introduction of a different drug regimen should preferably be done only after four to eight weeks after cessation of other chemotherapeutic drugs the patient was receiving. However, this may not necessarily be the practice in institutions where support systems such as laminar airflow rooms or cell separators (to obtain white cells and subsequently transfuse into leukopenic patients) are available.

12. Psychological and mental status: Willingness and cooperation of the patient are crucial in achieving the goals of chemotherapy. If the patient is emotionally unstable and nonreceptive, it has been found that the incidence of nausea and vomiting as ill effects of chemotherapy are increased.

13. Other considerations: It is important to realize that it is difficult to determine optimum dose schedules or regimen because of other factors that affect the patient's response to therapy, such as the length of the cell cycle, the proliferation fraction, changes that occur resulting from a decreasing or increasing mass, and the transit time through each cell phase.[13,14]

Principles of Combination Chemotherapy

To minimize toxic effects, relieve symptoms, and produce remission, a single drug which is active and effective is used alone. In combined chemotherapy, drugs that are biochemically synergistic in effect are used. Other principles that should be adhered to are:

1. Use drugs with different mechanisms of action.[7]
2. Use drugs that produce toxicity in different organ systems.[7]
3. Use drugs whose toxicity occur at different times following administration.[7]
4. Use drugs in repeated brief courses in order to minimize immunosuppressive effects that might otherwise occur.[7]
5. Recruitment: This is a treatment device whereby one drug is given to reduce tumor size and another drug is given to eliminate cells brought into cycle as a result of the first drug. It has been found that in general, when a high dose of the first drug is given and is followed immediately by a high dose of the second drug, the drug regimen may cause more harm to the host than the tumor itself.[15] Thus, a one-week interval between drug administration is recommended.
6. Sequential use of surgery, radiation therapy, or both may be necessary to relieve cell overcrowding in high-density

tumors so that cells can become proliferative and consequently sensitive to chemical treatment.[14]

In summary, the purpose of combination chemotherapy is to achieve the maximum therapeutic effect without precipitating severe toxicity. A good example of this is the COAP regimen, a combination of cyclophosphamide (Cytoxan), vincristine sulfate (Oncovin), cytosine arabinoside (Cytosar), and prednisone. The efficacy of COAP results from its ability to affect cells during every phase of the cell cycle and thereby achieve what no one drug could accomplish if it were administered alone.

ADJUVANT THERAPY AND
INVESTIGATION THERAPY

The new trend in cancer chemotherapy is adjuvant chemotherapy. This entails early drug treatment for patients with minimal disease to prevent spread of the disease. The specific objective is to remove the microscopic sites of metastatic cancer, or "micrometastases," that are believed to be present in most solid tumors such as those of the breast, colon, and lung. Adjuvant therapy is highly advantageous right after surgery since the patient is in a better state of health and can tolerate the drugs better. An example of this is the National Surgical Adjuvant Breast Project begun in 1971. This project involved the study of women with surgically removed primary breast carcinoma and with pathologically positive axillary nodes. A control group of 108 were given surgery alone and a study group of 103 women were given a drug, L-phenyl-amine mustard (L-PAM) following surgery. There was 22% cancer recurrence in the control group compared with only 9.7% in the study group. Another example is the study made by Bonadonna and his colleagues in Milan, Italy since 1973 wherein the CMF regimen (cyclophosphamide, methotrexate, and 5-fluorouracil) was used. There were 385 patients: 207 of them were given 12 monthly cycles of CMF and 179 received no further treatment after radical mastectomy. After 36 months, 45.7% of the patients who did not receive CMF had recurrence of the disease compared to only 26.3% of those who had adjuvant chemotherapy with CMF. In the same study, it was found that this regimen was particularly effective in premenopausal women.

Nursing Implications of
Adjuvant Chemotherapy

1. Recognition of specific concerns, misunderstandings, or questions of the patient so that these can be addressed. For example, a patient may comment: "I knew someone who

had chemotherapy and became more ill rather than get better from the drugs." Undoubtedly, this comment indicates the need for information to be provided to the patient regarding side effects of chemotherapy, the benefits of chemotherapy, and most important of all, the measures that will be undertaken to help the patient who states: "Why should I still have chemotherapy when I already had surgery? I thought the disease has been removed by my doctor." This patient needs reassurance that although the surgery was successful, adjuvant chemotherapy is one way of preventing spread of the disease.

2. Provision of adequate information to the patient with regard to:

   a. Series of tests to be done to rule out presence of metastases: This may include blood tests (CEA), x-rays, liver and bone scans, and mammography of remaining breast. Negative results from these tests mean that the patient does not have signs of the disease and therefore is a good candidate for adjuvant chemotherapy.

   b. Proposed treatment schedule: The drugs that will be given and their possible side effects should be explored. A written instruction about the regimen and side effects should be given to the patient (see Figure 3).

   c. Methods of relieving side effects of drugs: Various methods can be used, such as taking antiemetics orally or rectally, relaxation techniques to cope with nausea and anxiety, increased intake of clear fluids to alleviate pain caused by dry retching and to prevent hemorrhagic cystitis, and timing of injections, preferably given in late afternoon or evening so anti-emetics may be taken before bedtime, thereby promoting sleep and rest. In some clinics adjuvant chemotherapy is given preferably on Friday afternoon so patients can have help from family members on the weekend, thereby facilitating the patient's ability to cope with side effects of the drugs. This is especially beneficial for a working person. To relieve the metallic taste, patients should be advised to chew mints or cinnamon-flavored gum while receiving treatment. Some patients may even experience body odor the day following treatment. This can be minimized by using a little perfume or talc.

3. Encourage supportive care from family members and staff.

4. Obtain dietary history so that the patient's preferences, meal patterns, and food association can be determined.

5. Provide a physically clean and comfortable environment that is odor free.

Name of patient: _____ Date: _____

I. Purpose of adjuvant chemotherapy: _____

_____
              (State purpose in layman's terminology.)

II. Drugs that will be used: _____

_____
              (Specify drugs as ordered by physician.)

III. Method of administration: _____

_____
   (Describe in nontechnical terms how drugs will be given.)

IV. Treatment schedule: _____

_____

_____
   (Indicate how often each drug will be given and when given.)

V. Precautions/side effects: _____

_____

_____
(List any precautions the patient should know which may interfere with treatment and any side effects most likely to be experienced from the drugs.)

VI. Nursing orders: _____

_____

_____
(State specific instructions for patient to do to alleviate ill effects of adjuvant chemotherapy.)

                              _____
                              Primary nurse's signature

Figure 3: Information Sheet for Patient Receiving Adjuvant
          Chemotherapy. (A copy of this information sheet is
          to be given to the patient and/or family. Original
          copy is part of the patient's medical record.)

6. Adjustment of the patient's meals after therapy (such as giving liquids with dry carbohydrates initially and then progressively increase food intake as tolerated) reduces the possibility of nausea and vomiting.
7. Acknowledgement of the patient's food craving so that he can be given what he desires to eat has been found to help reduce the degree of nausea.
8. Serve meals that are attractive and of sufficient quantity and quality, thereby promoting nutritional status necessary for effective chemotherapy.
9. Establishment of patient support groups can provide opportunities to discuss common problems, ways of coping with the therapy, and learning from each other. These groups can be established in clinics, either formally or informally. The nurse may designate a specific day of the week and the time for patients to come together formally as a group, or patients who have the same schedule of treatment can informally meet as a support group during the time of their scheduled treatment with the nurse as a facilitator of group interaction.

Investigational therapy involves the administration of an investigational drug. It is important to realize that strict protocols are adhered to in giving investigational therapy such as:

1. Criteria for selecting patients
2. Requirements for monitoring patients
3. Overall treatment plan included in written guidelines
4. General directives to the investigators including data collection and evaluation in order to identify and document objective parameters of tumor response
5. Informed consent: The investigator explains to the patient both the potential value and possible risks of the drug. Thus, the patient can make a decision whether to have the drug or not.

It is equally essential to note that only qualified oncologists can prescribe investigational cancer drugs to ensure the patient's safety. Moreover, investigational drugs are put through a drug evaluation process in three phases:

Phase I: This involves patients with advanced disease for which conventional anticancer measures are not suitable. Toxicity and dosimetry are defined by data collected during this phase.

Phase II: The antitumor activity for the drug is determined in this period by conducting tests on patients with advanced disease. Tumor masses are measured and x-ray studies are taken so that a determination of efficacy of the drug is obtained before proceeding to Phase III.

Phase III: This entails testing on a large scale, since at this period much is already known about the drug's efficacy and toxicity.[16,17] The Cooperative Clinical Cancer Research Program of the National Cancer Institute conducts randomized trials comparing the results of Phase III drugs with other agents of known effectiveness. Once adequate data are available with regard to efficacy of the drug, then it can be approved for commercial use by the Food and Drug Administration.[17] In January 1980 for instance, the FDA hinted that it will allow laetrile tests to be done on cancer patients, according to a Chicago Sun-Times report.

REVIEW QUESTIONS

1. Describe the cell life cycle.
2. What is the mode of action of
    a. Antimetabolites
    b. Polyfunctional alkylating agents
    c. Hormones
    d. L-asparaginase
    e. Antifolics
    f. Antipurines
    g. Antipyramidines
    h. Hydroxyurea
    i. Procarbazine
3. Enumerate the toxic effects of
    a. Methotrexate
    b. Actinomycin-D
    c. Nitrogen mustard
    d. 5-Fluorouracil (5-Fu)
    e. Vincristine
    f. Prednisone
    g. TACE
    h. Halotestin
4. What is the nursing management of the toxic effects of the drugs referred to in Question 3?
5. Identify the types of resistance that can occur during chemotherapy.
6. Enumerate the goals of chemotherapy.
7. What are some of the factors that should be considered in the selection of appropriate drugs and/or regimen?
8. Identify at least three principles of combination chemotherapy.
9. What is meant by recruitment?

10. Define adjuvant chemotherapy.
11. Describe one example of adjuvant chemotherapy.
12. Enumerate the nursing implications of adjuvant chemotherapy.
13. Name the protocols that must be adhered to an investigational drug therapy.
14. What agency is responsible for randomized trials of investigational drugs?
15. Enumerate the phases involved in an investigational drug evaluation process.
16. Define "informed consent."

REFERENCES

1. Bouchard, R., Nursing Care of the Cancer Patient, C.V. Mosby Co., St. Louis (1972).
2. Brunner, L., et al., Textbook of Medical-Surgical Nursing, J.B. Lippincott, New York, pp. 185-188 (19
3. Livingston, B.M., Cancer Chemotherapy Research. Am. J. Nurs. 67(12) (December, 1967).
4. Galvey, R.B., Chemotherapy of Cancer. Am. J. Nurs. 60 (April, 1960).
5. Karnofsky, D.A., Mechanism of Action of Anticancer Drugs at a Cellular Level. Ca, 18(4):232-234 (July-August, 1968).
6. Karnofsky, D.A., Hormonal and Chemical Methods in the Treatment of Cancer. Postgrad. Med. 17(6) (June, 1955).
7. Krakoff, I., Cancer Chemotherapeutic Agents. Reprint from CA:208-219 (1973).
8. Marino, E.B. and LeBlanc, D.H., Cancer Chemotherapy. Nursing '75, 5:22-23 (November, 1975).
9. Peterson, B.H. and Kellog, C.J., Current Practice in Oncologic Nursing, C.V. Mosby Co., St. Louis (1976).
10. Rodman, J., Drug Therapy Today. Reprinted from RN Magazine (February, April, 1972) by Medical Economics Co., Oradell, N.J., pp. 20-34 (1972).
11. Skipper, H., Thoughts on Cancer Chemotherapy and Combination Modality Therapy. JAMA, pp. 1033-1034 (November 18, 1974).
12. Skipper, H., Factors Determining Cell Killing By Chemotherapeutic Agents in Vivo, Part I. Cyclophosphamide. Eur. J. Cancer, pp. 313-321 (August, 1970).
13. Hoffman, J. and Post, J., The Effects of Antitumor Drugs on the Cell Cycle. in Drugs and the Cell Cycle, (A.M. Zimmerman, et al. eds.), Academic Press, New York, pp. 219-247 (1973).

14. Wheeler, G.P. and Simpson-Herren, L., Effects of Purines, Pyramidines, Nucleosides and Chemically Related Compounds on the Cell Cycle. In Drugs and the Cell Cycle, (A.M. Zimmerman, et al., eds.) Academic Press, New York, pp. 249-293 (1973).

15. van Putten, L.M., Are Cell Kinetic Data Relevant for the Design of Tumor Chemotherapy Schedules? Cell Tissue Kinet, pp. 493-504 (September 1974).

16. Burkhatter, P. and Donley, D., Dynamics of Oncology Nursing, McGraw-Hill Co., New York, pp. 323-355 (1978).

17. Bingham, C.A., This Cell Cycle and Cancer Chemotherapy. Am. J. Nurs., 78:1200-1205 (July, 1978).

18. Tobey, R.A. and Crissman, H.A., Comparative Effects of Three Nitrosourea Derivatives on Mammalian Cell Cycle Progression. Cancer Res., pp. 460-470 (February, 1975).

19. Scogna, D.M., Chemotherapy-Induced Nausea and Vomiting. Am. J. Nurs., 79:1562-1564 (September, 1979).

20. Mayer, J., Nutrition and Cancer. Part I. Problems Due Directly to Tumors and Associated Diseases. Postgrad. Med., pp. 65-67 (October, 1971).

21. Cancer Chemotherapy. Intermed Communications, Inc., Jenkintown, Pennsylvania (1976).

22. Warren, B., Adjuvant Chemotherapy for Breast Disease: The Nurse's Role. Cancer Nurs., 2:32-37 (February, 1979).

23. Bonadonna, G., Rossi, A., Valagussa, P., et al., The CMF Program for Operable Breast Cancer with Positive Axillary Nodes - Updated Analysis on the Disease-Free Interval, Site of Relapse and Drug Tolerance. Cancer, pp. 2904-2915 (June, 1977).

24. Kellogg, C.J. and Sullivan, B.P. (eds.), Current Perspectives in Oncologic Nursing, C.V. Mosby Co.; Saint Louis, pp. 46-49 (1978).

25. Abelson, H.T., Methotrexate and Central Nervous System Toxicity. Cancer Treatm. Rep., 62(12):1999-2001 (December, 1978).

26. Guthrie, D., The Use of Cytotoxic Chemotherapy in Conjunction with Gynecological Surgery. Clin. Obstet. Gynecol., 5(3):709-727 (December, 1978).

27. Levine, N. and Greenwald, E.S., Mucocutaneous Side Effects of Cancer Chemotherapy. Cancer Treatm. Rev., 5 (2):67-84 (June, 1978).

28. Garattini, S. and Spreafico, F., Some Examples of Interactions Between Drugs in Cancer Chemotherapy. Antibiot. Chemother., 23:283-294 (1978).

29. Calabresi, P. and Parks, R., Chemotherapy of Neoplastic Diseases. (Goodman, L., and Gilman, A., eds.) The Pharmacological Basis of Therapeutics, 5th ed., Macmillan Co., New York, pp. 1248-1308 (1975).

30. Chabner, B., et al., The Clinical Pharmacology of Antineoplastic Agents, Part I. N. Eng. J. Med., 292(21): 1107-1112 (May, 1975).

31. Chabner, B., The Clinical Pharmacology of Antineoplastic Agents. Part II. N. Eng. J. Med., 292(22):1159-1168 (May, 1975).

32. DiPalma, J., Cancer Chemotherapy. RN, 39(4):85-88 (April, 1976).

33. Dole, D., Anthony, F., et al., Alternate Day Prednisone: Leukocyte Kinetics and Susceptibility to Infections. N. Eng. J. Med, 29(22):1154-1158 (November, 1974).

34. Hubbard, S. and De Vita, V., Chemotherapy Research Nurse. Am. J. Nurs., 76(4):560-565 (April, 1976).

35. Marino, E. and LeBlanc, D., Cancer Chemotherapy. Nursing 75, 5(11):22-23 (November, 1975).

36. McMullen, K., When the Patient Is on Bleomycin Therapy. Am. J. Nurs., 75(6):964-966 (June, 1975).

37. Patterson, B., The Quality of Survival in Response to Treatment. JAMA, 233(3):280-281 (July, 1975).

38. Somerville, E., The Nurse's Role in Cancer Chemotherapy. Proc. Nat. Conf. Cancer Nurs., American Cancer Society, New York, pp. 83-86 (1973).

39. Krim, M., Towards Tumor Therapy with Interferons. Part I. Interferons: Production and Properties. Blood, 55(5): 711-721 (May, 1980).

40. Penn, I., Malignancies Associated with Immunosuppressive or Cytotoxic Therapy. Surgery, 83(5):492-502 (May, 1978).

41. Greenberg, D.M., The Case Against Laetrile: The Fraudulent Cancer Remedy. Cancer, 45(4):799-807 (February, 1980).

CHAPTER 8
Immunotherapy

Immunotherapy is rapidly gaining popularity as a treatment modality for various kinds of neoplastic diseases. Optimism and enthusiasm have been incited by various and well-documented research findings as follows:

1. Cell growth inhibition by lymphocytes indicating a cell-mediated immune response
2. Immune response by tumor growths evidenced by the presence of tumor-specific and tumor-associated antigens
3. Depression of the genetic information by viruses
4. Immunodepression by carcinogens
5. Antigens which are normally "buried" or inaccessible are released by defective neoplastic cells
6. Normally sequestered antigens are released by lysis of neoplastic cells.

GOALS OF THERAPY

1. Challenge the immune system, thereby eliciting an efficient immune response
2. Augment the immune response to effect tumor destruction by conferring either active or passive immunity
3. Alter tumor cell surface to render them more immunogenic

MAJOR APPROACHES TO IMMUNOTHERAPY

1. Administration of treatment after surgical intervention, radiation, or chemotherapy
2. Administration of treatment in advanced diseases simultaneously or alternately with surgery, chemotherapy, or radiotherapy

It is widely advocated that immunotherapy should be an adjunctive treatment and, if possible, large tumors should be first reduced by another treatment modality in order to effect a more efficient and effective immune response. It is also believed or postulated that immunotherapy has the possibility of enhancing tumor growth.[14,15,16,17,20]

BASIC TYPES OF IMMUNOTHERAPY

1. Active immunization: specific stimulation of immune response (production of antibodies) with an antigen using:
    a. Whole tumor cell vaccines
        (1) Living tumor cells (i.e., autologous tumor cells of the host are injected intradermally in small doses at various sites), and allogenic tumor cells (mixture of tumor cells of the same type as the patient's tumor)
        (2) Inactivated tumor cells which are treated by such processes as freezing and thawing, irradiation, heat killing, or mitomycin C treatment.
        (3) Modified tumor cells, which are treated artificially to increase their antigenicity (i.e., addition of carrier protein, addition of haptens, plant lectins, and neuraminidase treatment).
    b. Extracts from sensitized lymphoid cells
        (1) Transfer factor
        (2) Immune RNA
    c. Vaccines composed of subcellular components
        (1) Crude cell extracts
        (2) Isolated cell membranes
        (3) Isolated tumor antigens

2. Nonspecific stimulation of immune response to a wide variety of antigens such as:
    a. BCG (Bacille bilie de Calmette-Guerin) vaccine[40,41]
    b. C-parvum (Corynebacterium parvum)
    c. DNCB (dinitrochlorobenzene)
    d. MER (methanol extracted residue of BCG)
    e. MUDR (5-mercapto, 2-deoxyuridine)
    f. HN_2 (nitrogen mustard)
    g. Thymosin (extract of the thymus gland)
    h. MBT (mixed bacterial toxins such as Serratia marcescens and Streptococcus pyogenes).

3. Passive immunization: Direct transfer of transient immunity from persons with established immunity is done by using antibodies or by other immunologically active cells.[21,22] Examples are:

a. "Educated" cytotoxins
b. Plasmapheresis*
c. "Antitumor serum
  (1) Allogenic antisera
  (2) Xenogenic antisera
  (3) Reconstituted autochthonous antisera
d. Lymphocyte therapy (dialyzable lymphoid or leukocyte extracts
  (1) Lymphocyte transfusion from allogenic, normal, or previously cured cancer patients or HLA-matched donors
  (2) Lymphocytes activated in vitro using tumor antigens or plant lectins.[14]
e. Bone marrow transplant: Bone marrow is obtained from a donor who is histologically identical with the recipient. Preferable donors are twins and siblings but nonrelated donors have been successfully tried.[6] The donor marrow cells are injected intravenously to the recipient through a filter. These marrow stem cells migrate into the patient's bone cavities and begin to grow, hopefully with the aid of rather vigorous preparation of the patient as follows:
  (1) Antiseptic or disinfectant baths prior to maintaining or placing patient in a "germ-free" environment
  (2) Gastrointestinal tract is "sterilized" with antibiotics
  (3) Immunosuppressants are administered, such as cyclophosphamide (Cytoxan) or antilymphocyte serum (ALS) and/or total-body irradiation to destroy all stem cells and lymphoid tissues in order to prevent rejection of the transplanted marrow cells.

---

* The term plasmapheresis is a technique first introduced in 1914 with the objectives of collection of plasma for fractionation into therapeutic components and therapeutic pheresis or plasma exchange. Therapeutic plasmapheresis is a procedure in which whole blood is removed and the red blood cells alone or in combination with other components are reinfused into the patient. Currently, plasmapheresis is performed to remove toxic or disease-causing substances from the plasma of patients. These substances consist of specific antibodies in excess, antigen-antibody complexes, or toxic metabolites.

4. Adoptive immunization: This also confers passive immunity and possibly subsequent active immunity accomplished by:
   a. Transfusion of allogenic blood leukocytes from donors primarily grafted with the recipient's tumor
   b. Cross-immunization conferred by first obtaining tumor cells and subcutaneously transplanting them from patient A to patient B and vice-versa followed by cross transfusions of lymphocytes from patient A and patient B

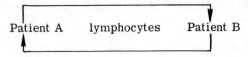

Patient A   lymphocytes   Patient B

METHODS OF ADMINISTRATION OF IMMUNOTHERAPY

1. Direct injection into tumor or tumor nodules
2. Oral administration
3. Aerosol inhalation (done postoperatively in lung cancer patients)
4. Intrapleural injection (postoperatively tried on lung cancers)
5. Scarification
6. Multiple puncture of the skin by using Heaf gun or tine technique
7. Intravenously
8. Subcutaneously

Some of the above-mentioned techniques will be discussed below.

Scarification Technique for BCG

An area on the upper arm or thigh is cleansed and shaved. A 2-inch (5-cm) square is scratched with the beveled cutting edge of (preferably) an 18-gauge needle done vertically then horizontally making a total of 7 to 10 lines of scratches on each direction. The needle should penetrate enough (2 mm deep) to cause oozing but not frank bleeding. A BCG filled syringe is used to spread a drop or two of the BCG on the scarified area followed by gentle massage of the medication using the shaft of the needle. The area is then allowed to dry. Some use the aid of a hair dryer set on cool to facilitate drying. This procedure is repeated until all the prescribed amount of BCG in the syringe has been used. The scarified area is then covered with a small Petri dish, plastic film, or Frisbee properly secured in place and left for 24 hours, then removed. After 48 hours, the scarified area is washed with soap and water and ointment or lotion is applied if skin irritation occurs.[2,3,13]

Tine Technique for BCG

A cleansed area, preferably on the forearm, is used. BCG is applied on the selected cleansed area then a 36-pronged grid square attached to a magnet is pressed through the BCG into the skin.[4]

Intradermal Injection Technique

A selected area, preferably the forearm, is used. Tumor cell vaccine in a small dose (usually 0.1 cc) is injected intradermally. For BCG, the freeze-dried BCG which is commercially prepared in a 1-ml vial is diluted and then kept in the refrigerator until one hour before use to assure potency. The diluent used is 1 cc of sterile water and no preservative added. The mixed solution will give approximately 0.1 cc for intradermal injection. Positive or negative reactions are observed after 48 to 72 hours.

BCG is an experimental therapeutic agent for cancer and still not cleared by the Food and Drug Administration as a cancer treatment.[5] Administration of vaccines do cause some known side effects which include: [4,5,13,28]

1. Painful or pruritic areas in or around test site
2. Localized abscesses
3. Ulceration
4. Fever and chills
5. Malaise
6. Adenitis
7. Intralesional side effects such as hyperpyrexia, hypotension, convulsions, and dusky skin color
8. Itching, scaling, or festering of the skin
9. Jaundice (usually temporary)
10. Elevated SGOT or/and alkaline phosphatase.

GENERAL NURSING CARE OF SIDE EFFECTS

1. As a preventive measure, antihistamine and acetaminophen (Tylenol) as prescribed are given before symptoms occur or prior to treatment.
2. Isoniazid (INH) 300 mg given daily may be prescribed for persistent symptoms.
3. Keep site clean, wash with soap and water at least twice a day or use hydrogen peroxide wash, dry, and apply dressing.
4. Ointments or soothing lotion are applied whenever necessary or as prescribed.

GLOSSARY

Active immunity: The individual manufactures antibodies against antigens.

Allogenic: Genetically dissimilar although of the same specimen.

Anergy: Inability to react to an antigenic stimulus.

Antibody: Protein substances produced by the body in response to a specific antigen.

Antigen: Any foreign substance (microorganisms, foreign proteins, etc.) which induces antibody formation.

Autochthonous: Derived from the same subject.

B cell: Lymphocyte that matures outside the thymus and produces humoral antibodies.

Blastogenic: Ability to initiate rapid mitosis of sensitized lymphocytes.

Blocking factor: Substance or an antigen that interferes with another antibody by occupying the combining sites of an antigen.

Cellular-mediated immunity: Production of antibodies primarily by T cells (specialized lymphocytes).

Complement: Proteins or enzyme precursors found in normal serum that interact with an antigen-antibody complex.

Humoral immunity: Production of antibodies, primarily by B cells.

Immunologic competence: Ability to detect and respond to foreign materials (antigens).

Immunodepressant: Substances that weaken or depress the efficiency and competence of the immune response.

Immunogenicity: Capacity to stimulate the formation of antibodies.

Lymphokines: Chemicals released by T cells which act on target cells.

Macrophage: Large cells derived from bone marrow stem cells and cells of the reticuloendothelial system which when stimulated become motile and ingest microorganisms and cellular debris.

Phagocytosis: Ingestion of microorganisms and other particles by the macrophage.

T cells: Specialized lymphocytes that mature in the thymus and are capable of killing tumor cells, tissue transplant cells, and viruses.

Transfer factor: A type of lymphokine which transforms non-sensitized T cells to sensitized T cells.

REVIEW QUESTIONS

1. What are the goals of immunotherapy?
2. Enumerate the basic types of immunotherapy.
3. What is active immunization? What is passive immunization?
4. Describe the preparation of a patient for bone marrow transplant.
5. List the various methods of administration of immunotherapy.
6. What are some of the general nursing care principles for the side effects of vaccination?
7. List some of the side effects of vaccination.

REFERENCES

1. Clinical Oncology for Medical Students and Physicians - A Multi-disciplinary Approach. Rubin, P. and Bakemeier, R., (eds.), 4th edition, American Cancer Society, New York (1974).
2. Isler, C., Newest Treatment for Cancer: Immunotherapy. RN, pp. 29-31 (May, 1976).
3. Cancer Immunotherapy Starts from Scratch. Med. World News, pp. 39-53 (February, 1973).
4. Bochow, A., Cancer Immunotherapy: What Promise Does It Hold? Nursing 76, pp. 50-56 (October, 1976).
5. Donley, D., Nursing the Patient Who Is Immunosuppressed. Am. J. Nurs., pp. 1619-1625 (October, 1976).
6. Donley, D., The Immune System: Matthew's Story. Am. J. Nurs., p. 1613 (October, 1976).
7. Holmes, D., et al., Immunotherapy of Malignancy in Humans - Current Status. JAMA, 32:1052-1055 (1975).

8. Terry, W., BCG in the Treatment of Human Cancer. CA, 25(4):198-203 (1975).
9. Silverstein, M.J. and Morton, D.L., Cancer Immunotherapy. Am. J. Nurs., pp. 1178-1181 (July, 1973).
10. DiLuzio, N., Globulin May be a Cancer Tip-Off. Med. World News, p. 22 (September 28, 1973).
11. Zamcheck, N. and Pusztaszeri, G., CEA, AFP, and Other Potential Tumor Markers. CA, 25(4):204-213 (July/August, 1975).
12. Zamcheck, N. and Pusztaszeri, G., Assaying CEA: Most Valuable in Monitoring for Metastases. Hosp. Prac., pp. 30-33 (February, 1974).
13. Peterson, B.H. and Kellog, C.J., Current Practice in Oncologic Nursing. C.V. Mosby Co., St. Louis, p. 63 (1976).
14. Radiation Therapy and Immunotherapy: The Value of Immunotherapy in the Control of Local and Regional Cancer. Cancer Symp. Suppl., 37(4):2108-2119 (April, 1973).
15. Kobayashi, H., A Prospect on Cancer Immunology. Hokkaido Igaku Zasshi, 54(6):549-577 (November, 1979).
16. Barber, H.R., Immunology in Tumor Therapeutics: An Overview. Del. Med. J., 52(4):117-209 (April, 1980).
17. Weiss, D.W., Tumor Antigenicity and Approaches to Tumor Immunotherapy: An Outline. Curr. Top. Microbiol. Immunol., 89:1-83 (1980).
18. Herberman, R.B., Holden, H.T., et al., Macrophages as Regulators of Immune Responses Against Tumors. Adv. Exp. Med. Biol., pp. 361-379 (1979).
19. Schechter, G.P., et al., Suppressor Monocytes in Human Disease: A Review. Adv. Exp. Med. Biol., pp. 283-298 (1979).
20. Richards, V., Cancer Immunology - An Overview. Prog. Exp. Tumor Res., pp. 1-60 (1980).
21. Pilch, Y.H., Mediation of Immune Responses to Tumor Antigens by Immune RNA. Prog. Exp. Tumor Res., pp. 163-177 (1980).
22. Spitler, L.E., BCG, Levamisole, and Transfer Factor in the Treatment of Cancer. Prog. Exp. Tumor Res., pp. 178-192 (1980).
23. Goodnight, J.E. and Morton, D.L., Immunotherapy of Cancer: Current Status. Prog. Exp. Tumor Res., pp. 61-88 (1980).
24. Math, E., Florentin, I., et al., Active Immunotherapy of Cancer for Minimal Residual Disease: New Trends and New Materials. Prog. Exp. Tumor Res., pp. 242-274 (1980).
25. Al-Sarraf, M. and Baker, L.H., Transfer Factor. Cancer Treatm. Rev., pp. 209 -215 (December, 1979).

26. Low, T.L., Thurman, G.B., et al., Current Status of Thymosin Research: Evidence for the Existence of a Family of Thymic Factors that Control T Cell Maturation. Ann. NY Acad. Sci., pp. 33-48 (1979).

27. Bartlett, G.L., Milestones in Tumor Immunology. Sem. Oncol., pp. 515-525 (December, 1979).

28. Milas, L. and Scott, M.T., Antitumor Activity of Corynebacterium Parvum. Adv. Cancer Res., pp. 257-306 (1978)

29. Morton, D.L., Changing Concepts of Cancer Surgery: Surgery as Immunotherapy. Am. J. Surg., 135(3):367-371 (March, 1978).

30. Holl, A.N. Sr., Clinical Significance of Circulating Immune Complexes. Effects of Plasmapheresis. Haematologia, (Budapest) 12(1-4):69-83 (1978-1979).

31. Isra-El, L., Edelstein, R., and Samak, R., Some New Approaches to Cancer Immunotherapy in Man. Immunotherapy of Human Cancer, Raven Press, New York, pp. 363-374 (1978).

32. Fahey, J.L., Principles of Immunology with Relevance to Immunotherapy. Immunotherapy of Human Cancer, Raven Press, New York, pp. 31-39 (1978).

33. Mastrangelo, M.J., Berd, D., et al., Limitations, Obstacles, and Controversies in the Optimal Development of Immunotherapy. Immunotherapy of Human Cancer, Raven Press, New York, pp. 375-394 (1978).

34. Gall, S.A., Immunotherapy for Gynecologic Malignancies. Immunotherapy of Human Cancer, Raven Press, New York, pp. 303-319 (1978).

35. Math, E.G., Immunotherapy: Experimental and Rational Basis. Immunotherapy for Human Cancer, Raven Press, New York, pp. 5-27 (1978).

36. Sinkovics, J.G., Immunotherapy of Human Tumors. Pathobiol. Ann, pp. 241-284 (1978).

37. Hortobagyi, G.N., Richman, S.P., et al., Immunotherapy with BCG Administered by Scarification: Standardization of Reactions and Management of Side Effects. Cancer 42(5): 2293-2303 (November, 1978).

38. Morton, D.L. and Goodnight, J.E. Jr., Clinical Trials of Immunotherapy: Present Status. Cancer, 42(5):2224-2333 (November, 1978).

39. Streilein, J.W., Immunotherapy for Cancer. Surg. Gynecol. Obstet. 147(5):769-782 (November, 1978).

40. Shin, H.S., Johnson, R.J., et al., Mechanisms of Tumor Immunity: The Role of Antibody and Nonimmume Effectors. Progr. Allergy, pp. 163-210 (1978).

41. Baldwin, R.W. and Pimm, M.V., BCG in Tumor Immunotherapy. Adv. Cancer Res., pp. 91-147 (1978).

42. Broder, S., Muul, L., et al., Suppressor Cells in Neoplastic Disease. J. Nat. Cancer Inst., 61(1):5-11 (July, 1978).

43. Goldstein, A.L., Thurman, G.B., et al., Hormonal Influences on the Reticuloendothelial System: Current Status of the Role of Thymosin in the Regulation and Modulation of Immunity. J. Reticuloendo. Soc., 23(4):253-266 (April, 1978).

44. Rochman, H., Tumor Associated Markers in Clinical Diagnosis. Ann. Clin. Lab. Sci., 8(3):167-175 (May-June, 1978).

45. Murphy, S. and Hersch, E., Immunotherapy of Leukemia and Lymphoma. Semin. Hematol., 15(2):181-203 (April, 1978).

46. Goodnight, J.E. Jr. and Morton, D.L., Immunotherapy from Malignant Disease. Ann. Rev. Med., pp. 231-283 (1978).

47. Ruma, T.A., Therapeutic Pheresis and Plasma Exchange. Clinical Diagnosis and Management by Laboratory Methods (Henry, J., et al., eds.) W.B. Saunders Co., Philadelphia, pp. 1483-1489 (1979).

CHAPTER 9
Radiation Therapy

Radiation therapy can either be external or internal. In the former, x-rays or gamma rays are delivered to the specific body area affected by cancer. In the latter, an isotope is placed intracavitarily or interstitially in the cancerous lesion.

The goals of radiation therapy are curative, palliative, or as adjunct to other therapies in the hope of effecting remission. In breast cancer, radiation therapy has been found to be palliative in that it reduces bone pain from bony metastases. In many cases of stage I or II Hodgkin's disease, radiation has been found to be curative.

Notwithstanding the desirable effects of radiation therapy, it is common knowledge that normal cells may also be destroyed in the therapeutic process, especially in the gastrointestinal and urinary tracts. Hence, fear of radiation is basic in a patient who is to undergo this type of therapy. Moreover, the importance of protecting those individuals who come in contact with sources of radiation cannot be overlooked.

NATURE OF RADIATION

In order to fully understand the concept of radiation therapy, a knowledge of the nature of radiation is essential.

An atom can either be stable or unstable. It is stable because of the effects of the neutrons on the protons. When it is unstable, the nucleus gives up energy in the form of rays or particles - alpha (α), beta (β), and gamma (γ) in order to become more stable. This phenomenon of disintegration of the atom and emission of radiation (energy) is referred to as radioactivity. An isotope is an element whose nucleus contains a constant number of protons but differing number of neutrons, thereby changing its weight. The optimal ratio between protons and neutrons in a chemical element is one that is stable. It is possible, however, to make this stable chemical element unstable through the use of nuclear reactors and high speed particle accelerators. For instance, Cobalt-59(^{59}Co) can be bombarded with additional free neutrons so that it absorbs an extra neutron, thereby becoming Cobalt-60 (^{60}Co), which is unstable. An unstable radioactive isotope can then emit particulate radiation (small fragments of the nucleus having mass and size) and electromagnetic radiation ("rays" that have no mass). The particulate radiation types are represented by alpha and beta particles, which are actual parts of radioactive atoms. These particles can break away and travel at high speeds and with great energies.

X-ray is one of the basic types of electromagnetic radiation. It consists of rays or waves of very high electric energy traveling at very high speeds. The electromagnetic radiation from natural or artificially created radioactive isotopes is called gamma radiation.

The various types of radiation act upon living tissues by altering the atoms in the chemical systems of the cells, a process known as ionization. The effect of ionization is dependent upon the amount (dose) of radiation given. The overall damage or destruction of tissue varies with dosage, intensity of radiation (gamma rays being the most penetrating), and the nature of the site to be irradiated.

RADIOACTIVE DECAY OR DISINTEGRATION

The rate at which atoms emit their radiation (disintegrate or decay) is called the half-life. This is the time (hours, days, months, or years) required for one-half of the atoms of a particular radioactive material to decay or be reduced to half their initial activity. The half-life of iodine-131 (^{131}I), for example, is slightly more than eight days, whereas that of radium-226 (^{226}Ra) is over 1600 years. Radioisotopes which are administered in open, unsealed form have a relatively short life and are essentially inactive after the desired therapeutic effects have been achieved. Isotopes of longer life are administered intracavitarily in sealed containers and removed for storage and use some other time. Among the unsealed radioisotopes are iodine-131(^{131}I), gold (^{198}Au), and phosphorus-32 (^{32}P). The sealed radioisotopes include radium, radon, cobalt-60 (^{60}Co), cesium-137 (^{137}Cs), iodine-125 (^{125}I), cesium-131 (^{131}Cs), and iridium-192 (^{192}Ir).

EFFECT OF RADIATION
ON BODY TISSUE

Since ionizing radiation is harmful to normal living tissue, it is important that the factors which influence the risk of tissue damage be noted.

1. Dose: A prescribed dose causes less tissue destruction, especially if administered in small amounts over a long period of time, than when given all at once.
2. Cell susceptibility: Rapidly dividing cells with no specialized function are more sensitive than slowly dividing cells and highly differentiated cells (e.g., lymphocytes and germ cells are more sensitive than nerve cells or muscle cells). The law of Bergonie and Tribondeau classifies various cells in order of sensitivity to radiation, with the most sensitive cells listed first as follows:
   a. Lymphocytes
   b. Erythroblasts
   c. Myeloblasts
   d. Epithelial cells:
      (1) Basal cells of the testes
      (2) Basal cells of intestinal crypts
      (3) Basal cells of ovaries
      (4) Basal cells of the skin
      (5) Basal cells of secretory glands
      (6) Alveolar cells of the lungs and bile ducts
   e. Endothelial cells
   f. Connective tissue cells
   g. Tubular cells of the kidneys
   h. Bone cells
   i. Nerve cells
   j. Brain cells
   k. Muscle cells.
3. Area of body exposure: The larger the area exposed to irradiation, the greater the effects.
4. Biological variability: Susceptibility to radiation varies from one individual to another. A healthy person, for instance, is more responsive to the desired effects of radiation than an unhealthy person.
5. Oxygenation: Increased tissue oxygenation, i.e., through the use of hyperbaric oxygen, enhances the effects of radiation treatments.

EXTERNAL RADIATION THERAPY

The principle used to determine the kind of x-ray apparatus to be used in the treatment of various kinds of tumors is the wavelength and penetrating power of a particular type of x-ray. Soft x-rays which have longer wavelengths are generally used in treating superficial cancers and for diagnosis. Hard x-rays (shorter wavelengths) are generally used for the treatment of deep-seated tumors. X-ray machines generally used are in the 30 to 120 kv range. The linear accelerators are powerful and can deliver up to 33 meV.

In external radiation therapy, fractionation (doses are not given in a single application, but in daily or less frequent fractions which are distributed over a total treatment regimen of several weeks) is believed to be more efficacious than one-time treatment. The rationale for this is that such a mode of treatment regimen allows for the normal cells to recover in between treatments while still achieving a progressive biologic damage to the tumor cells. The tumor cells are killed by the divided doses in the premitotic stage.

Leukemias, lymphomas, and teratomas are most likely to respond to x-radiation therapy. X-ray therapy has been very effective in the treatment of carcinoma of the larynx, the nasopharynx, the tongue, the lip, the skin, and in lymphomas, particularly Hodgkin's disease. The radiocurability of malignant tumors is high if the tumor is localized. However, many of the most radiosensitive tumors are not localized when the patient is seen for the first time. Consequently, the tumors are not cured as often as indicated by their radiosensitivity. When a tumor is situated such that the surrounding tissues can tolerate large doses of irradiation, then it has a good chance of being cured.

NURSING CARE PRINCIPLES IN
EXTERNAL RADIATION THERAPY

There are certain principles of care of the patient who is to receive external radiation therapy which should be done to insure effectiveness of the therapeutic process and to decrease the fear associated with radiation.

1. Inform the patient that he will not feel the penetration of the rays.
2. Remove any pins, buttons, pens, or any metal objects on the patient's body prior to therapy, since these will interfere with therapy.

3. Inform the patient of the exact area for irradiation which may have to be marked with indelible ink by the radiologist. This should not be washed off unless instructed to do so by the radiologist.
4. Reinforce the physician's explanation of the purpose, effects, and procedure involved for the treatment regimen.
5. Inform the patient of the possibility of the following untoward effects of radiation therapy:
   a. Skin reactions: radiodermatitis, radioepithelitis due to loss of epidermal cells (may be noticed after first therapy), dry skin and scaling, weeping skin
   b. Systemic reactions: nausea, vomiting, fever, loss of appetite, and a feeling of extreme malaise lasting for a few days or weeks
   c. Bladder irradiation: hematuria may be a manifestation
   d. Drop in blood count.
6. If untoward effects occur, specific nursing intervention can be started as indicated in Table 6.
7. Answer all of the patient's questions as honestly as you can. The use of professional resources is helpful when experiencing difficulty in dealing with the patient's responses to therapy.

RADIOISOTOPE THERAPY

There are several methods used in radioisotope therapy. These are teletherapy (tele-distance), external mold therapy, interstitial isotope therapy, intracavitary, and internal irradiation. Each of these methods has its own advantages and disadvantages as well as its specific usage. A simplified description of each method and how it works will be discussed below.

Teletherapy

Teletherapy uses gamma rays emitted by a radioactive source kept in a shielded unit placed at a certain distance from the patient. The teletherapy unit allows the continuous emission of radiation and therefore must be shielded by heavy shutters or a retractable device. The advantages of this method include: reduction of undesirable skin effects, the unit does not depend on electronic circuitry, and there is minimal involvement of the bone or cartilage. Among its disadvantages are that the radioisotope must be replaced after its half-life, it is not possible to vary the amount of radiation emitted from the source, and the cost of shielding is high. Cobalt-60 (^{60}Co) has been used for this purpose as it is roughly comparable to a 2 million electron volt (2-meV) x-ray machine.

Table 6: Nursing Management of Untoward Effects
of Radiation

Problem (Untoward effect)	Nursing Management
Radiodermatitis	No ointments, lotions, cosmetics, or depilatories should be applied to site of radiation unless prescribed by the physician
Radioepithelitis, due to loss of epidermal layers, occurring between 3-6 weeks after first treatment	Avoid vigorous rubbing of skin Vitamins A and D may be applied as prescribed by the physician
Weeping skin	Antibiotic lotion may be applied as prescribed by the physician Steroid cream may also be applied as per physician's orders Expose skin to air Gently wash skin with plain warm water, pat dry, and apply cream No powder or alcohol-based ointment should be used Apply baby oil
Skin irritation, dry skin, and scaling	Avoid friction, extremes of temperature, and exposure to sunlight
Nausea and physiological vomiting, loss of appetite	Give high-protein, high-carbohydrate, fat-free, low-residue diet to reduce bulk and yet maintain calories Patient should not eat before treatment

Table 6 (cont'd)

Problem (Untoward effect)	Nursing Management
	Patient should be given small, frequent, and attractively served feedings instead of 3 large meals
	Give patient plenty of nourishing fluids to replace fluid and electrolyte loss from vomiting
	Avoid foods that induce or aggravate nausea
	An elemental, high nitrogen diet (Vivonex) may be given. This is a low residue, easily absorbed, diet supplement which helps maintain nutrition and fluid intake
Feeling of extreme malaise	Give patient sedative as prescribed to promote rest and relaxation
Anemia	Watch for pallor, complaints of fatigue
	Give patient foods that are high in iron content
	Allow patient to have adequate rest periods
Bleeding, especially in conjunction with chemotherapy	Watch for any hematuria or nose bleed and report to the physician

External Mold Therapy

In this method the radioisotope is packaged and screened within an appropriate container and subsequently applied directly to a skin surface of the lesion. This is valuable in the treatment of carcinoma of the lip, ears, scalp, mouth, larynx, and penis. Among the radioisotopes used in this fashion are cobalt-60 (^{60}Co), radioactive tantalum-182 (^{182}Ta), radioactive strontium-90 (^{90}Sr), and Yttrium-30 (^{30}Y). Tantalum-182 is a flexible wire which can be bent to conform to anatomic variations and may be applied in the form of a ring to the exterior surface of a retinoblastoma involving the eyeball and optic nerve. Strontium-90 and yttrium-30 are pure beta emitters which can be used in external molds for shallow irradiation of eye neoplasms. For skin malignancies, radiophosphorus (phosphorus-32 or ^{32}P) has been used by cutting and molding it to the size and shape needed to be applied over the skin lesion.

Intracavitary Isotope Therapy

A radioactive substance in a capsule or radioactive liquids placed inside a balloon are put within a cavity of the body such as the uterus, the maxillary sinus, or the bladder. Cobalt-60 in a capsule may be placed into the body of the uterus, the cervical canal, or into a maxillary sinus. Colloidal gold (^{198}Au), radioactive sodium (^{24}Na), and radioactive bromine (^{82}Br) have been placed in balloons within the bladder for beta irradiation of the internal bladder wall to a depth of a few millimeters.

Interstitial Isotope Therapy

Radioisotopes in the form of needles can be directly implanted within a tumor tissue. These include Cobalt-60, Cesium-137 (^{137}Cs), Iridium-192 (^{192}Ir), Gold-198, Radon-222 (^{222}Rn), Tantalum-182, and Iodine-125 (^{125}I). The implantation of radon seeds, needles, tubes, or wires is done in the operating room under aseptic conditions. Sometimes a radioisotope solution can be injected directly into a tumor and the surrounding tissues as in the case of ^{198}Au.

Internal Irradiation

This is achieved by oral or intravenous method. Intravenous injection of sodium phosphate (^{32}P) has been effective in the treatment of myelogeneous leukemia. For patients with hyperthyroidism, solution of radioiodine (^{131}I) has been given orally as treatment.

NURSING CARE PRINCIPLES
IN RADIOISOTOPE THERAPY

General Principles of Care of the
Patient with Radioisotope

1. A patient who receives a therapeutic dose of a radioisotope
    temporarily becomes a source of radiation. Therefore,
    certain precautionary measures need to be undertaken to
    avoid radiation exposure hazards.
    a. A wrist band with a radioactive symbol should be worn
       by the patient.
    b. A special radiation instruction sheet should be developed
       and displayed at the patient's room, preferably on the
       door. There should be appropriate radiation tags on the
       patient's chart cover, the nurse's notes and physician's
       records to alert all of the health team members of the
       need for observing radiation precautions.
    c. The special radiation instruction sheet should include the
       type of radioactive source used, time of insertion, an-
       ticipated time of removal, precautions to be followed,
       and who to notify in case of an emergency such as dis-
       lodgement of the radioactive substance or when in doubt
       about the management for any kinds of procedures to be
       done while caring for the patient.
    d. The use of a special private or single room which is fully
       equipped with all the necessary equipment needed by the
       patient is advisable in order to insure safety among other
       patients, hospital staff, and others. It should be noted
       that patients with sealed radiation should not be put to-
       gether in one room because this would increase the dose
       that each patient would be receiving during therapy.

2. The amount of radioactivity the nurse can receive in work-
    ing close to a patient with radiation depends on the distance
    from the patient (doubling the distance from a radiation
    source cuts the intensity received to one fourth), the amount
    of time spent with the patient in actual contact, and the de-
    gree of shielding provided.

3. The greatest amount of radiation is present during the first
    24- to 72-hour period of therapy. It is important to do only
    what is essential for the patient at this period. Hence, giv-
    ing a daily bath is not essential since prior to therapy a com-
    plete bath is given.

4. Visitors should stay at least 6 feet away from the patient's bed and stand behind a shield, if available, so that the shield is between the visitor and the patient.

5. Pregnant women should not be assigned to care for patients with sealed radiation. If a nurse who happens to take care of a patient with radium implant is unaware that she is pregnant, there is no real cause for alarm. In the United States, a fetus can receive as much as 500 mrem, which is far greater than one would expect to see even for an entire year of caring for a patient with radiation provided the proper precautions were carried out. Extant literature reveals that in certain hospitals with oncology sections, the highest dose for any nurse for one year has been 340 mrem.

Specific Nursing Care Principles in
Caring for a Patient with Internal Radiation

The specific problems of radiation therapy can best be understood in terms of those emanating from sealed radiation sources and of those resulting from nonsealed sources.

Sealed internal radiation includes radium, radon, iridium, or gold seeds. Initially this is controlled at the time of application by its being encased in a nonradioactive metallic covering. Thus it cannot directly contaminate any other object or tissue, even though it continues to radiate. The casing material absorbs practically all the alpha radiation and most of the beta rays, hence the only hazardous radiation left is gamma radiation. Because of this built-in control, there is no reason for the nurse to fear such a patient since internal radiation cannot be transferred to her or another person without actual contact. Nevertheless, the nurse should not spend time with the patient unnecessarily while giving basic care, since the radiation remains with the patient.

The following are factors to observe in caring for the patient with sealed radiation.

1. When the patient has an internal radiation near the mouth, the nurse should give good and frequent oral care.

2. Measures should be undertaken to prevent displacement of the radiation substance, such as gentle handling of the patient, avoiding abrupt position change or movement, instructing the patient to avoid sneezing or straining, and checking for a distension of the bladder or constipation so

that measures may be instituted to prevent straining of patient or unnecessary movements.

3.   Watch for any dislodgement of implants. If there is an unusual dislodgement of the radium needle or other sealed substance which is radioactive, the nurse must not pick it up with her hands; instead, she should use a long-handled forceps or tongs and then put the radioactive substance in a sealed container in the patient's room. The incident is then promptly reported to the radiologist in charge of the therapy.

4.   Any dressings or bandages as well as linen from the patient should not be discarded until the nurse is sure that they are no longer a source of radiation. A radiograph or survey meter may be used for ascertaining extent of radioactivity and/or absence of it.

5.   Maintain a distance from the source of radiation. The intensity of the radiation decreases by the square of the distance between the nurse and the source. For example, if a nurse stands three feet from the source (patient) and moves back 3 more feet (double the distance) the radiation drops by a factor of 9 (3 squared).

6.   Use a lead shield whenever possible when caring for the patient.

7.   The less time the nurse spends near the patient, the less radiation she is going to receive. In order to reduce time, carefully plan what has to be done, organize and assemble everything needed to carry out procedures to be performed, and bring equipment needed at the bedside before carrying out the planned care for the day. As a guideline, it is important to realize that if a nurse stands 3 feet behind a shield for 42 hours and 30 minutes, she gets the same amount of radiation as when she would stand 6 feet behind a shield for 110 hours. In direct patient care, the amount of time which can be spent safely in close contact with the source (while wearing a shield) is only 6 hours and 40 minutes at any given time. It is important to realize that the effect of radiation is cumulative, based on time and distance maintained while being with the patient. The amount of radiation is measured in millirems (mrem). By law (State and Energy Research and Development Administration Regulation) people who work near radiation sources may receive no more than 1,250 mrems every three months

to the whole body. This is measured through a film badge or a pocket dosimeter.

8. The patient with radium implant is to remain within his room until the removal of the implant, which is usually done by the radiologist in the radiology department. After removal of the radium implant, a check should be made by a radiograph to insure that all radioactive materials have been removed. Thereafter, the radiation precautions are discontinued.

9. If a patient has a permanent implant, as in the case of bladder carcinoma when radon seeds are used, the patient remains on radiation precautions until discontinued by the radiologist. All urine and bed clothes are checked for possible lost seeds. In effect, when caring for a patient with sealed internal radiation, the nurse should:
    a. Follow radiation instruction precautions
    b. Refrain from staying within 3 feet distance from the patient longer than is necessary to provide the required nursing care
    c. Never pick up dislodged radioactive sources with her hands. Only long-handled forceps should be used and the radiologist should be notified immediately in case of dislodgement.

Unsealed internal radiation: In this type of radiation, the radioactivity may be widely spread in the patient's body, depending upon the type of isotope's biologic pattern of distribution. It may be localized or diffused in the body tissue or fluid. The most commonly encountered and most widely used radioactive substance is radioactive iodine. The radiation from a patient who is receiving radioactive iodine does not constitute exposure hazard when both time and distance precautions are observed. Nonetheless, it circulates in the bloodstream and is excreted by the kidneys. Therefore, both blood and urine of the patient contain radioactivity. It may also be secreted by the sweat glands and is sometimes contained in the vomitus of a patient who has recently received an oral dose.

The following are factors to observe in caring for the patient with unsealed internal radiation.

1. All contaminated materials and equipment used by the patient should be thoroughly washed before being reused. Careful handwashing is essential after taking care of the patient.

2. Wound dressings and bedclothes used by the patient who received small tracer doses should be wrapped well with paper or nonradioactive linen (so that no possible contamination is left exposed) and subsequently stored until safe for disposal.

3. If a patient received a large dose of radioisotope, stricter precautions should be observed. Bedpans, for instance, should be marked and used only for the same patient with radiation and should never be handled without rubber gloves. All dressings and bedclothes should also be handled with gloves during the first two or three days after the administration of the radiation dose, then treated as described earlier for tracer-dose patients.

4. The first three days after radioactive iodine therapy is the time for strict adherence to radiation precautions, since it is during this period that radiation is at its maximum hazard. After 8 days, the radioactivity declines to one-half and the precautions can usually be relaxed.

5. Radioactive phosphorus is also a source of unsealed internal radiation. Similar precautions are to be observed as in iodine radiation except that elimination is primarily in the feces rather than in the urine. Unlike iodine, radioactive phosphorus does not emit gamma radiation. Consequently, the patient is no hazard as an external source.

REVIEW QUESTIONS

1. What are the two types of radiation therapy?
2. Define isotope, ionization, and half-life.
3. What factors influence the risk of tissue damage during radiation therapy?
4. Enumerate six nursing principles in the care of a patient with external radiation.
5. What are the side effects of radiation therapy?
6. Describe the specific nursing intervention for the various side effects of irradiation.
7. List the various methods used in radioisotope therapy.
8. What are some of the general principles of care of the patient with radioisotope therapy?
9. Define millirem. How many millirems can be legally allowed every three months for a person working with radiation sources?
10. How much time can a person spend safely in close contact with the source of radiation?
11. Enumerate some specific nursing care principles in caring for a patient with sealed internal radiation. What are the principles for a patient with unsealed internal radiation?

REFERENCES

1. Brunner, L., et al., Textbook of Medical-Surgical Nursing. J.B. Lippincott Co., New York (1975).
2. Breeding, M.A. and Wollin, M., Working Safely Around Implanted Radium Sources. Nursing 76, pp. 59-63 (May, 1976).
3. Elliott, St. John, C., Radiation Therapy: How You Can Help. Nursing 76, pp. 34-41 (September, 1976).
4. Shafer, K., et al., Medical-Surgical Nursing, C.V. Mosby Co., St. Louis (1971).
5. Fletcher, G., Radiotherapy: An Ideal Teammate for Cancer Surgery. Nursing Times, pp. 26-32 (May, 1974).
6. Peterson, B.H. and Kellog, C.J., Current Practice in Oncologic Nursing, C.V. Mosby Co., St. Louis (1976).
7. Smith, D.W. and Hanley, C.P., Care of the Adult Patient. J.B. Lippincott Co., New York (1975).
8. Adelstein, S.J., The Risk: Benefit Ratio in Nuclear Medicine. Hosp. Pract., 8:141 (January, 1973).
9. Arena, V., Radiation Accidents: What You Need to Know About Them. RN, p. 42 (September, 1973).
10. Barnes, P. and Reiss, D., Textbook for Radiotherapy. J.B. Lippincott Co., Philadelphia (1972).
11. Buschke, F. and Parker, R., Radiation Therapy in Cancer Management. Grune and Stratton, New York (1972).
12. Rummerfield, P.S. and Rummerfield, M.J., What You Should Know About Radiation Hazards. Am. J. Nurs., p. 780 (April, 1970).
13. Behnke, H. (ed.), Radiation Therapy - A Treatment Modality for Cancer. In: Guidelines for Comprehensive Nursing Care in Cancer, Springer-Verlag, New York (1973).
14. Craytor, J. and Fass, M., The Patient in Radiation Therapy. In: Ch. 6, The Nurse and the Cancer Patient: A Programmed Textbook, J.B. Lippincott, Philadelphia (1972).
15. Kaplan, H.S., Historic Milestones in Radiobiology and Radiation Therapy. Semin. Oncology, 6(4):479-489 (December, 1979).
16. Shaw, M.T., Spector, M.H., and Ladman, A.J., Effects of Cancer. Radiotherapy and Cytotoxic Drugs on Intestinal Structure and Function. Cancer Treatm. Rev., 6(3):141-151 (September, 1979).
17. Breeding, M.A. and Wollin, M., Working Safely Around Implanted Radiation Sources. Nursing '76, pp. 58-63 (May, 1976).
18. Leigh, H., et al., Denial and Helplessness in Cancer Patients Undergoing Radiation Therapy: Sex Differences and Implications for Prognosis. Cancer, 45(12):3086-3089 (June, 1980).

CHAPTER 10
Surgical Intervention and Multimodal Treatment

According to statistics revealed in extant literature on cancer, 80 to 85% of curable cancers are treated by surgery. Those cancers which are localized to a primary region and have not spread beyond the regional lymph nodes are effectively treated with surgical intervention. On the other hand, for those that have spread beyond the primary site, surgery is only a means of palliation.

The objectives of palliative surgery include: promoting a more comfortable existence, relieving clinical symptoms, and preventing deterioration of the clinical manifestations of the disease, such as preventing additional symptom formation.

TYPES OF CANCER IN WHICH SURGERY IS THE TREATMENT OF CHOICE

1. Breast cancer
2. Lung cancer
3. All gastrointestinal cancer - cancers of the esophagus, stomach, biliary system, large and small bowel, and the pancreas
4. Cancer of the endometrium when preoperative radiation is given
5. Carcinoma of the cervix in situ
6. Ovarian cancer
7. Most head and neck cancers with cervical metastases
8. Certain radioresistant cancers of the head and neck, such as cancers of the thyroid and salivary glands
9. Soft tissue sarcoma and melanomas
10. Renal cancer

CURATIVE SURGICAL PROCEDURES THAT MAY BE DONE AS TREATMENT FOR CANCER

1. Incisional biopsy: This procedure determines the presence of sarcoma which may then indicate the need for radical

excision of the entire tumor and surrounding lymph nodes.

2. Local excision of tumors: Wide local excision may be adequate treatment in certain low-grade tumors. Tumors that can be treated in this manner are basal cell carcinomas, mixed tumors of the parotid, adamantinomas, and leiomyomas.

3. Excision with wide margin: When a tumor has spread widely into normal appearing surrounding tissue, then excision of the tumor with very wide margins may be done in order to excise any tumor cells that have gone beyond the primary lesion. This is effective in the treatment of esophageal, gastric, and bladder cancers. It is important to note that cancer of the esophagus spreads 10 to 20 cm above or below the gross limits of the primary tumor. Hence, the need for wide-margin excision.

4. Block dissection: This is the most important surgical principle in treating tumors that metastasize to regional lymph nodes. A block dissection is done of the tumor itself, all of the intervening tissue, and the primary node-bearing areas, if at all possible. The lymph nodes farthest from the tumor are dissected first and then the surgeon proceeds toward the tumor. Although some tumors may not have regional node involvement, routine node dissection is recommended for tumors that frequently metastasize to regional nodes. This procedure has high applicability to cancers of the breast, stomach, bowel, thyroid, some head and neck cancers, and skin malignancies.

5. Radical operations: Perhaps this procedure is one that should be done only after a careful and thorough assessment of the reality of possible cure or effective palliation. The physical and psychological trauma of body disfigurement, the psychosocial impact of the effects of the surgery on the patient's self-concept, ego, and body image, and the economics of the situation need to be taken into consideration when a decision has to be made on whether to do surgery or not. Nonetheless, there has been some degree of success from some radical operations. Hence, weighing the beneficial effects and adverse effects of radical surgery needs a multidisciplinary approach and collaboration in the decision-making process.

6. Resection of metastases: After treatment of a primary tumor, if a solitary metastasis appears with no clinical evidence of other metastases anywhere else in the body, then

a resection of the solitary lesion can be justifiably done. For example, a solitary metastasis in the lung, liver or brain can be resected. Most often, the possibility of other metastases is ruled out prior to resection in order to insure that the lesion is a solitary one. The diagnostic procedures done to rule out metastases include metastatic survey, scalene biopsy, bone marrow aspiration, liver scan, and laparotomy.

7. Colonoscopic surgery: Removal of carcinomatous tissue in the colon is done via a colonoscope, as in colonoscopic polypectomy.[6]

8. Cytoreductive surgery: This is done on inoperable cancer in conjunction with a planned treatment program of combined chemotherapy, radiotherapy, and immunotherapy. The surgery involves devascularization of the tumor mass.[7]

PRECAUTIONS TO PREVENT TUMOR
CELL SPREAD DURING SURGERY

In surgical intervention, it is important for the nurse to realize that the curative resection of cancerous tissue can also spread the disease. Hence, adequate precautions to prevent cancer cell spread need to be observed.[5]

1. In preparing the skin for surgery, avoid vigorous scrubbing of the area where the lesion is located.
2. If an ulcerating lesion is present at the site of the incision, this is covered with antiseptic through an impregnated sponge and left untouched while the surrounding skin is prepped. Afterwards, the sponge is removed and a sterile, dry protective pad is placed to protect the surrounding skin.
3. All instruments that come in contact with the tumor are washed, resterilized, and returned to the sterile field.
4. In a positive breast biopsy, a completely new set up is used when mastectomy is to be done. The patient is reprepped and redraped, and the surgical team don sterile gowns and gloves.
5. During a radical surgery the wound may have to be irrigated with distilled water or cancericidal agent prior to closure of the wound. Sodium oxychlorosene (Clorpactin) and nitrogen mustard are being used experimentally for this purpose to inhibit growth of any remaining cancer cells.

6. All tumors should be palpated gently.
7. Protective pads are placed on edges of wounds. Bowel lumens are ligated above and below the tumor and arteries and veins of a tumor are ligated before operative manipulation.

SURGICAL STAGING PROCEDURES

Staging is the determination of the extent and location of any metastases. This is a new and important concept for surgeons which greatly affects the efficacy of surgical intervention. The surgeon works with radiologists, biochemists, and hematologists to determine the "stage" of the cancer which will influence the type of surgical procedure to be done.

Some examples of regularly done staging procedures follow.

1. Esophagus: Esophagoscopy is done with biopsy. Exploratory laparotomy is done to evaluate metastases to the liver and coeliac nodes for lower-third lesions.
2. Metastatic cervical lymph nodes from unknown primary source: Multiple blind biopsies of the pharynx are done.
3. Lung: Bronchoscopy and bronchial brushing are done, then scalene node biopsy and mediastinoscopy followed by thoracotomy.
4. Hodgkin's and some non-Hodgkin's lymphomas: A tumor biopsy is followed by exploratory laparotomy with splenectomy and biopsy of the liver, then retroperitoneal nodes and iliac marrow.
5. Testis and selected cases of cervix (Stage 1), of prostate, and of bladder: Exploratory laparotomy and retroperitoneal exploration for evaluation of lymph nodes and liver are done. For positive para-aortic lymph nodes at laparotomy or on lymphangiogram, a scalene node biopsy is performed.
6. Breast cancer: Triple node biopsy is not largely done if simple mastectomy is done.[1]

SPECIAL SURGICAL TECHNIQUES AND EXPERIMENTAL PROCEDURES

Some special surgical procedures which are now being reintroduced as alternative treatment methods are described below.

1. Electrosurgery: This involves the use of high-frequency current applied by needle, blade, or disk electrodes. This has been used for certain cancers of the skin, oral cavity, and rectum.[2]

2. Cryosurgery: This utilizes a probe containing liquid nitrogen which is applied to a tumor. It is useful in treating cancers of the oral cavity, brain, and prostate.

3. Chemosurgery (Moh's technic): This utilizes an escharotic paste in combination with multiple frozen section examinations to achieve a surgical margin. This is effectively used in skin cancer treatment.

4. Laser therapy is not recommended as a means of treatment even though it has been tried.

5. Isolation perfusion: The arterial and venous supply to an extremity are cannulated, the limb excluded from the body by a proximal tourniquet, and the extremity perfused with oxygenated blood containing a chemotherapeutic drug through a pump-oxygenator. Control of some melanomas, sarcomas, and cancers of the digits has been achieved with salvage of the extremity.[3]

6. Intra-arterial infusion: This involves the administration of a high concentration of chemotherapeutic agent directly to the organ or part which is cancerous. This is done by insertion of a teflon catheter by a surgeon (or sometimes the radiologist under fluoroscopy) into the appropriate artery and the drug is pumped in steadily for several weeks through the catheter. Although not widely applicable, rare dramatic cures of advanced oral carcinoma have been seen.

Among the experimental procedures being done for cancer treatment are tumor transplant, organ transplant, and bone marrow transplant.

1. Tumor transplant: Tumor tissue is removed surgically from patient A and implanted in the thigh of patient B and vice versa to "sensitize" one patient's lymphocytes to the other patient's tumor. Several days later, lymphocytes are transferred daily from one patient to the other (via leukopheresis) for two weeks. It is hoped that sensitized lymphocytes from patient A will make cellular contact with patient B's tumor, causing death of the tumor cells and vice-versa.

2. Bone marrow transplant: This is done for selected patients with acute leukemia or bone marrow aplasia as a result of other illness or treatment such as chemotherapy or irradiation. About 300 to 600 cc of bone marrow are surgically removed from a donor under general anesthesia using multiple aspirations of the anterior and/or posterior iliac crest. The aspirate is then filtered and given to the patient

intravenously. Prior to infusion, tests must be done to insure histocompatibility between the patient (recipient) and the donor to prevent serious or fatal graft versus host reaction. The most desirable donors are identical twins or siblings with close tissue match.[4]

3. Organ transplant: A donor organ is transplanted to replace a diseased organ, such as in providing a hemografted donor kidney for a patient with bilateral hypernephromas.

MULTIMODAL TREATMENT

Today there is increasing evidence that a combination of treatment modalities has been very effective in the management of cancer patients. It should be recognized that surgery and radiotherapy can cure only if the cancer is localized within the treatment field, whereas chemotherapy has greater applicability in that it affects cancer cells anywhere in the body. Chemotherapy is more effective in the treatment of microscopic foci of cancer than in large, bulky disease, and it is very effective in disseminated cancer.

1. Where surgery is the mainstay of therapy, preoperative radiation has been used with improved long-term results. This procedure is believed to decrease the viability of the tumor cells, particularly those at the periphery of the spreading tumor. Thus, preoperative radiation therapy lessens the chance for recurrence or spread of these cells either during or following surgery. The range of radiation used is from a low of 2,000 rads to a moderate 4,500 rads. Another effect of preoperative radiation is to destroy the peripheral extensions of a tumor and increase its resectability.[5] This is most effective in certain head and neck cancers and in large cancers of the rectum.
2. Postoperative radiation therapy is believed to prevent recurrence of the disease and has been used primarily for breast cancer with axillary node involvement.
3. Radiotherapy for postoperative residual cancer has been curative in some cases. The residual cancer must be localized to a small field and be radiosensitive.
4. Radiation for late recurrences after surgery is primarily for palliation of late symptoms, such as small skin recurrences following a mastectomy.
5. In some cases, tumors that fail to respond favorably to radiation are cured by surgical intervention. Curative radiotherapy has been used while surgery was used to control metastases.

6. Chemotherapy, either preoperatively or postoperatively has been used to eradicate circulating cancer cells.

7. Combined surgery and radiotherapy in full measures is useful in the treatment of advanced carcinoma which cannot be treated effectively by surgery or radiotherapy alone. It is also useful in cancers of the oral cavity.[8]

8. Combined surgery, chemotherapy, and radiotherapy is used totally to treat Wilms' tumor, embryonal rhabdomyosarcoma, testicular carcinoma, and retinoblastoma.

9. Immunotherapy as an adjunct to surgery has had limited success, as in BCG vaccination of certain melanomatous skin deposits. As previously stated in Chapter 8, immunotherapy stimulates the host immunity.[9,10]

10. Radiofrequency therapy is a new therapy for tumor eradication. This involves the transfer of radiofrequency (RF) energy (for heating tissues locally) into the cancerous tissue. It has been found in animal studies that such RF heat eradicated the animal cancers without destruction of normal tissue. The basis for RF heating treatment is that the blood circulation in cancer tissues is sluggish and therefore by heating the cancerous tissue, the rise in temperature can cause necrosis of tissue since the impaired circulation impedes the cooling effect of the circulatory system which would otherwise normally take place.[11]

The decision to resort to multimodal treatment is influenced by certain factors.

1. The surgery is expected by the surgeon to be followed by irradiation, e.g., in the treatment of neuroblastoma.

2. The radiotherapist expects the case to be followed by surgery.

3. Certain advanced Stage III and IV carcinomas.

4. Clinical experience of the surgeon indicates the need for combination therapy.

REVIEW QUESTIONS

1. What types of cancer are likely to be cured most effectively by surgery?

2. Name two objectives of palliative surgery.

3. Describe the various surgical procedures that may be done for cancer treatment.

4. Enumerate the precautions needed to prevent spread of cancer cells during surgery.

5. What is a tumor transplant? What is a bone marrow transplant?

6. Define staging, electrosurgery, and cryosurgery.
7. Describe isolation perfusion and intra-arterial infusion.
8. What is a multimodal cancer treatment?
9. Name some examples of combined cancer therapy.
10. What factors influence the decision to use multimodal treatment for a cancer patient?

REFERENCES

1. Rubin, P. and Bakemeier, R. (eds.), Clinical Oncology for Medical Students and Physicians, The University of Rochester School of Medicine and Dentistry, published by the American Cancer Society, New York (1974).
2. Madden, J.L. and Kandalhaft, S., Clinical Evaluation of Electrocoagulation in the Treatment of Cancer of the Rectum. Am. J. Surg., 122:347-352 (1971).
3. Laurence, W., Current Status of Regional Chemotherapy. NYS J. Med., 63:2359-2382 and 2518-2534 (1963).
4. Isler, C., The Cancer Nurses - How the Specialists Are Doing It. RN, p. 10 (February, 1972).
5. Alston, F., Prevention of Cancer Dissemination During Surgery. RN, p. 35 (February, 1972).
6. Overholt, B., Colonoscopy. CA, 25(2):74-81 (March/April, 1975).
7. McBride, C., Trends in Surgery: Operating on the "Inoperable." Med. Opinion, 4(4):20-25 (April, 1975).
8. Peterson, B.H. and Kellog, C.J., Current Practice in Oncologic Nursing. C.V. Mosby Co., St. Louis (1976).
9. Smith, D.W. and Hanley, C.P., Care of the Adult Patient. J.B. Lippincott Co., New York (1975).
10. Shafer, K., et al., Medical-Surgical Nursing. C.V. Mosby Co., St. Louis (1971).
11. LeVeen, H.H., et al., Tumor Eradication by Radiofrequency Therapy. JAMA, 235(20):2198-2200 (May 17, 1976).

PART IV
Psychosocial Aspects of Cancer Nursing

CHAPTER 11
Coping With Fear

In cancer nursing, it is important to recognize that there are several phases of the disease process, viz. the prediagnostic phase, diagnostic phase, initial treatment phase, followup phase, recurrence and retreatment phase, and the terminal-palliative phase. Throughout these phases there are several fears that the patient and his family experience. During the prediagnostic phase, the fear of the unknown and the fear of having cancer permeate the individual's thinking and psychological reaction to the occurrence of any of the danger signs of cancer. To cope with these fears, the person either overreacts to the situation by needing constant reassurance that he does not have cancer or denies that he has cancer and delays seeking medical attention. In either case, the nurse can help the patient in this dilemma by allowing him to verbalize his fears and by being sensitive to the patient's psychological reactions to his fears. If the concern for the presence of cancer is unfounded as per medical evaluation, then reinforce the physician's reassurance of the patient that he does not have cancer. If the patient chooses to deny, the nurse should be cognizant of the positive value of allowing the patient to cope with his fear by denial. Sometimes denial assists the patient in being able to continue to live his life with hope. In this case, it should be allowed. However, if the denial becomes a detriment in seeking medical evaluation and treatment, the nurse can help the patient work through his denial by making him recognize the importance of prevention. The patient should not be forced to relinquish the coping mechanism of denial.

In the diagnostic phase, the patient's initial reaction is predominantly that of disbelief. This is gradually replaced by fear of death, fear of pain, and fear of the consequences of the disease. The fear of death is largely a result of the fatality associated with cancer and partly due to the fact that to date there is no known single or specific cause of cancer. In view of the patient's fear of death, he may or may not go through the stages of the dying process as described by Elisabeth Kubler-Ross, i.e., denial, anger, bargaining, depression, and acceptance.[1] Denial is an adaptive pattern of behavior, since it enables the patient to regain control of himself after the initial shock or numbness at the time of diagnosis. During this stage, the nursing intervention should focus on assisting the patient to cope with the psychological stress to his ego by allowing him to deny his illness. According to Bunch and Zabra, denial may be the patient's most effective coping response which constitutes feelings of sadness, anger, despair, hope, caring, sympathy, and empathy.[2]

Extant literature reveals that there seems to be a general consensus among health professionals that a patient should be told when he has cancer. Those who strongly contend that the patient should be told of the cancer diagnosis feel that it is the patient's human right to know about his illness. Recently, in a study made by Gottheil, et al., they have concluded that it seems questionable whether the knowledge that one is dying should be considered a human right and whether the sharing of such knowledge is necessarily human.[3] There are those professionals who believe that telling the patient he has cancer will better prepare the patient for the subsequent treatment of the disease, since the patient and his family can have time to grieve, can ask questions, and be given answers which would allay their fears and anxiety. In the light of these considerations, it is important for the nurse to realize that the question of revealing the diagnosis is a medical decision. Hence the nurse should not volunteer information except as planned and as a result of initial discussion with the patient's physician. Preferably a multidisciplinary approach should be used in dealing with the question of whether or not to tell the diagnosis to the patient. Knowledge of the patient's past behavior under stress, his self-concept, and the kind of family relationships he has should be taken into consideration in making the decision of revealing the diagnosis. There are patients who wish that family members should not know about their illness because they want to spare them the agony of the fatalism of cancer. Likewise there are family members who do not wish the patient to know the diagnosis. In these two extremes of denial the nurse can contribute to the decision-making process of the health team by sharing her own assessment and observations of the patient and the family members so that the health team can arrive at a plan of action to deal with such extreme reactions. Utilizing the nursing process, the nursing intervention should focus on:

1. The ego strengths of the patient and family members in terms of intellectual and emotional maturity as evidenced by their shared recollection of past successful handling of

stress; successful social, marital, and family relationships.

2. The ability of the patient to comprehend the situation and
    his reactions to diagnostic procedures. The age of the pa-
    tient influences his perception of death. According to Nagy,
    the psychological reactions demonstrated by the patient and
    his family such as anxiety, fear, denial, hysteria, hostil-
    ity, or anger may be seen mostly in adult behavior. How-
    ever, in children it is contended that realistic concept of
    death is lacking until the patient is nine years of age, that
    fear of separation characterizes the preschool child, and
    fear of mutilation characterizes the school-age child.[9]
3. The patient's self-concept and body image.

Thus, whether to tell or not to tell the patient that he has cancer necessitates consideration of the following:[7,11,15]

1. Whether the patient can acknowledge the fact of cancer on a
    conscious level; to determine this, the nurse should listen
    and observe the patient's reactions.
2. Knowledge of when the patient and/or the family has been
    told of the possibility of cancer.
3. Cognizance of the fact that the patient's reaction to the di-
    agnosis of cancer will depend on his ability to adapt to situ-
    ations of threat based on chronologic age, emotional matu-
    rity, established patterns of behavior in reaction to stress,
    family relationships, and his belief about cancer.

According to Kubler-Ross the patient does not fear the actual
fact of death nearly as much as he fears the process of dying,
the isolation, and the loss of dignity.[2] With this contention, the
nurse can help alleviate these fears by communicating to the patient a feeling of confidence and trust that the treatment team
will do everything possible to care for him during his illness.
The nurse should convey to the patient that there is reason for
hope during this phase of the disease process.

The fear of pain is one of the most acute and imminent fears experienced by both patient and family. The nurse can reassure
the patient's family that he will be kept comfortable with personalized care and medication. The patient's fear of the consequences of his illness can best be allayed by allowing him to verbalize his feelings, listening to the patient, and encouraging him
to share his feelings about death and dying. The patient should
be informed of the diagnostic procedures that will be done and
how he may be affected by such procedures. Through sharing
of information, the patient is more likely to be cooperative in

undergoing diagnostic tests and fear of the consequences of the tests would be minimized.

During the initial treatment phase the patient's major fears would be fear of anesthesia and fear of bodily disfigurement if the treatment plan is surgical; fear of being harmed when he is to be irradiated; fear of the toxic effects of drugs in intensive chemotherapy; and fear of the outcome of the specific treatment modality.

Fear of anesthesia can best be handled by having the anesthesiologist or certified nurse anesthetist (CRNA) talk with the patient. The anesthesiologist's or CRNA's explanation can be reinforced by the nurse. In some hospitals, patients are allowed to tour the operating room, recovery room, and intensive care unit so that the patient becomes acquainted with the environment wherein he will be cared for. The nurse should reassure the patient that modern technological advancement in medicine makes anesthesia a relatively safe procedure.

Fear of body disfigurement or mutilation is greatly influenced by the patient's self-concept and body image. Body image is our appearance and how we perceive our own function, sensation, mobility, and our feelings as well as how we think we are. It is a combination of our "ego identity" (our social self) which includes our moods, social state, profession, beliefs, values, goals, other people's opinion of us, and how we feel as a person.[4] Hence, our body image constantly changes. According to Shilder, it is the image of our body which we form in our mind, or the way in which our body appears to us; it is a mental picture which is ever changing with no end point in its development.[12] On the other hand, Schonfeld contends that body image is a complicated constellation of phenomena both conscious and unconscious which involves actual subjective perception of the body's appearance and function and the internalized psychologic factors arising out of the individual's personal and emotional experiences.[13] Both Murray and Blaesing speak of body image in terms of perceptions. For the former, body image is part of self-concept, which like other self-perceptions, is a product of relevant experiences with others and is primarily the result of others' reactions to the self.[10] For the latter, body image is the total of all conscious and unconscious information, feelings, and perceptions about the body as different and apart from all others.[14] Clearly body image is something that is uniquely personal, psychological, perceptual, social, emotional, and experiential. As such, it is helpful to synthesize the characteristics of body image.[12]

1. It is a psychologic entity derived from past experiences and current sensations.
2. It is a mental picture of the body and may not be consonant with actual body structure and function.
3. It is built up through the years from physiologic, psychologic, and social components organized by the central nervous system.
4. The self-picture is made up of a variety of personal characteristics; some parts of the body become invested emotionally with greater significance than other parts, often unrelated to structure and function.
5. The attributes of the "self" differ with respect to how central they are to the "essential me." For instance, events involving the face and torso are more closely associated with self-essence than the appendages. There is less connection with body image when an attribute is looked upon as a tool rather than when it is viewed as a characteristic. For example, false teeth may be a tool for eating or may be thought of as an important part of one's face or age.
6. The ideal body image is formulated from the individual's attitude toward his body, which is derived from his identification with bodies of other individuals: sexual identification, type of work (one's very essence may be felt to be a nurse, physician, lawyer, actress, artist, etc.), and society's reactions as well as the individual's own interpretations of such reactions from others. Thus each person is a product of his times and the society in which he lives.
7. It is perceptual, it depends upon the person's perception of his self-esteem and worth, and how others perceive him as well.

Undoubtedly, cognizance of the above-mentioned characteristics of body image is essential in making a meaningful assessment of the patient's body-image concept so that appropriate intervention can be planned and implemented when it is disrupted. Body-image disruption can occur as a result of several factors.

1. It may result from neurologic diseases affecting sensory and motor systems.
2. It may result from failure to accept the body as it is and adapt to it. There may be a conflict between perceived body image and that maintained by the ego. For example, the woman who has a mastectomy may not be able to accept it because she views the removal of her breast as mutilation and thus she is no longer a woman.
3. It may be caused by decompensation resulting from the body-image disturbances as scapegoat for other problems.

For instance, a person who views himself as a failure because of his physical appearance and not necessarily due to lack of perseverance to succeed.

4. It may be caused by inappropriate body image resulting from unmet needs and developmental tasks. For example, seeing physical changes with exaggeration or chronic self-pity, egocentricism, and persistent defeatism.

5. It may result from specific conditions such as feelings of being dirty, progressive deformities, dual change in body structure and function, sensation of size change, depersonalization resulting from drugs, stress, anesthesia, immobility, sensory deprivation and loss of body boundaries.

When the patient has body-image disruption, identification of his coping mechanisms is necessary to plan therapeutic intervention. Common ego mechanisms utilized when there is disruption of body image are regression, isolation, compartmentalization, and denial. It is important to realize that unless regression is massive, the patient should be allowed to regress to a certain degree. Care should be exercised, however, to prevent the emotional isolation of the patient from significant others. Observation of the onset of loneliness and depression is crucial, since these can lead to the possibility of suicide. In a 1978 study of 41 patients at the University of California in Los Angeles, it was found that one in four women undergoing mastectomy have considered suicide.[16] In case of compartmentalization, the patient deals with one thing at a time and is therefore rigid, repetitive, and resistive. If this occurs, it makes cooperation for needed therapy very difficult. As previously mentioned, denial is positive when it allows the patient to achieve a higher degree of ego integration more so than if he remains open to the stressor. However, it is best to eventually work through the denial towards acceptance of the body-image disruption for better self-concept. This can be achieved through empathy and understanding of the patient's reactions and coping mechanisms.

Understanding of body image would not be complete without consideration of the body-image theory which has been expounded at great length in the literature. For our purposes, a brief description of this theory and its applicability in the care of patients with fear of body disfigurement is therefore fundamentally necessary.

The body-image theory suggests that we have body boundaries. The way we react to our body boundaries depends upon what type of barrier we set ourselves. If we have a high barrier, we tend to perceive our boundary with definitiveness and clarity; we have definite goals, we are independent, forceful and communicative, and our psychological reaction to stress is more through peripheral manifestations (skin and muscles) such as neurodermatitis and arthritis. On the other hand, if our barrier is low we perceive our body boundaries with more indefinitiveness; we tend to be more passive, less achievement oriented, less goal striving, and we demonstrate physiological response to stress internally as in the development of peptic ulcers or ulcerative colitis.

Applying the above concepts to the care of the patient who fears the disfigurement he will have as a result of surgery, the nurse can best help the patient by being attuned to the kind of barrier manifested by the patient. In the patient with a high barrier, the nurse should allow him to verbalize his feelings and then listen to his concerns in order to alleviate anxiety. The nurse may prepare the patient psychologically through the use of diagrams or pictures of patients who had surgery similar to what will be done to him. For example, when a patient is to have a colostomy done, the nurse should show visual aides to clarify some of his conception about how the colostomy will look and how it will affect his body image. In the case of the patient with a low barrier, the nurse should be the initiator in the communication process and encourage the patient to talk about his fears and concerns. The nurse should reassure the patient of the advantages of surgery. Feelings of acceptance and understanding of the patient should be conveyed. In both cases, it is important to instill confidence and trust in the professional skills of the treatment team. When the patient is confident that everyone will do the best possible to help him, there will be more hope and less fear of being mutilated.

Postoperatively the nurse can help the patient cope with his altered body image through an accepting, warm, and empathetic attitude. The patient should be helped in making a satisfactory adjustment to his altered body image. For example, the patient with ostomy surgery should be allowed to let the nurse know how he feels. The nurse should spend time with the patient and make him feel at ease by relating to him as a person and as a professional willing to care for him the way he is. The nursing care plan of the ostomy patient should include ways of aiding the patient's ability and readiness to confront his stoma in order to begin integrating its appearance and function with his self concept and body image.

Another important concept for the nurse to understand and subsequently use in helping the patient cope with fears of body disfigurement or mutilation is that of adaptation. Under a stressful situation, a person adapts to it according to the nature of the stress, the meaning of the stressful situation to him, the ego strengths and coping mechanisms he can effectively use in a healthy or unhealthy manner, the primary or secondary gains he will derive from the situation, and the help available to him.

Applying this concept of adaptation in the care of the patient with fears of body disfigurement, the nurse can help the patient by being cognizant of the latter's adaptive behavior. Any misinformation should be discussed so that the patient can understand what is being done and the reasons behind treatment modalities he is likely to receive. Verbal and nonverbal cues should be noted so that an appropriate nursing care plan can be developed to meet the patient's needs. For instance, in the care of an ostomy patient the nurse can feel the nonverbal response of the patient toward the sight of the stoma. The nurse can help the patient by encouraging him to talk about the stoma, touch it, or look at it. If the patient is not willing to see the ostomy, he should not be forced to confront it. Instead, the nurse should gradually encourage verbalization about the stoma such as asking the patient questions like: "Have you seen what it looks like?" If the patient says no, then she can respond by saying: "Let's both look at it." The nurse's acceptance of the patient's altered body image will assist him in coping with his fear of being rejected.

To assist the patient in readapting to his lifestyle after surgery, rehabilitation should begin from the time of diagnosis. When the patient is told how long he will be hospitalized, when he will be discharged, and what to expect after discharge, then his fear of being alienated from society will be greatly decreased.

If the mode of treatment for the patient is intensive chemotherapy, the nurse should recognize the patient's fears of becoming impotent (in males), fear of alopecia, and fear of being very sick from the drugs. [7] The nurse can help the patient cope with these fears by explaining to him the side effects of the drugs prior to therapy and what can be done to minimize any side effects he may develop. The nurse should reassure the patient that alopecia is temporary and stress the fact that there will be regrowth of hair.

In the followup phase of the patient's illness, fear of recurrence of symptoms and possible metastasis is intensified. Continued reassurance and emotional support is essential at this phase.

If the nurse cannot handle the patient's fear, she should initiate referral to the appropriate professional who can assist him to cope with his concerns.

In the terminal phase, the patient's fears are compounded. He fears pain, loneliness, lack of fulfillment or meaning in his life. We have already discussed how to help the patient with these fears. In addition, the nurse should realize that leaving the patient alone can intensify the feeling of pain. Therefore, primary care nursing should be implemented if not already in progress. To help the patient cope with loneliness, the nurse should spend as much time as possible with him and the family should also be encouraged to do the same. This is especially important in the care of the dying child. Parents should be allowed to remain with the child even at night. They should be encouraged to participate in the daily care such as feeding the child, playing with him, and reading him stories from his favorite book. This will make the child feel a sense of security and the mother will feel she has done something meaningful for her child.

REVIEW QUESTIONS

1. Identify the fears of the cancer patient during the
   a. Prediagnostic phase
   b. Diagnostic phase
   c. Initial treatment phase
   d. Followup phase
   e. Terminal phase.
2. Enumerate the nursing care principles that can be applied in the care of the patient during the above-mentioned phases.
3. Whose responsibility is it to reveal the patient's diagnosis of cancer?
4. What factors should the nurse assess and evaluate that would prove useful in the decision-making process of whether or not to tell the patient he has cancer?
5. Describe the body-image theory. How can it be used in the care of the dying patient?
6. What factors influence a patient's adaptation to stress?
7. How can the nurse assist an ostomy patient cope with his altered body image?
8. Enumerate at least five characteristics of body image.
9. What factors can cause disruption of body image?
10. What coping mechanisms are used by the patient with disturbed body image?
11. Identify the proper nursing intervention when the patient utilizes various defense mechanisms to cope with his disrupted body image.

REFERENCES

1. Kubler-Ross, E., On Death and Dying. Macmillan Co.,
   p. 39 (1969)
2. Bunch, B. and Zahra, D., Dealing with Death - The Unlearned Role. Am. J. Nurs., pp. 1486-1488 (September,
   1976).
3. Gottheil, E., et al., Truth and/or Hope for the Dying Patient. Nursing Digest, pp. 12-14 (March/April, 1976).
4. McCloskey, J.A., How to Make the Most of Body-Image
   Theory in Nursing Practice. Nursing 76, pp. 68-72 (May,
   1976).
5. Fink, S., Crisis and Motivation: A Theoretical Model.
   Arch. Phys. Med. Rehab., 48:592-597 (1967).
6. Gallagher, A.M., Body Image Changes in the Patient with
   a Colostomy. Nurs. Clin. North Am., 7(4):669-676 (December, 1972).
7. Brunner, L.S. and Suddarth, D.J., Textbook of Medical-
   Surgical Nursing. J.B. Lippincott, New York, pp. 106-
   113 (1975).
8. Rubin, P. and Bakemeier, R. (eds.), Clinical Oncology
   for Medical Students and Physicians. The University of
   Rochester School of Medicine and Dentistry, New York,
   published by the American Cancer Society, pp. 109-116
   (1974).
9. Nagy, M.H., The Child's View of Death. In: The Meaning of Death, (H.F. Feifel, ed.) The McGraw-Hill Book
   Co., Inc., New York (1959).
10. Murray, J., Principles of Nursing Interventions for Adult
    Patients with Body-Image Changes. Nurs. Clin. North Am.,
    7(4):697-707 (December, 1972).
11. Corbei, M., Nursing Process for a Patient with Body-Im-
    age Disturbances. Nurs. Clin. North Am., pp. 155-163
    (March, 1971).
12. Shilder, P., Image and Appearance of the Human Body.
    International Universities Press, New York (1951).
13. Schonfeld, A., Body Image in Adolescents: A Psychologi-
    cal Concept for the Pediatrician. Pediatrics, pp. 845-855
    (May, 1963).
14. Blaesing, S., The Development of Body Image in the Child.
    Nurs. Clin North Am., pp. 597-607 (December, 1972).
15. Schoenberg, B., et al., (eds.), Psychosocial Aspects of
    Terminal Care. Columbia University Press, New York,
    p. 211 (1972).
16. Craven, R.F. and Sharp, B., The Effects of Illness on
    Family Functions. Nursing Forum, XI(2):186-193 (1972).

CHAPTER 12
Coping with Death and Dying

THE DYING PATIENT AND THE NURSE

Numerous books and articles have been written about death and dying. Undoubtedly, the nurse who keeps herself abreast with current nursing and other health professional literature is familiar with what has been said. Perhaps what needs to be done now is to synthesize some of the key ideas already expounded within a psychosocial and philosophical framework which can be useful for the nurse in caring for the dying patient.

Bunch and Zahra contend that dying is as much a psychosocial reality as a biological one.[1] Hence, the nurse needs to relate with the dying as persons with needs and concerns. This means that she has to be open to the dying person's personal response to death. Moreover, the nurse has to acknowledge her own personal feelings about death and the dying process so that she can be more sensitive to the patient's needs.

Although recent studies of the Kubler-Ross proposed five-stage model of the dying process suggest that the validity of such a model is questionable in terms of objective measurement rather than clinical insight,[2] our own personal experience and those of other colleagues tend to validate the Kubler-Ross model. Nonetheless, what is more important than whether or not the patient goes through the five stages of dying is the fact that the dying patient reacts to his death in a variety of ways. The patient's reactions to the fatality of his illness can be: hysteria (as manifested by crying, screaming, mutism, or unresponsiveness), denial, anger, bargaining, depression, acceptance, resignation, and hope.

According to Glaser and Strauss, the dying patient can experience four levels of awareness, viz., closed awareness, suspected awareness, mutual pretense awareness, and open awareness.[20] During the stage of closed awareness, the family and the staff know that the patient is dying but the patient does not.

As a result of this, mutual support is not possible, thereby creating stress among staff and family members alike in that a decision has to be made whether or not to let the patient know he is dying. When the patient reaches the stage of being suspicious of what the staff and family know that he is not aware of, then a different type of stress ensues, i.e., feelings of being always cautious so that the patient's suspicions cannot be confirmed. At times, this leads to defensiveness that may hinder the grieving process. When both the patient and the family as well as the staff know that the patient is dying and yet pretend it is not the case, then poor communication and professional distance maneuvers can occur. The nurse may find herself spending less time with the patient for fear of being confronted to talk about his dying or she may use talkativeness as an excuse to deal with own feelings of inability to communicate to the patient what really is going on. Clearly, open awareness is the stage that is most therapeutic in that open communication, emotional support, and sharing of information permeate the patient, family, and staff interactions. In this case, the patient can have control over his destiny, can participate in the decisions made that affect him, and can be helped to grieve toward a peaceful death.

Knowledge and recognition of these levels of awareness are important in the management of the dying patient. The nurse can identify the problems resulting from such a level of awareness and then plan and implement nursing intervention to resolve such problems.

Anticipation of the possible reactions of the dying patient to the process of dying is essential for holistic care. These reactions can vary according to chronologic age. The child under five years of age views death as reversible. The 5- to 10-year old personifies death; thus it can be imagined as a separate person. After the age of 9 or 10, the child sees death as final. Hence, themes of inevitability and universality appear in their descriptions.[21] For the adolescent, death represents a lack of fulfillment. He seldom thinks about death since his preoccupation is the present "now."[22] For the middle-aged adult, fear of death and more so of the dying process is a core reaction. The elderly experiences not only anticipatory grieving over death of self but also bereavement on the continuous loss of personal relationships. More than death, however, the elderly fears isolation, humiliation, loneliness, and rejection. As the elderly approaches the dying process, he is willing to tolerate deterioration, but at some point death becomes preferable to life.[23]

It would be most beneficial for both the patient and the nurse if their individual reactions to the patient's dying could be identified and acknowledged. The result would be a more therapeutic nurse-patient relationship. Some nurses may find caring for the dying patient a most challenging role; others may find it difficult to relate to the dying patient. Hence, if the nurse is cognizant of her own feelings and capabilities, she can plan her nursing care better. If the nurse recognizes the patient's need to cry, she should make the patient feel it is all right to cry. On the other hand, if the nurse feels like shedding her tears when her patient dies, she also should allow herself to cry. It is only human to be deeply touched by the loss, especially if the nurse has put a great deal of loving care in her working relationship with the patient.

Should the dying patient persist in denying her death, such denial can be expressed in some other forms of behavior such as anger, hostility, resentment, despair, hope, or excessively demanding behavior. Whatever the reactions may be, especially when it is negative, the nurse should accept the patient's behavior and find ways of helping to cope with her own feelings.

When the patient despairs, the nurse should provide emotional support and compassion. Moreover, the nurse should help the patient verbalize his feelings, prevent further regression by involving the patient with his self-care and other activities compatible with his condition, and promote reintegration of the patient's ego. Sometimes the use of human touch, holding the patient's hands, can be very reassuring since such action can convey warmth, empathy, and the feeling of caring.

In the case of excessively demanding behavior, the nurse can best help the patient by recognizing that behind the demanding behavior may be fear of loneliness, fear of isolation, and fear of being left alone when he dies. We have discussed earlier how to cope with these fears. In addition, the nurse should be relieved of additional routine tasks so that she can spend more time with the patient during his impending death.

Depression in the dying patient may be an expression of "my will would not work," and the patient withdraws from any meaningful interaction. Often, underlying the depression is a feeling of hostility which may not be outwardly expressed. When this happens, the patient may refuse to eat or drink anything, may not be cooperative in going through certain necessary treatment, and may feel the futility of any further treatment. There is a severe stress on the patient's ego and a loss of the sense of "futureness." In this case, the nurse can help the patient by initially showing interest in him and providing emotional support so that he can open up and verbalize his feelings. The nurse should listen to the patient and refrain from giving false reassurance. It is helpful to make the patient feel some sense of control over his remaining life. Thus, the patient should not be hurried when he is supposed to do something; he should be treated accordingly at his own level of functioning. Finally, the dying patient can be assisted to find hope for a peaceful death. This can be achieved by respecting the patient's individuality and providing reassurance that he has lived a meaningful existence. The essence of a lived existence is making the most of what life has to offer within one's own capabilities, ego strengths, values, and limitations. If only the dying patient can view his past and present as a "lived" existence, then the peace of death can be attained.

All of the above-mentioned nursing care interventions can be carried out most efficaciously if the nurse has come to grips with her own feelings about death and dying. As Sonstegard and Hansen said, working with the dying patient need not be a morbid experience. Rather, it can be a growing experience both personally and professionally.[3] Personal growth, for example, can be attained through working with the dying patient's hostility and emotional outbursts, as these behaviors necessitate tolerance, understanding, patience, and acceptance. Professional growth results from the continued efforts of the nurse to provide clinical expertise, emotional support, comfort, and compassion.

In some instances, the nurse may also find caring for the dying patient very depressing, especially when the patient is a child. Somehow it is much more difficult to cope with youthful death since the idea of the child not having had the chance to live life long enough becomes unbearable. The nurse should seek professional support from her peers or colleagues, from others she can relate to, even her own superior. The nurse needs to ventilate her own feelings and frustrations so that she can better adapt to the situation. In staff clinical conferences, the feelings and concerns of the health team members should be openly discussed so that group support can be elicited. A multidisciplinary approach to special problems of both the staff and patients is most effective, since input from various disciplines promotes a much broader perspective. There are nurses who are slightly hesitant to seek available resources when faced with problems that they find difficult to handle on their own. Perhaps this is due to fear of being stereotyped or being labelled as inadequate. It is important that such hesitancy be resolved through an increased awareness of one's own limitations and subsequently accepting one's inadequacies. The person who learns most is the one who is willing to admit that he does not know.

There are times when the nurse's initial reaction to the dying patient may be that she does not want to see him go through a painful death or that she experiences fear since the patient's death reminds her of the reality that the same thing may eventually happen to her. When this occurs, peer support and open communication with health team members can be very helpful.

A very important challenge of cancer nursing is being able to meet the needs of the dying patient through the process of caring. This caring entails not just physical care, but also and most important of all, emotional care. But caring is not easy because it requires strength of character, fortitude to see human pain and agony without losing hope, and an enduring patience and empathy. When the patient states: "I am afraid to die," emotional support can be given through an honest response such as "I am also afraid of dying." To provide emotional care, listen and spend time with the dying patient. Ascertain at what stage of the grieving process the patient is at and identify feelings that may be covert so that these can be articulated. If the patient is in the stage of denial, unless a more effective coping mechanism is feasible, he should be allowed to deny his illness and then be gradually assisted to work through his feelings towards acceptance of his impending death. Adverse behavioral manifestations should be shared among health team members, discussed, and utilized in planning appropriate therapeutic intervention. During the stage of anger, it may be very difficult for the nurse to maintain self-control so that withdrawal from the patient does not ensue. Thus, opportunities to discuss the patient's angry behavior and outbursts should be provided for during staff conferences or in consultation with experts. Appropriate responses by staff members can be determined by the team and the experts in order to facilitate the emotional adaptation between the patient and the health team members.

When the patient is in the bargaining stage and is able to live long enough to attain what he bargained for, he is likely to forget whatever he promised to do as part of the bargain. Thus, if he has promised to donate part of his money to a certain charitable institution in exchange for a prolonged life so that he could live through Christmas when his sons would come home from another state, this may not be fulfilled. Nevertheless, he should not be reminded of this promise nor urged to fulfill it; no one has a right to impose an obligation to comply with his promise.

In the process of grieving, the patient may cry and become depressed. It is important to realize that it is at this moment that the nurse can be most supportive by staying with the patient and perhaps holding his hands in silence. The human touch conveys a feeling of warmth and understanding which cannot be expressed through verbal communication. When the patient reaches the stage of acceptance, family members can assist the health team in facilitating death with dignity and peace. Family members should be allowed to stay with the dying patient during his last moments. Preferably, provisions should be made for them to stay nearby so that they can be summoned immediately when imminent death is approaching and thus be at the bedside when the patient dies. Spiritual care should be provided through a chaplain or a minister. In some cases, the patient or family may wish to bring in their own priest or minister rather than the hospital's chaplain. Arrangements should then be made to ensure attainment of this wish. If the patient is a Catholic, Extreme Unction may have to be administered as the patient desires. In this regard, the nurse should be cognizant of the fact that some patients may view the last sacrament of extreme unction as the ultimate prelude of earthly existence, and some may not have accepted the reality of impending death. Whenever this happens, extreme unction should not be imposed upon the patient. The decision to receive extreme unction should be made by the patient when he feels ready for it. In a similar vein, nurses who have a different religious orientation from that of the dying patient should not impose their own religious beliefs on the patient. At times the nurse may be asked to perform acts that may not be within the realm of her professional domain, but of necessity must nevertheless be complied with. I recall a personal experience as a staff nurse in an Australian hospital when I was asked by a dying patient for a priest. It was about three o'clock in the morning and I called for the priest to come immediately. As I stood by the patient's bedside, I realized that her final moments were fast approaching and I felt so alone. I kept looking at the entrance to the unit for the priest to arrive as I really did not know what to do. Then the patient said: "I need a rosary to take with me to my grave." I told her that I did not have a rosary but that I had a scapular of Our Lady of Mt. Carmel which I have been wearing around my neck since a freshman in high school. She pleaded for me to give it to her and although I felt it difficult to part with my scapular, I had no choice but to give it to her. Within seconds after she held the scapular in her feeble hands, she expired. I felt obligated to let her have my scapular instead of a rosary and I informed the family of her death wish. They were very grateful and assured me that the scapular would be buried with the patient. In retrospect, I realized that I had been able to help the patient have a peaceful death, especially since the priest was not able to be at the bedside when she expired. This experience enhanced my awareness of the need for spiritual care for the dying patient and the necessity to perform certain acts, out of the ordinary at times, in order to attain desirable goals. In this singular experience, the goal was death with peace and spiritual fulfillment.

In an earlier chapter, we discussed the issue of whether or not to tell the patient he has cancer. In this chapter, a similar issue is whether or not the patient should be told that he is dying. The primary responsibility for letting the patient know he is dying belongs to the physician. However, there are some physicians who may feel uncomfortable telling the patient of his imminent death. In this regard, the nurse should try to establish open lines of communication with the physician and offer to be present when the patient is told of his prognosis so that someone will be available to give emotional support after the doctor tells him of his impending death. The manner of telling the patient that he is dying should not be blunt; rather it should be factual such as: "You are seriously ill and the chances of survival for people with this disease are minimal, although there are available treatment possibilities." Moreover, the patient is best told of the fact that he is dying when he is ready. But how does one know when the patient is ready? One way of ascertaining this is to be alert when the patient brings up the topic of dying itself. It should be emphasized that even though a patient may not be told that he is dying, he has a sense of what is really happening and can assess his prognosis. Thus, we may only be kidding ourselves.

DYING AT HOME VERSUS DYING IN AN INSTITUTION

Most health professionals would agree that the primary goal of caring for the dying patient is death with peace and dignity. In this regard, the dying patient should preferably be given the opportunity to die at home, in familiar surroundings, rather than in an institution. Unfortunately, statistics reveal that in 1976, out of two million people who died in the United States, 70% died in institutions.[24] In view of this, hospice care has become increasingly popular in the United States within the last two years. Historically, hospices were shelters which were used by travellers to the Holy Land during the crusades. Today, hospices are programs which seek "to provide medical and social support necessary for patients and families to go through the process of dying in a manner they would consider dignified."[25] The key concept of hospice philosophy is to maintain the patient in his home among his family as the most normal way for him to live the rest of his life. The focus of nursing care in hospice is one of care rather than cure. This caring is on a humanistic, holistic level through meeting the patient's emotional and physical comfort needs. Holistic care entails meeting the physical, spiritual, psychological, emotional, sociological, and intellectual needs of the patient in order to constitute his wholeness as a human person. In Chapter 15, we shall discuss more intensively the hospice care of the oncology patient.

ETHICAL-MORAL CONSIDERATIONS

As mentioned earlier, the nurse must come to grips with her own feelings and fears about death and dying in order to be therapeutic. At this juncture, there are other important considerations to be confronted by the nurse. For instance, the issue of euthanasia may present a great deal of difficulty for the nurse. While one nurse may view death as a valuable end to the patient's pain and suffering, thereby making her feel that euthanasia is justifiable, another nurse may be strongly against it because of religious convictions. To date, there are no specific rules to be applied in making ethical decisions affecting the dying patient. Primarily, each patient is a unique individual whose needs are different from others. Thus, the decision to prolong life and for how long depends upon this awareness of the unique human dimension of health care.

To assist the nurse in coping with ethical and moral dilemmas, it is useful to go through a values clarification process. But before one can go through such a process, it is essential to attain a basic understanding of what is a value and what is values clarification.

According to Simon, "values are a set of personal beliefs and attitudes about the truth, beauty, worth of any thought, object, or behavior. They are action oriented and give direction and meaning to one's life."[26] Williams defines value as a conception of desirable states of affair utilized in selective conduct as criteria for preferences or choices as justification for proposed or actual behavior.[27] We contend that value is a code of conduct, ideals, beliefs, customs, criteria, or standards which influence one's judgement in making a decision to act or not to act and in choosing for or against any object, idea, or state of affairs based upon what is personally and socially acceptable. Moreover, one's values constitute an integral part of the personality's integrity and worth. As such, values are derived from life's experiences from early childhood to adulthood formed by cultural, social, religious, and moral background and philosophy of life.

Thus, it is understandable for Orientals to manifest a high degree of respect for any person in authority as a result of cultural upbringing. For example, it is unacceptable for a young Oriental to call an older person on a first name basis, although this practice is culturally acceptable in American society. In terms of philosophical orientation, an existentialist is more likely to make his ethical decision on the basis of what is humane and meaningful in the here and now of the present, while the pragmatist is likely to decide on the basis of what works or functions well. A person who subscribes to the utilitarian theory makes his decision on the basis of the maximum ends or goals achieved which justify the means used in attaining the goals.

Values clarification is then a dynamic process by which we can sort out the ethical and moral issues we are confronted with and hopefully enable us to make the decisions which we can live with comfortably. There are several steps involved in this process, viz., choosing freely from distinct alternatives, careful consideration of the consequences of each alternative, being proud and happy about the choice, affirming it publicly, acting on the choice so that it becomes part of one's behavior, and then repeating the choice at some other time or occasion.[28] In effect, when one goes through the above-mentioned steps, then a belief, attitude, or choice becomes a value. Let us apply this valuing process in the following clinical situation:

Mrs. Cynthia Graves, age 65, is dying of metastatic cancer. She is very emaciated and is suffering constant severe pain. The physician's order reads: Give meperidine HCl (Demerol) 100 mg for severe pain prn., IM. Janet Smith, is a 23 year-old registered nurse who is a newly hired staff nurse assigned to care for Mrs. Graves. At 7:15 a.m., Janet gave Mrs. Graves Demerol 100 mg intramuscularly. At 8:00 a.m. Mrs. Graves requests another pain medication. Janet gave Mrs. Graves Graves another Demerol. She feels it is too soon and may cause Mrs. Graves to be addicted to Demerol. When she checks with the charge nurse, she is told to go ahead and give it anyway. Janet still hesitates to give the medication and is perturbed by the attitude of the charge nurse.

The valuing process would require Janet to choose freely from either giving Mrs. Graves the Demerol or not. She is told to give it anyway by the charge nurse but she decides not to do so because she is not happy about the consequence of possible drug addiction. Thus, it may be said that Janet holds a certain value about drug addiction. Unfortunately, it is obvious that Janet's value about drug addiction is derived from a limited knowledge and experience about pain management in cancer patients which has influenced her valuing process. Nonetheless, this clinical situation further validates what has been stated earlier that values are derived from life's experiences. Thus, we contend that a great deal of life experiences enriches one's value system. For the health care giver, ethical and moral decisions can be made more comfortably through consultation with others who can share their values derived from a wealth of experience in caring for the dying patient.

Thus far, the psychosocial reality of death and dying has been explored. Equally important for the nurse is a philosophical approach to the concept of death. Philosophically, death can be viewed in terms of a phenomenology of death. This entails an immediate and experiential encounter with death. Such an encounter makes one feel that death is not just a biological finality but that it is still a process of living in the present, the existential here and now. Within this philosophical framework, the nurse should care for the dying patient not as a physical being awaiting annihilation but as a person living his life in the present, living in and with others in the world. This means that the patient's life has meaning in relation to others in the world and not apart from others in the world. As such, the goal of nursing care should be to assist the patient to adapt to his maximum level of functioning. The nurse should help the patient live each day in a meaningful interaction with others rather than in isolation. In light of this, the nurse who cares for the dying patient need not be grim in appearance, nor need be too serious or sad looking. She needs to be herself and relate with the dying patient no differently from others who are well. There seems to be a tendency for nurses to behave differently when caring for the dying patient. Even the nurse's sense of humor should not be lost. In fact, it should be maintained in an appropriate way such as in focusing on the little but meaningful and successful adaptations and accomplishments of the patient. Each day the patient lives can be experienced as moments more precious than the last. The patient may live today as if it was the last day.[4]

The nurse should also note that the dying patient has a need to feel himself in control of his destiny. This need can be met by allowing the patient certain freedom of mobility and activity which she can handle without causing undue stress or fatigue. In effect, the patient is enabled to live the remaining days of his life in a meaningful and peaceful experiential encounter.

THE DYING PATIENT'S
FAMILY AND THE NURSE

Just as the dying patient experiences the grieving process, so does the patient's family. The nurse can be most helpful to the patient's family if she can identify the family members' individual needs. Hampe's study suggests that the grieving person's needs are:[5]

1. Those that center on relations with the dying
    a. To be with the dying person
    b. To feel helpful to the dying person
    c. To be assured of the patient's comfort
    d. To be informed of the patient's condition
    e. To be aware of the patient's impending death
2. Those that center on himself
    a. Need to ventilate own feelings
    b. Need to receive comfort and support from others
    c. Need to receive acceptance and support from the health team.

The family should be allowed to participate in the care of the patient, especially in children, in order to decrease feelings of isolation. The nurse should accept the family's reactions to the patient's impending death and subsequently provide emotional support. In case of deterioration of the patient's condition, the family should be notified so that they may be able to spend time with the patient in his last moments. There have been cases where the loss of a loved one while not in attendance triggered a great deal of guilt feelings and depression. To prevent these serious sequelae, the nurse should inform the family at the first sign of deterioration of the patient's condition. If the physician has ascertained that the patient may not last longer than a few days, then the nurse should make the family aware of the possibility that the patient may succumb to his death any time in the next few days. This will alert the family to make necessary arrangements at home or at work so that they can be with the patient.

The sociocultural aspects of death and dying cannot be overlooked as they play a vital role in the adaptations of the family to the dying process. There are those who view death as finality; others believe that there is life after death and therefore it is not so bad that their loved one will be reaching the life of the beyond. Some find value in death itself and still others view dying as just a temporal aspect of life and death as a continuum. Whatever the meaning of death may be to a particular culture or society, it should be respected by the nurse no matter how strange it may seem.

It is suggested that after the patient's death, the family should be contacted within a week or two to see if they have any final questions and concerns which they need to discuss in order to resolve their feelings of loneliness, guilt, or anger. Support to the family at this point in time is crucial in their successful readaptation to their new lifestyle. Share with the family members the following resources available to assist them in coping with death and dying.

Make Today Count: This group helps cancer patients cope with their feelings. Their motto is: "Don't think of the future. Just get the most of each minute of each day."
Contact: Orville Kelly
        218 S. 6th Street
        Burlington, Iowa 52601

Widow-To-Widow: This is a consultation center that helps widows set up groups to cope with their new situation and problems.
Contact: Widow Consultation Center
        136 E. 57th Street
        New York, New York 10022

Parents Without Partners: Their goal is to bring children to healthy maturity and overcome problems of being an isolated parent in society.
Contact: Parents Without Partners
        7910 Woodmont Avenue
        Washington, D.C. 20014

Euthanasia Educational Council: Copies of the living will, a request for the cessation of heroic measures and even for the hastening of death under appropriate circumstances, are available (see Figure 4).
Contact: Euthanasia Educational Council
        250 West 57th Street
        New York, New York 10019

INNOVATIVE APPROACHES TO CARE OF THE DYING PATIENT AND HIS FAMILY

Several institutions have developed and implemented a number of innovative approaches in the care of the dying patient and his family, which have been published in various journals or periodicals. A synthesis of several of these innovative interventions and ideas follows.

A LIVING WILL

To my family, my physician, my lawyer, my clergyman, to any medical facility in whose care I happen to be, to any individual who may become responsible for my health, welfare, or affairs:

Death is as much a reality as birth, growth, maturity, and old age - it is the one certainty of life. If the time comes when I, _____ , can no longer take part in decisions for my own future, let this statement stand as an expression of my wishes while I am still of sound mind.

If the situation should arise in which there is no reasonable expectation of my recovery from physical or mental disability, I request that I be allowed to die and not be kept alive by artificial means or heroic measures. I do not fear death itself as much as the indignities of deterioration, dependence, and hopeless pain. I therefore ask that medication be mercifully administered to me to alleviate suffering, even though this may hasten the moment of death.

This request is made after careful consideration. I hope you who care for me will feel morally bound to follow its mandate. I recognize that this appears to place a heavy responsibility upon you, but it is with the intention of relieving you of such responsibility and of placing it upon myself in accordance with my strong convictions that this statement is made.

Signed _____

Date _____
Witness _____
Witness _____
Copies of this request have been given to _____

Figure 4: A Sample Copy of a Living Will. (Reprinted with permission from Concern for Dying, 250 West 57th Street, New York, N.Y. 10701)

1. A primary care nursing model has been developed to ensure that there is always a staff nurse accountable for meeting the needs of the dying patient.
2. Special sensitivity training programs have been organized for staff and even volunteers to enhance their ability to listen to and discuss the patient's fears and concerns as well as their own feelings.
3. Group therapy sessions have been organized for patients, relatives, and members of the health team. These sessions

4. A bereavement clinic for surviving family members can provide emotional support in working through the grieving process.
5. Staff educational programs can help when centered on discussion and understanding of the patient's Bill of Rights (as proposed by the Southwestern Michigan Inservice Education Council, shown in Figure 5) and implications for patient care. Annas has proposed the following rights of the terminally ill:[29]
   a. Right to know the truth
   b. Right to confidentially and privacy
   c. Right to consent to treatment
   d. Right to choose a place to die
   e. Right to choose the time of death.
6. Joint conferences between nurses and physicians in order to plan the most effective management of the patient's course of illness are recommended.
7. Acknowledgement should be made of the increasing numbers of people who are expressing a wish to choose the manner and time of death as part of the philosophy of care. The Euthanasia Educational Council has developed the Living Will (see Figure 4) which when signed allows the omission of extraordinary life-saving measures to prolong life[37].
   It should be noted that in 1976 the California Legislature passed the Natural Death Act, giving individuals the legal right to choose to avoid the use of extraordinary measures prolonging life.
8. Effective pain management can be attained through a pain-relief modality that promotes maximum comfort which may include any combination of medication, relaxation techniques, acupuncture, biofeedback, surgical intervention, etc. A more extensive discussion of pain management is found in Chapter 14.

SUPPORTIVE CARE OF THE DYING PATIENT AND HIS FAMILY

In order to provide the maximum supportive care of the dying patient and his family, the following measures should be undertaken:

1. Allow the patient to care for self as much as possible.
2. Have family members participate in the care of the patient.
3. Explain all tests, procedures, and treatments and the possible ill effects of therapy.
4. Inform the patient of the goal of treatment, whether to add to the quality of his life or just to prolong life.

I have the right to be treated as a living human being until I die.

I have the right to maintain a sense of hopefulness, however changing its focus may be.

I have the right to be cared for by those who can maintain a sense of hopefulness, however changing this might be.

I have the right to express my feelings and emotions about my approaching death, in my own way.

I have the right to expect continuing medical and nursing attention, even though "cure" goals must be changed to "comfort" goals.

I have the right to participate in decisions concerning my care.

I have the right not to die alone.

I have the right to be free from pain.

I have the right to have my questions answered honestly.

I have the right not to be deceived.

I have the right to have help from and for my family in accepting my death.

I have the right to die in peace and dignity.

I have the right to retain my individuality and not be judged for my decisions, which may be contrary to the beliefs of others.

I have the right to discuss and enlarge my religious and/or spiritual experience, regardless of what they mean to others.

I have the right to expect that the sanctity of the human body will be respected after death.

I have the right to be cared for by caring, sensitive, knowledgeable people who will attempt to understand me.

Figure 5: The Dying Person's Bill of Rights. (Reprinted with permission from Southwestern Michigan Inservice Education Council)

5. Visiting should be allowed, including children, during hours other than the regularly scheduled hospital visiting period.
6. Encourage the patient to ask questions and express needs to the health team.
7. Involve other health disciplines in the care of the patient and family, such as the clergy and social services.
8. Assist the patient to make peace with himself so that he can live the rest of his life with hope.
9. Post-mortem care is just as important for the patient's dignity after death. Thus, tapes, tubes and other equipment used should be removed gently from the patient to prevent tissue damage and wash patient as needed, especially if there are any body discharges. Allow relatives to see the patient after death as they wish, although note that decomposition occurs after only an hour.
10. Continuity of care for the family members, especially of the bereaved spouse after burial and for several weeks thereafter, is essential.
11. Provide for physical comfort as much as possible during the painful course of the disease through timely administration of pain medication and assessment of the patient's reactions and response to pain management.
12. Allow the patient to decide for himself where to die. It is suggested that home care may be an alternative to hospitalization if the cure-oriented treatment has been discontinued, the patient wants to be home, the family wants to have the patient at home, the family has the ability to care for the patient, the health care team members can be on call for the family in case of problems, and the patient's physician is willing to be an on-call consultant.[30]
13. Accept the patient's wish to complete a living will. Knowing his wishes makes the inevitable action not less awesome, or even less difficult, but perhaps less lonely. And if the living will becomes commonplace, the decision will rest where it rightfully belongs.[31]
14. Respect the dying patient's Bill of Rights.
15. Holistic care should be given to the patient.

REVIEW QUESTIONS

1. How can the nurse relate to the dying person's death as a reality?
2. What are some of the patient's reactions to the fatality of cancer as a disease?
3. Identify some nursing care principles that should be applied in assisting the cancer patient to cope with denial, despair, depression, and excessively demanding behavior.

4. How can caring for the dying patient be a personally and professionally rewarding experience?
5. How can the nurse cope with her own feelings about the dying patient?
6. Describe the philosophical approach to death and dying.
7. How can the nurse assist the patient live a meaningful day-to-day existence?
8. Identify the needs of the grieving person. How can the nurse meet these needs?
9. Describe the therapeutic intervention that would meet the dying patient's emotional needs in each stage of the grieving process.
10. How should the dying patient be told that he is dying?
11. What is the key concept of hospice philosophy?
12. Define value and values clarification.
13. Enumerate the steps in the value clarification process.
14. List three resources available to family members and the dying patient to assist them in coping with death and dying.
15. Identify at least four innovative approaches to care of the dying patient and his family.
16. Enumerate the patient's Bill of Rights according to Annas.
17. Compare the dying person's Bill of Rights as proposed by the Southwestern Michigan Inservice Education Council with that of Annas' Bill of Rights.
18. Discuss the implications of the living will.
19. Enumerate at least six supportive care measures for the dying patient and his family.
20. Identify the criteria that should be met in determining home care as an alternative to hospitalization of the dying patient.

REFERENCES

1. Bunch, B. and Zahra, D., Dealing with Death - The Unlearned Role. Am. J. Nurs., pp. 1486-1488 (September, 1976).
2. Schulz, R. and Aderman, D., Clinical Research and the Stages of Dying. Nursing Digest, pp. 47-48 (January-February, 1976).
3. Sonstegard, L., Hansen, N., et al., The Grieving Nurse. Am. J. Nurs., pp. 1490-1492 (September, 1976).
4. Hendrickson, S., A Philosophy of Death Made Personal. Am. J. Nurs., p. 1290 (January, 1976).
5. Hampe, S.O., Needs of the Grieving Spouse in a Hospital Setting. Nurs. Res., 24(2):113-115 (March/April, 1975).
6. Williams, J., Understanding the Feelings of the Dying. Nursing 76, pp. 52-56 (March, 1976).
7. Krant, M.J., In the Context of Dying. In: Psychosocial Aspects of Terminal Care (Schoenberg, B., et al., eds.)

Columbia University Press, New York, pp. 201-209 (1972).

8. Maddison, D. and Raphael, B., The Family of the Dying Patient. In: Psychosocial Aspects of Terminal Care (Schoenberg, B., et al., eds.) Columbia University Press, New York, pp. 185-200 (1972).

9. Davitz, L., Yasuko, S., and Davitz, J., Suffering as Viewed in Six Different Cultures. Am. J. Nurs., pp. 1296-1297 (August, 1976).

10. Marks, M.J.B., The Grieving Patient and Family. Am. J. Nurs., pp. 1488-1490 (September, 1976).

11. Schneiden, E.S., You and Death. Psychology Today, pp. 43-45 (June, 1971).

12. Seligman, M.E.P., Submissive Death: Giving Up Life. Psychology Today, pp. 80-85 (May, 1974).

13. Papoff, D., What Are Your Feelings About Death and Dying? Nursing 75, pp. 39-50 (October, 1975).

14. Wentzel, K., The Dying Are the Living. Am. J. Nurs., pp. 39-50 (June, 1976).

15. Klagsburn, S.C., Communications in the Treatment of Cancer. Am. J. Nurs., pp. 944-948 (May, 1971).

16. Barckley, V., Families Facing Cancer. Cancer News, American Cancer Society (Spring/Summer, 1970).

17. Verwoerdt, A., Communication With the Fatally Ill. CA, 15:105-111 (1965).

18. Burton, G., Families in Crisis - Knowing When and How to Help. Nursing 75, pp. 36-37 (December, 1975).

19. Peterson, B. and Kellogg, C., Current Practice in Oncologic Nursing, C.V. Mosby Co., St. Louis (1976).

20. Glaser, B. and Strauss, A., Awareness of Dying. Case Western Reserve University, Cleveland, p. 11 (1969)

21. Nagy, M., The Child's View of Death. In: The Meaning of Death (Feifel, H., ed.), McGraw-Hill Book Co., New York, pp. 81-96 (1965).

22. Kastenbaum, R., Time and Death in Adolescence. In: The Meaning of Death (Feifel, H., ed.), McGraw-Hill Book Co., New York, p. 104 (1965).

23. Gonda, T., Coping with Dying and Death. Geriatrics, p. 71 (September, 1977).

24. Fulton, R. (ed.), Death and Identity. Charles Press Publ., Inc., Bowie, MD, p. 4 (1976).

25. Rovinski, C.A., Hospice Nursing: Intensive Caring. Cancer Nursing, 2(1):19 (February, 1979).

26. Simon, S.B., et al., Values Clarification: A Handbook of Practical Strategies for Teachers and Students. Hart Publishing Co., New York, p. 174 (1972).

27. William, R., American Society, Alfred Knoph, Inc., New York, pp. 452-500 (1970).

28. Simon, S.B., et al., American Society, Alfred Knoph, Inc., New York, p. 38 (1970).
29. Annas, G., Rights of the Terminally Ill Patient. J. Nurs. Admin., p. 42 (March-April, 1974).
30. Martinson, I., et al., When the Patient is Dying, Home Care for the Child. Am. J. Nurs., p. 1817 (November, 1977).
31. Schorr, T., The Right to Die. Am. J. Nurs., p. 53 (January, 1976).
32. Goffnett, C., Your Patient's Dying, Now What? Nursing 79, 9(11):27-32 (November, 1979).
33. Keeling, B., Giving and Getting the Courage to Face Death. Nursing 78, 8(11):38-41 (November, 1978).
34. Paige, R.L., Living and Dying. Am. J. Nurs., pp. 2171-2172 (December, 1978).
35. Wiley, L. (ed.), The Other Side of Death. Nursing 78, 8(12):42-45 (December, 1978).
36. Sharer, P., The Shock of Sudden Death. Nursing 79, 9(1):20-21 (January, 1979).
37. McGrory, A., A Well Model Approach to Care of the Dying Client, McGraw-Hill Book Co., New York, p. 77 (1978).

CHAPTER 13
Sexuality and the Cancer Patient

Human sexuality is an integral part of the wholeness of the person. Fonseca states: "Just as man is more than the sum of his parts, so too human sexuality is more than isolated physical acts. It is a powerful and purposeful aspect of human nature that is expressed in everyday life."[1] According to Masters and Johnson, sexuality is a dimension and an expression of personality.[2] Sexuality is then an integrated, individualized, and unique expression of self.[3] Thus, sexuality is not to be equated to sex in that the latter refers to the physical act of making love while the former refers to the integration of the somatic, emotional, intellectual, and social aspects of one's personhood into one's identity and lifestyle.[4] Moreover, sexuality tends to be the expression of one's need for companionship, communication, love, concern, vitality, energy, pleasure, enjoyment, belongingness, and fulfillment.

The patient with cancer experiences a significant disruption of his sexuality. From the time of diagnosis, through the treatment process, and until the time of death, the disruption of a person's sexuality can result in impaired sexual functioning; strained interpersonal relationships; feelings of uncertainty and depression; fear of rejection; feelings of being less than a complete person; and feelings of guilt, isolation, and inadequacies as a sexual partner. In view of all of these untoward effects, it is essential to explore the impact of sexuality disruption in the cancer patient and the resultant nursing care implications.

IMPACT OF SEXUAL DISRUPTION
AT TIME OF DIAGNOSIS

The impact of sexual disruption at the time of diagnosis will depend upon several factors such as whether or not the patient will be told he has cancer, the knowledge of the patient about cancer prognosis and treatment, the beliefs of the patient about cancer itself, and the reactions of both the patient and family to the diagnosis. As we have already indicated, it is preferred

134

that the patient should be told that he has cancer. In the female, a diagnosis of cancer of the uterus may generate guilt feelings out of having had affairs with several men and/or abortion, or increased sexual activity which the patient believes to be instrumental in irritation of the uterus, thereby resulting in cancer. If the female has a spouse or sexual partner, the diagnosis of cancer of the uterus may cause decreased frequency of sexual contact or abstinence because of anxiety about touching cancer and contracting it or the fear of harming the patient. Moreover, the couple may experience negative feelings about each other and weakened interpersonal relationships. In case of grief or depression, the sexual drive or patient's libido may be impaired. The anxiety of grim prognosis can decrease sexual responsiveness and expression of one's individual needs to the point of isolation and hopelessness or suicide.

The reaction of the family members to the patient's diagnosis of cancer may be excessive concern and solicitousness or rejection. Both of these reactions are normal but pose difficulties for the patient and the nurse. Experts in psychiatry and clinical psychology contend that where there has been close family relationships in an atmosphere of love and affection, the patient is likely to receive support and understanding. However, if the family has been hostile or ambivalent towards the patient before the diagnosis, there is an out-and-out rejection of the patient. In some cases, the family is so overwhelmed by the diagnosis of cancer that it seems to completely fall apart.

The patient's reaction to the diagnosis can be shock or denial. Moreover, depending upon the site affected by the cancer, the patient's emotional reaction can be highly varied, according to the significance, special meaning, or value held by the patient regarding the body part involved. For example, cancer of the penis can cause profound anxiety and depression due to inability to continue active participation in coitus despite normal libidinal desires. The patient may fear aggravation of his condition if he continues to have sexual intercourse. On the other hand, if the patient is a male and has not had satisfactory sexual relationships prior to the diagnosis, then the illness itself may be a temporary excuse for avoiding the sexual partner.

Nursing Care Implications

1. Understanding of the family members' reactions to the patient's cancer diagnosis is essential in order to provide the necessary support and help needed by the patient.
2. Exploration of the patient's and family members' feelings about cancer and its meaning or significance to them should

be done in order to have a data base upon which to plan the
therapeutic intervention necessary to meet their emotional
needs.

3. Acceptance of the beliefs of the patient about cancer, no
matter how outlandish they may be, is essential in promoting trust and confidence in the health team's efforts to help
the patient. A gradual clarification of the erroneous beliefs through patient education can be done during the treatment regimen.

4. Awareness of the rational basis, parapsychological, or
supernatural (an act of God) factors underlying the patient's
or family's beliefs can be helpful in understanding the fear,
anxiety, loss of control, anger, and hostility that permeate
their behavioral response to the diagnosis of cancer.

5. Recognition of the significance of religion, the patient's
concept of God, and his spiritual beliefs to his state of health
can enhance the emotional comfort and psychologic well-
being of the patient.

6. Knowledge of when the patient has been told of the diagnosis
is important in order to provide guidance and assistance in
building his hope for the future.

7. Caution regarding possible projection of the nurse's feelings or perceptions about the diagnosis should be exercised
so that interference with the patient's and family members'
ability to cope and adjust to cancer and subsequent treatment can be prevented.

IMPACT OF SEXUAL DISRUPTION
DURING THE COURSE OF TREATMENT

It is during the course of treatment that sexual disruption can
be most devastating to the patient and family. The patient's reactions to his treatment regimen can be fear of loss of job because of the length of hospitalization and thereby loss of finances
needed to pay the necessary bills; fear of mutilation, pain,
death, bodily disfigurement; loss of femininity or masculinity;
fear of the effects of chemotherapy; and hopelessness. The overwhelming anxiety and fears experienced by the patient can even
impair his decision-making ability to the point of being suicidal.
The disease itself and the rigors of treatment modalities instituted can cause mental and physical fatigue which inhibit sexual
responsiveness.[5] In some cases, the prolonged separation of
the patient from the sex partner can cause him to seek substitu-
tion in sexual outlet through autoerotic behavior such as mas-
turbation or sexual advances on the nurse.[6] There may also be
feelings of infidelity on the part of the partner due to inability to

satisfy sexual needs.[7] For the aged patient, feelings of loneliness, depression, and increased need for companionship intensify as the treatment regimen continues.

Surgical intervention can cause serious consequences on the
patient's sexuality. For the patient with cancer of the prostate
who undergoes orchiectomy and estrogen therapy, impotence -
the lack of ability to achieve erection, the inability to maintain
erection, or inability to ejaculate - can occur.

For the female who has a mastectomy, there is gross impairment of self-concept and body image. The patient may experience feelings of rejection, feelings of mutilation, feelings of
destroyed or decreased femininity, and fears of being unattrac-
tive, unacceptable to the partner, as well as decreased sexual
stimulation during foreplay because of the lost breast as an
erogenous zone.[8] In some cases, the mastectomy may cause
complete cessation of all intimate sexual contact.[8] In the
American Cancer Society Gallup poll of 1974, it was found that
51% felt they would lose their sense of femininity after mastectomy, especially among women aged 18 to 34 years; 51% of single women felt that chances of being happily married decreased
after mastectomy; 36% had persistent concern about cancer recurrence; and 32% had problems with emotional adjustment.[10]
Sexual intercourse may be avoided because the patient feels un-
attractive to her partner or the partner himself may avoid sex
out of fear of unwittingly causing injury to the operative site.[7]
If there is pain or discomfort, sexual expression may be im-
peded to the point of avoidance of any enjoyment of sexual intimacy. In situations where prior to the mastectomy the patient
did not attach any special significance to sexual intimacy, the
surgery itself may provide an excuse to avoid sexual intercourse with the partner. The gravity of the above-mentioned
outcomes of mastectomy depend to a great extent to the female
patient's own body image and unique way of expressing her sexuality, self-worth, and identity. However, societal pressures
can contribute to the stress and effects of mastectomy in view
of the commercialized significance placed on the breast.

Hysterectomy, the surgical removal of the uterus, can cause
several psychological and emotional reactions that impede sexual expression and responsiveness. In a similar vein, the uterus
may have a special meaning and significance to the female patient. The uterus may be valued as a symbol of femininity,
child-bearing ability, center of the woman's strength and energy, or as a very important part of the woman's sexuality. As
a result of these values, the patient undergoing hysterectomy

may grieve, experience depression, decreased sexual responsiveness, and can fear loss of sexual attractiveness which may
cause the partner's decreased interest. As previously stated,
the hysterectomy patient may have guilt feelings arising from
illicit sexual relations and abortions. This reaction is primarily due to the recent findings that a history of early sexual intercourse increases the risk of development of cervical cancer.
If oophorectomy is done with hysterectomy, there may be decreased lubrication and thinning of the vaginal canal unless estrogen therapy is instituted. This can cause dyspareunia and
eventually vaginismus which impedes sexual pleasure. Signs
and symptoms of premature aging as well as induced menopausal symptoms may occur which can be very distressing to
the patient. With the loss of childbearing capability, the patient may feel less than a complete female. The absence of
menstruation leads to anxiety, menstruation being viewed as a
necessary mechanism for periodic cleansing of the body.[7] The
patient's partner may react to the surgical procedure with
avoidance of sexual intercourse due to an assumption that resumption of sexual activity can harm the operative site and may
cause pain and discomfort. The partner may also believe the
patient is too weak inside and therefore resumption of sexual
intercourse is not the right thing to do.

For the ostomy patient, several severe consequences can have
a great deal of impact on the patient's sexuality. For the enterostomal patient, there may be isolation out of fear of fecal
spillage, fear of social rejection, feelings of unacceptability,
decreased self-worth or self-esteem, feelings of mutilation,
and feelings of rejection and impotence. The Orbach and Tallent
studies revealed that men felt a stoma as representing castration and the initial bleeding of the stoma as feminization, while
women felt sexually violated.[5]

In another study regarding sexual practices of 211 males and
198 females aged 17 to 87, 78% had experienced no interference
with presurgical sex practices; 89% enjoyed sexual intercourse
preoperatively and 85% postoperatively; 90.5% had excellent to
average marital relationships preoperatively as opposed to 86%
postoperatively; 21% experienced a decrease in sexual responsiveness; and 22% had an increase in sexual interest postoperatively. Interestingly, 75.8% of male samples were able to
maintain an erection postoperatively as opposed to a 92.6% preoperatively. In the 41 to 60 year old group, this was more profound; 87% of the total sample were able to achieve orgasm
postoperatively, which was only 3% fewer than preoperatively.
The frequency of both multiple orgasm and extramarital affairs

decreased postoperatively, although sexual interest was present and pursued by a majority of patients postoperatively.[11]
Most investigators found that sexual function and interest probably decreased during the first year after surgical intervention.

Among male ostomates, Sutherland's study revealed that out of
29 subjects, 14 became completely impotent, five had marked
impairment of erection, and seven had only slight or no changes
in potency.[11] Psychologically, the ostomate experienced dissat-
isfaction, degradation, inadequacy, and decreased rapport with
the spouse. Other effects of surgical intervention among male
ostomates are humiliation, fear of rejection, and feelings of
unacceptability. For female ostomates, cessation of sexual intercourse may occur, which is usually initiated by the female
herself. At times, misconceptions regarding fertility and sterility can ensue among female ostomates, such as the belief that
pregnancy is no longer possible after an ostomy operation.

Nursing Care Implications

The following nursing care interventions can be most therapeutic for the male cancer patient who has undergone surgical intervention.

1. Assess preoperative sexual activity and or marital relationship in order to determine ways of assisting the patient's postoperative adaptation to the possibility of impotence.
2. Explore the patient's concept of the impact of his surgery
   on his body image, self-esteem, and financial or social responsibilities preoperatively so that positive coping mechanisms can be identified and strengthened.
3. Encourage open communication with spouse or partner and
   include both in developing a care plan that can best meet
   their psychosocial needs. Discussion of the possibility of
   sexual dysfunction following a colostomy, ileostomy, or
   other ostomy procedure should take place with both partners so that suggestions of other means of stimulation such
   as manual or oral may be practiced if acceptable to both.
4. Clarify any misconceptions and provide opportunities to discuss the patient's fears. For example, the patient may
   think that having an ostomy can cause complete impotence.
   This is not necessarily true. Impotence occurs as a result
   of severed neural pathways and may be due to emotional
   stress, fear of accidents of spillage, or fear of inability to
   achieve sexual gratification for the partner.
5. Encourage to resume sexual activity when strength has been
   regained and discomfort has diminished. Give helpful hints

about body hygiene so that sexual intimacy can be better achieved. These hints may include bathing and care of the ostomy prior to intimate contact and wearing a protective covering over the stoma.

6. Postoperatively, explore his feelings about the stoma, its effects, and the partner's response to the patient's ostomy. Assist the patient to accept his ostomy by gradually encouraging him to look at his colostomy or ileostomy and involving him in ostomy care. Responses like: "Have you looked at your stoma yet? Why don't we look at it together?" can be helpful initially. If the patient refuses to look at the stoma, then plan a definite time with the patient when he may be ready to visualize it, such as: "Why don't I come back this afternoon about 2:00 p.m. and we can look at it together?" Ask the patient if he wishes his partner or a close relative to see the stoma also and to explain its appearance and subsequent care.

7. Provide emotional support to the patient and his partner through a nonjudgmental and accepting attitude.

In the female cancer patient, there are several nursing interventions specific to the type of surgical intervention performed on the patient. For our purposes, specific interventions for the mastectomy, hysterectomy, and ostomy patient are summarized in Table 7.

Response of the patient towards surgical intervention depends to a large extent on his or her self-concept. Thus, the loss of a body part or bodily function generates varying reactions relative to the meaning and effects of such loss. Moreover, the patient whose bodily image is impaired by radical surgery has to go through an adjustment process which may entail anger, guilt, denial, despair, or depression.

Special problems that occur in the laryngectomy patient which can grossly affect his sexuality include:

1. Feelings of inadequacy due to low-pitched esophageal speech which may be viewed as offensive

2. Embarrassment from frequent burps which lead to the patient's tendency to speak softly and possibly inaudibly to others

3. Perception of laryngectomy stoma as a social disaster which leads to inability to socialize with others.

Table 7: Specific Intervention for Mastectomy, Hysterectomy, and Ostomy Patients

Type of Surgery	Nursing Intervention
Mastectomy	Preoperatively, explore the patient's body image concept, particularly the value she assigned to her breasts in order to gather information about the impact of mastectomy on her sexuality.
	Assess preoperative practices in her sexual relationships with partner in order to promote better adaptation to the effects of mastectomy. For example, if she usually undresses herself in front of her husband or partner, she should be encouraged to continue the same postoperatively.
	Discuss with the patient and partner their fears and concerns preoperatively.
	Encourage preoperative and postoperative visits by a recovered mastectomy patient to lend emotional support and discuss concerns about effects of surgery.
	Assist the male partner in expressing his feelings so that he can be more supportive to the patient. If the male partner conveys untoward feelings such as shock, nonverbally or inadvertently, this may cause the female partner to feel rejected or feel less of a woman. Determine if the partner has fear of possibly hurting the spouse during intercourse and suggest to them the use of a soft pillow to cover the operative site as a protective device.
	Take a sexual history as it relates to sexual roles and identity, sexual function, and sexual problems. On the basis of data collected, clarify misconceptions and plan for sexual counseling as indicated. An assessment of preoperative marital relationships is essential to decrease difficulties in postoperative adjustment.

Table 7 (Cont.)

Type of Surgery	Nursing Intervention
	Allow both patient and her spouse or partner privacy and time to grieve or accept the change. Reinforce the feeling that mature love is based on mutual respect for one's strengths and weaknesses and the acknowledgement that physical attributes, such as the appearance of a lost breast, should not interfere with the loving relationships of both partners.
	Use of the Reach to Recovery Manual and identification of a recovered model of a former mastectomy such as Mrs. Ford or Mrs. Rockefeller can be most supportive.
Hysterectomy: Bilateral oophorectomy	Assess the patient's self-concept, particularly the meaning of the uterus to her. To some females the uterus can be a symbol of femininity, childbearing ability, or as a means of cleansing the body through the excretory function of the uterus.
	Discuss concerns about lessening of sexual desire and diminution of the ability to respond sexually.
	Encourage expression of feelings regarding the partner's possible tendency to look for another woman.
	Reassure the patient that in due time she will be able to resume daily activities that are not strenuous and maintain a relatively normal lifestyle.
	Assist the patient to cope with feelings of guilt arising from past illicit affairs and abortions.

Table 7 (Cont.)

Type of Surgery	Nursing Intervention
	Discuss the implications of premature menopausal symptoms and give information on what to expect and the availability of medication to alleviate these symptoms.
	Assess the effects of the surgery on the patient's biologic, sociologic, and psychological or emotional well-being. Discuss the possibility of having drainage per vagina, what biologic functions will cease postoperatively, such as the ability to conceive and bear children, and clarify concerns about ability to engage in sexual activity postoperatively.
	Explore with the patient her fears so they can be alleviated, such as fear of loss of bladder and bowel control associated with the surgery.
	Identify the modes of adaptation preoperatively and support those healthy coping mechanisms.
	Discuss conjointly with partners the treatment plan preoperatively and postoperatively. Encourage their active participation in the decision-making process of what care plan need be developed and implemented.
	Reassure both partners that sexual relations are still possible postoperatively.
Ostomy	Discuss the implications of the surgery with the patient and partner.
	As previously stated, the care of the male ostomate also applies here. Additionally, for the female ostomate the use of lacy covers over the ostomy bag can be suggested.

Table 7 (Cont.)

Type of Surgery	Nursing Intervention
	Suggest the use of a protective covering such as a stoma seal, if possible. Moreover, suggest emptying of the stoma bag prior to coitus in order to promote comfort.
	Encourage an open discussion of both the patient and spouse's fears and/or concerns and assist them to cope with these through clarification of misconceptions, reassurance, and emotional support.

To assist the laryngectomee in coping with the above-mentioned reactions, a recovered laryngectomy patient should be sought to visit the patient postoperatively to give support and convey a feeling of social acceptance. For specific care of the laryngectomy patient, see Chapter 30.

In a patient who undergoes vulvectomy and clitorectomy, psychic trauma can occur from the surgical absence of genitalia, which leads to feelings of inadequacy to participate in sexual intercourse or to enjoy it. Clitoral stimulation may not be achieved and sexual intercourse may not be satisfying.[7] When the female patient has invasive carcinoma of the cervix, partial vaginectomy may be done, which results in shortening of the vaginal vault. This can decrease the depth of penile penetration and therefore can be unsatisfying to the patient and her partner. Similarly, in radiation therapy, stricture of the vaginal outlet can cause inadequate penetration. Another problem that can ensue is dyspareunia (painful intercourse) due to scarring. This has a tremendous impact on the patient since she may interpret the pain erroneously as recurrence of malignancy. It is important to clarify the patient's misinterpretation and encourage altered coital positions and techniques that can be tolerated by both partners.

Another modality of treatment that can cause alterations in the patient's sexuality is chemotherapy. If the cancer patient is depressed as a result of his malignant disease, an antidepressant may be ordered by the physician. The tricyclic compounds which include imipramine (Tofranil), amitriptyline (Elavil),

nortriptyline (Aventyl) and protriptyline (Vivactil) can cause
male impotence. Another drug that is used in cancer management which affects male patients is the antiandrogen steroid
cyproterone acetate, which is primarily used in cancer of the
prostate. This drug can cause decreased libido and potency.
As previously stated in Chapter 14, marijuana has also been
used in the management of pain in the cancer patient. It is in-
teresting to note that marijuana is considered by many to be a
sexual stimulant. However, its effects are primarily from relaxation and eradication of inhibitions regarding sexual activity
and may be influenced by the dose, the circumstances under
which it is smoked, and the personality of the user. Interestingly, there is also evidence that marijuana smokers have a
higher incidence of decreased libido and impaired potency than
nonusers.[12]

It should be noted that most of the chemotherapeutic agents used
in cancer treatment can cause oligospermia (low sperm count)
or azospermia (absence of sperm in the semen). In the female,
temporary or permanent sterility can occur depending upon the
drug dosage and length of chemotherapy. In a study of 116 men
who received chemotherapy for lymphoma, it was found that
spermatogenesis can return after discontinuation of chemotherapy.[13] Chemotherapy has a potential for mutagenic and teratogenic effects. Mutagenic effects are those of a chemical that
may be responsible for fetal abnormalities because of its effect
on the development of sperm or ova. Teratogenic effects refer
to fetal abnormalities caused by the drug as well as fetal death
after conception. In view of these effects of chemotherapeutic
agents used in cancer management, the administration of anticancer drugs to a female patient can be of grave concern since
she can become pregnant or may be pregnant at the time of the
commencement of chemotherapy. In the male, the concern is
the inability to have adequate sperm count for successful fer-
tilization of the ovum, particularly if the patient desperately
wants a child. Moreover, there is also the concern of possible
fetal abnormalities which can be very emotionally and psychologically traumatic for the male who wishes to have a child, as
well as for the partner.

To assist couples in coping with these dilemmas of parenthood
during cancer chemotherapy, the life's goals of both partners
should be explored so that they can have a better perspective of
what they really want of their sexual relationship.[18] An assessment of their readiness for parenthood should be done through
discussion of the current concerns relative to the effects of chemotherapy. Information specific to the various drugs and their
effects should be shared with the couple. Folic acid antagonists

have been implicated as causing spontaneous abortions, fetal abnormalities, or both, especially if administered between the fourth and twelfth weeks of gestation. Alkylating agents are thought to cause abortion if given in the first trimester of pregnancy, although they do not seem to cause fetal abnormality.

It is essential to assist the couple to understand their roles and responsibilities by discussing with them their concerns, uncertainties, and motivation for wanting to have a child. In so doing, the couple can achieve realistic expectations for themselves and for their child. Introduce the concept of parenting as distinct from mothering or fathering. The former refers to sensitivity to the future generation, respect for the dignity of children, kindliness, protectiveness, and continuity of care.[14] Moreover, parenting entails a mutual sharing of responsibility for the physical, social, and economic needs of the family members. Through an awareness of the implications of parenting, the couple may become more realistic in deciding their life's goals.

SEXUAL COMMUNICATION PROBLEMS AND SPECIFIC INTERVENTIONS

There are several problems that can occur between the patient with cancer and his or her partner that result from inadequate or poor sexual communication patterns. These dysfunctional communication patterns are listed below.

1. Failure to verbalize assumptions which leads to false or incorrect expectations.[15] For example, the patient with a mastectomy may assume that her partner no longer considers her attractive. As a result, she withdraws from any meaningful interaction with her partner. If her assumption had been shared with her partner, she could have validated it and perhaps found it to be erroneous.
2. Overprotection of one partner from the information that he or she is assumed to be unable to handle, resulting in lack of participation in the decisions affecting the care and management of the cancer patient.[15] For example, the patient may not wish his partner to know of the cancer diagnosis or vice versa. When this happens, both the patient and his partner are deprived of the emotional support needed to grieve and to cope with the emotional impact of the diagnosis.
3. Silent collusion on the part of both partners in order to avoid talking about unpleasant topics, thereby creating an atmosphere devoid of meaningful interaction.[15] For example, in the dying process, if both partners avoid talking about the

patient's impending death, they cannot find peace in themselves and are likely to experience bitterness due to their failure to go through the grieving process as discussed in Chapter 12.

4. Reading whatever is in the mind of the partner and always anticipating what is to be said next can prevent articulation of one's true feelings and deeper sentiments. For example, if a male cancer patient begins to communicate his need for pain medication and the partner has already anticipated what he wanted to say, the patient may decide then to refrain from asking since it may be viewed as a weakness on his part to be getting pain medication so frequently; it is not consistent with his view of masculinity.

5. Failure to recognize nonverbal cues of communication can impair communication between partners. For example, in the semiconscious patient who is dying, the inability of the partner to communicate through the use of touch can be attributed to lack of verbal response from the patient. When this occurs, the dying patient is deprived of the emotional support he needs to attain a peaceful death.

To assist both partners in resolving the above-mentioned communication problems that affect their sexual relationships, the following steps can be implemented.

1. Discuss with both partners the importance of open communication.

2. Elicit information on the reasons for the overprotectiveness of one partner about sharing what is happening to the patient and assist both to gradually come to grips with the reality of the situation. This can be achieved by identifying their coping mechanisms first and then strengthen those that would enable them to face the reality of their situation.

3. A multidisciplinary health care team approach can be beneficial in breaking the barriers to open communication through the particular contribution of the various disciplines. The social worker can assist in the social concerns of the patient, the minister can promote the patient's readiness to face death, the nurse can be most supportive through her frequent understanding interaction with both partners, and the physician can assist both partners in understanding the disease process, the treatments to be instituted, and the effects of therapy.

4. Assessment of the premorbid self-concept of the patient and taking a sexual history can be most beneficial in enabling the patient to share his true feelings and sentiments with his partner.

5. Encourage the partner to hold the patient's hands to communicate warmth, love, and empathy.

REVIEW QUESTIONS

1. Define sexuality.
2. Discuss the impact of sexuality disruption on the patient at the time of diagnosis of cancer disease.
3. What are some of the reactions that family members can have towards the patient's diagnosis of cancer?
4. Enumerate seven nursing care implications of sexuality disruption at the time of diagnosis.
5. List the sexuality problems that occur in each of the following patient treatment modalities:
   a. Mastectomy
   b. Hysterectomy
   c. Ostomy
   d. Laryngectomy
   e. Radiation therapy
   f. Chemotherapy.
6. List five specific nursing interventions in the care of the patient with sexuality problems in each of the treatment modalities mentioned in Question 5.
7. Discuss the sexual communication problems of the cancer patient and his or her partner and give specific interventions for each problem.

REFERENCES

1. Fonseca, J.D., Sexuality - A Quality of Being Human. Nursing Outlook, p. 25 (November, 1970).
2. Masters, W.H. and Johnson, V.E., Human Sexual Response, Little Brown & Co., Boston, p. 301 (1966).
3. Morrison, E.S. and Borosage, V. (eds.), Human Sexuality: Contemporary Perspectives, Mayfield Publishing Co., Palo Alto, CA (1973).
4. Maddock, J.W., Sexual Health and Health Care. Postgrad. Med., 58:52-58 (1975).
5. Woods, F., Human Sexuality in Health and Illness, C.V. Mosby Co., St. Louis, pp. 140-142 (1975).
6. Bouchard, R. and Owens, N., Nursing Care of the Cancer Patient, C.V. Mosby Co., St. Louis, p. 38 (1976).
7. Haswell, G., Chronic Illness and Sexuality. In: Human Sexuality for Health Professionals (Barnard, M., et al., eds.), W.B. Saunders, Philadelphia, pp. 222-234 (1978).
8. Burkhatter, P.L. and Donley, D., Dynamics of Oncology Nursing. McGraw-Hill Co., New York, pp. 261-262 (1978).
9. Katchadourian, H.A. and Lunde, D.T., Fundamentals of Human Sexuality. Holt, Rinehart, and Winston, New York (1972).

10. Women's Attitudes Regarding Breast Cancer. Occup. Health Nurs., 22:20-23 (February, 1974).
11. Dlin, B.M., et al., Psychosocial Response to Ileostomy and Colostomy. AORN Journal, pp. 77-84 (November, 1969).
12. Kolodny, R.C., Masters, W.H., et al., Depression of Plasma Testosterone Levels After Chronic Intensive Marijuana Use. N. Eng. J. Med., 290:872-874 (1974).
13. Sherins, R.J. and De Vita, V.T., Effect of Drug Treatment for Lymphoma on Male Reproductive Capacity. Ann. Intern. Med., 79:216-220 (August, 1973).
14. McBride, A.B., The Growth and Development of Mothering. Harper and Row, New York, p. 129 (1974).
15. Hohmann, G., Psychosocial Aspects, Treatment, and Rehabilitation of Spinal Injured Person. Paraplegic Life (May/June, 1977).
16. Gress, L., Human Sexuality and Aging. In: Human Sexuality for Health Professionals (Barnard, M., ed.), W.B. Saunders, Philadelphia, pp. 222-234 (1978).
17. Dericks, V., Nursing Care of the Patient with an Ostomy. American Cancer Society, Professional Education Publication.
18. Acosla, K. and Sommerfeld, D., Helping People with Cancer Consider Parenthood. Am. J. Nurs., pp. 1580-1582 (September, 1979).

CHAPTER 14
Pain and Cancer

Cancer is often equated to pain. The malignancy per se does not necessarily cause pain. In fact, one of the characteristics of a malignant tumor of the breast, for example, is a painless, fixed, encapsulated growth. Physiological causes of pain due to tissue injury, compression, pressure, metabolic waste, and other pain-causing chemicals do exist in most types of cancer. This chapter provides an overview of the concept of pain, explores related theories of pain, pain assessment, and management of the cancer patient in pain.

PAIN AS A CONCEPT

The concept of pain is as varied as there are individuals experiencing it in various contexts, threshold and endurance levels, and personality characteristics. From a psychologist's viewpoint, pain and its processes have a physiological and psychological aspect. Pain can transcend both the physical and psychological; it is an actuality inseparable from the person experiencing it and thus encompasses both objective and subjective correlates. Interestingly, pain can be a way of life to some individuals by making the experience of pain as a "career," or it can be a transient temporal experience associated with loss of something valued. In any case, the experience of pain is real and it is whatever the person in pain says it is. Pain can serve a definite normal function - that of protection and/or adaptation.[1,2,16,17]

A person's concept of pain is highly individualized. It is determined by the total biophysical, psychological, social, cultural, and spiritual self. Research on pain has revealed the following factors which synergistically form one's concept and expression of pain:

> The meaning attached to pain-producing situations (e.g., threat to body image and/or self-concept)

The perceived relevance of spatial-temporal aspects which are internal or external to the individual

The attention or cognitive states (e.g., knowledge of amount of information given relative to potential pain producers)

Past experiences in coping with pain

Cultural and subcultural influences (e.g., pain augmenters or enculturation of American males as "pain reducers")

Personality characteristics

Disease and symptom states

Psychological states and ego strengths

Social and economic status and lifestyle.

PAIN THEORIES

It would be remiss not to include in this chapter a few of the well-known pain theories since they offer significant concepts to foster our understanding of the pain concept. However, discussion of these theories becomes necessarily limited to the bare essentials of the specific theory within the format of this reference text. Nonetheless, it is hoped that the following presentation of the pain theories can augment one's knowledge of the pain concept.

Specificity Theory

This theory is a very simplistic, single-tract, response theory. It is considered the traditional-classical theory of pain described by Descartes in 1644. This entails the presence of a stimulus that triggers a specific skin receptor which carries the message directly into an alarm system in the brain, thus evoking a response. This is precisely why this theory derives its name of "pushbutton or an alarm bell theory."[15] This theory has since been modified through research. The physiological and psychological assumptions of the theory now contend that a mosaic of pain receptors in the body carries messages to a pain center in the brain. The stimuli elicit a chain of responses from the stimulation of the pain receptors to the transmission of the impulse by peripheral nerve fibers and through the spino-thalamic tract in the spinal cord to a pain center in the thalamus, thereby producing a sensation of pain. As a sensation, it presumes the psychological aspect of pain.[10]

Pain and Summation Theory

Goldscheider in 1894 proposed that the critical determinants of pain are the central summation of and the intensity of the stimuli. This theory purports that pain occurs " . . . when the total output of the cells exceeds a critical level," which ensue from excessive receptor stimulation from nonnoxious causes or noxious (pathological) states.[15] Derivations of this theory are the central and peripheral pattern theories. The former asserts that pain occurs due to a specific neural mechanism for the summation of stimuli while the latter asserts that pain results from a patterning of peripheral nerve impulses which is interpreted as pain in the brain center.

Sensory Interaction Theory

This theory is related to the central summation theory. It purports that pain impulses are carried by small-diameter nerve fibers which are normally inhibited by large-diameter fibers. The ratio of small to large fibers determines the presence and intensity of pain. Livingston (1943) was the first to propose that pain syndromes occur from pathological stimulation of peripheral sensory nerves producing activity in a closed circuit of neuron pools in the spinal cord which are centrally interpreted as pain by the brain.[11] This theory thus extends into the emotional-affective aspects of pain, i.e., emotional states evoke neural activity in the neuron pools.

Affect Theory

In this theory, pain is conceived not only as sensation but also as an emotion or as an emotional quality which permeates life's experiences. Specifically, an object is never perceived with absolute indifference and there is a continuum of feeling in any conscious experience. The inherent concept in this theory alludes to the cognitive, sensory, and emotional processes involved in the expression of pain behavior.

Gate Control Theory

In 1965, Melzack and Wall proposed a more comprehensive theory incorporating specificity, pattern theories, and psychological processes in concert during a pain experience. This theory asserts that pain impulses from peripheral receptors pass through a gating mechanism in the dorsal horn of the spinal cord. The three spinal cord systems function in the following manner: cells in the substantia gelatinosa act as the control mechanism, dorsal column fibers projecting towards the brain act as the central control, and central transmission cells (T cells) activate neural mechanisms which culminate in the perception and response to the stimuli. The input as it goes through the cord is subject to this gate-control system. The impulse carried by the small nerve fibers is transmitted into the T cells which, if unblocked, leave the gate open, thereby allowing the stimulus to pass through the system into the thalamus and cerebral cortex. It is proposed that the dorsal horn T cells can be stimulated to close the gate to further incoming pain stimuli by a descending blocking action. The totality of this control system is affected by anxiety, anticipation, memory, attention, information, cognitive dissonance, and other cerebral processes giving meaning to the pain experience.[18]

To summarize, pain is a matrix of interrelated referents: physical, behavioral, personal and attitudinal which are expressed as a complex and composite experience. Pain behaviors and pain quality are deterministically related to the whole biological, social, psychological, and spiritual self. Pain theories range from the specificity theory to the coded patterning, and differentiated nerve pathways, adequacy and intensity of stimuli, as well as the spinal cord system control mechanisms, and all have a powerful impact on our understanding of the pain concept and the implications for pain management.

ASSESSMENT OF PAIN

The efficacy of pain management depends to a large extent upon a systematic assessment of clinical pain. Several investigators such as McCaffrey (1977), Copp (1974), Crue (1970), Jacox (1977), Fagerhaugh and Strauss (1977), Graffam (1979), Neal (1978), Storlie (1978), Zborowski (1964), Sternbach (1974), and Meissner (1980) advocated the use of parameters and measurements of pain. Based on the individual's adaptation and coping mechanisms, the subjective account of pain, observable cues of pain, the use of measuring instruments (e.g., color scale, affective rating scale), and clinically inferred causes (e.g., pathologic and nerve-irritating chemicals), the diagnosis of pain can be made which reflects the sum total of all the aforementioned factors and provides direction to the measurement of the pain experienced by the patient.[9] A graphic portrayal of the variables interacting in pain assessment is provided in Figure 6.

MANAGEMENT OF THE PATIENT IN PAIN

Management of the patient in pain is based upon the specific variables mentioned in Figure 6. The ultimate objective is relief of physical, mental-spiritual, and socio-ethical concerns

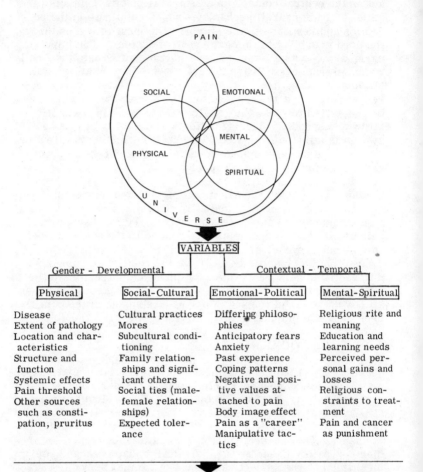

Energy Sources + Personal Gains - Deficits and Personal Losses = Pain Experience
= Diagnosis

Figure 6: Pain assessment showing the universe of pain and
critical interacting elements within the domain. (The
variables derived from the elements are considered
within the contextual-temporal-gender-developmental
process. Analysis should reveal the person's energy
sources and personal gains. Subtracting from it the
deficits and personal losses equals the pain experience (net effect) which equals the diagnosis of pain.)

through a multidisciplinary systematic approach. The pain therapy team should consist of nursing, medical and surgical oncologist, radiation and chemotherapist, clinical pharmacologist,
psychiatrist, social worker, theologians or ministers, and significant others. Coordination and sharing of the specific goals
of the pain therapy team members constitute the core of effective pain management. The mode of pain therapy may be directed towards both the elimination of causes and control of pain
by manipulating the patient's internal resources and external
environment.[3,5,6,10,20,24] To eliminate the physiologic
causes, the following approaches may be used:

1. Surgical removal of or reduction of the pain-producing pathology and resection of nerve roots by rhizotomy or cordotomy
2. Radiation treatment
3. Chemotherapy
4. Administration of sclerosing chemicals
5. Sex hormone therapy.

The control of pain may be achieved by a combination of pain-
eradicating methods and one or more approaches aimed at cognitive and behavioral manipulation by the patient and the pain
therapy team. Some of the methods of control supported by research are operant conditioning, hypnosis, relaxation techniques,
imagery, displacement and conversion, biofeedback, electronic
stimulation of nerve pain pathways, and drug therapy using analgesics, narcotics, heroin, and marijuana.[25,27]

Britain popularized the use of Brompton's cocktail which uses
heroin. This mixture has been modified for use in the United
States by substituting heroin with morphine or methadone.[7,23]
The Val-Steck elixir is a modification of the Brompton's cocktail.
This consists of 1 mg of methadone (instead of morphine) per
milliliter of the elixir, 10% ethyl alcohol, and syrup for flavor
containing raspberry and peppermint. Cocaine when used with
it increases the potency of the mixture and decreases sedation
from the methadone. Chloroform water and a phenothiazine,
which are used with heroin in the Brompton's cocktail are omit-
ted. The elixir is prescribed and given every four hours. The
initial dose is usually 10 to 20 ml although the patient's age,
body size, and renal function may indicate lower dosage. Another modification of the Brompton's cocktail is the use of morphine sulfate at varying dosages of 5 to 10 to 100 mg, cocaine
(10 mg), thorazine or compazine (5 mg), flavoring syrup (5 ml),
95% ethyl alcohol (5 ml), and chloroform water (20 ml). One
important aspect of the treatment regime is the administration
of the mixture on a regular schedule rather than on a p.r.n.

basis in order to achieve optimum effect. Pain memory disappears with the use of heroin and a regular four-hourly administration precludes the occurrence of pain perception. Other important considerations in pain management include: (1) Research findings indicate that natural morphine-like substances occur in organ cells and endomorphine is present in the pituitary, and that one-third of patients do not respond to exogenous morphine. (2) Drugs vary in their biotransformation, metabolic excretion, peak effect, and duration, as well as side and toxic effects. (3) Although pain is an adaptive response (in that it gives biologic signals), it may not signal the accurate degree of pain intensity. (4) Cross tolerance to all narcotics is not necessarily complete. (5) The immediate parenteral or intravascular administration of drugs for pain relief should be followed by oral route doses in order to maintain the efficacy of the drug effects. (6) When the patient has pain, it is believed that the nature of the pain is 90% continuous and only 10% instant.

Recently, the use of marijuana in pain management was tested through the courts. On January 1, 1980, the state of Texas passed a law that allowed a judge to issue an order permitting the use of marijuana in the management of a cancer patient. Nevertheless, further research has to be done relative to the beneficial effects of controlled substances in order to meet the expectations of state and federal laws.

The role of the nurse in pain management can be defined in terms of her concept of pain and personal philosophy of life. Since pain is deeply intertwined with every aspect of human experience - in one's state of being and becoming, living, suffering, and dying - the approach to the management of pain in the cancer patient necessarily becomes more heuristic and humanistic. To ensure this kind of approach, the following principles should be considered:

1. Two individuals' perception of the same stimulus cannot be identical.
2. Self-description of pain, which can be a better indicator of the degree and intensity of pain than autonomic responses to noxious stimuli, should be validated.
3. The meaning of pain in a given culture or subculture is subject to variations within and among individuals.
4. Pain augmenters (pain intensifiers) have relatively low tolerance to pain.
5. Age and sex influence pain experience and response.
6. Anxiety states influence pain tolerance and response and also intensify the pain experience. [12]

7. Behavioral patterns, though similar, may have different meaning to individuals in different ethnic groups.
8. Pain, if viewed as a simplistic stimulus response, becomes equated with the amount of pathology and the amount of pain; thus it equals the amount of pain medication.
9. The effects of any drug therapy are influenced by blood levels, route of administration, and timing of administration.
10. Pain complaint and/or pain avoidance are influenced by individual motives and value systems.
11. Physiological indicators of pain (e.g., changes in blood pressure, respiration, perspiration, temperature, pupillary responses, motor responses) should be used as cues in patients who are unconscious or alert but do not communicate the nature of their pain experience.
12. Previous coping mechanisms to the pain experience should be assessed. Substitute ineffective adaptations with alternative effective mechanisms when the time and situation prove conducive and the patient is ready.
13. Instruments in measuring clinical pain are useful only when used in combination with prudent judgment.
14. Ethical, moral, and legal implications take precedence in situations beyond the individual's domain of control.

Clinical assessment of the patient's pain have been made through different methods such as simple descriptive scales, numerical scales, and visual analogue or graphic representation. The instruments that have been used successfully in clinical pain assessment include:[3]

>Pain checklists
>McGill-Melzack pain questionnaire
>Stewart pain-color scale
>Stewart's pain circle
>Sternbach's pain ratio scale
>Sternbach's tourniquet pain test
>Johnson's two-component scales.

In any event, pain management involves assessment of the patient's condition, the precipitating factors that influenced the occurrence of the pain, the adaptive behavior of the patient relative to his pain and its management, and the professional's philosophical and ethical orientation. It is important to realize that evaluation of the efficacy of the pain medication regimen has a great deal of impact on the achievement of the ultimate goal of pain management, viz., a relatively comfortable condition with the least amount of pain and suffering.

REVIEW QUESTIONS

1. Discuss the relevance of the four theories of pain.
2. List patient and environmental variables of pain.
3. Describe two major approaches to pain elimination and control.
4. List six instruments in clinical pain measurement.
5. Discuss the nursing implications of the methods of clinical pain measurement.
6. Enumerate 10 principles in the assessment of the pain syndrome.
7. What is the ultimate objective of pain management?
8. Discuss the effective use of the Brompton's cocktail and Val-Steck elixir in pain management.

REFERENCES

1. Baer, E., et al., Inferences of Physical Pain and Psychological Distress: 1. In Relation to Verbal and Nonverbal Patient Communication. Nurs. Res., 19(5):388-392 (1970).
2. Bonica, J.J., et al., (eds.), Recent Advances on Pain: Pathophysiology and Clinical Aspects. Charles C Thomas, Springfield, ILL (1974).
3. Bonica, J.J., Cancer Pain: A Major National and Health Problem. Cancer Nursing, pp. 313-316 (August, 1978).
4. Crue, B.L (ed.), Pain and Suffering: Selected Aspects. Charles C Thomas, Springfield, ILL (1970).
5. Crue, R.L. (ed.), Pain: Research and Treatments. Academic Press, New York (1975).
6. Davidson, P. and Neufeld, R.W.J., Response to Pain and Stress: A Multivariate Analysis. J. Psychosom. Res., 18:25-32 (1974).
7. Davis, J.A., Brompton's Cocktail: Making Good-Byes Possible. Am. J. Nurs., 4:611-612 (April, 1978).
8. Fagerhaugh, S.V. and Strauss, A., Politics of Pain Management: Staff-Patient Interaction. Addison-Wesley, Menlo Park, CA (1970).
9. Graffam, S.R., Nurse Response to the Patient in Distress. Development of an Instrument. Nurs. Res., 19(4):331-336 (1970).
10. Jacox, A., Pain: A Source Book for Nurses and Other Health Professionals. Little, Brown and Co., Boston (1977).
11. Livingston, W.K., Pain Mechanics. McMillan, New York, (1943).
12. Mastrovito, R.C., Psychogenic Pain. Am. J. Nurs., pp. 514-519 (March, 1974).

13. McCaffrey, M., Nursing Management of the Patient in Pain. J.B. Lippincott Co., Philadelphia (1972).
14. Meissner, J.E., McGill-Melzock Pain Questionnaire. Am. J. Nurs., pp. 550-551 (January, 1980).
15. Melzack, R., The Puzzle of Pain. Basic Books, Inc., New York (1973).
16. Melzack, R. and Torgerson, W.S., On the Language of Pain. Anesthesiology, 34(1):50-59 (1971).
17. Neal, H., The Politics of Pain. McGraw-Hill, New York (1978).
18. Siegle, D.S., The Gate Control Theory. Am. J. Nurs., pp. 498-502 (March, 1974).
19. Smith, M., The Nature of Pain With Some Personal Notes. Nurs. Clin. North Am., pp. 621-629 (December, 1977).
20. Sternbach, R.A., Pain Patients: Traits and Treatments. Academic Press, New York (1974).
21. Storlie, F., Pain: Describing It More Accurately. Nursing 72, pp. 15-16 (June, 1972).
22. Straus, A., et al., Pain: An Organization-Work-Interactional Perspective. Nursing Outlook, pp. 560-566 (September, 1974).
23. Valentin, S., et al., Pain Relief for Cancer Patients. Am. J. Nurs., pp. 2055-2056 (December, 1978).
24. Zborowski, M., People in Pain. Jossey-Bass, Inc., San Francisco (1969).
25. Eland, J.M., Living With Pain. Nursing Outlook, pp. 430-431 (July, 1978).
26. Graffam, S., Nurse Response to Patients in Pain: An Analysis and an Imperative for Action. Nursing Leadership, pp. 23-25 (September, 1979).
27. Benoliel, J.Q. and Crowley, D.M., The Patient in Pain: New Concepts. Nursing Digest, pp. 41-48 (Summer, 1977).

CHAPTER 15
Hospice Care Concept

The hospice care concept mirrors a health care delivery model especially designed to provide holistic, humanistic, and interdisciplinary care of the dying patient and his family. The interpretation and operation of a hospice care program may vary, but certain guidelines or criteria have been formulated by various advocates of the program. Such guidelines and criteria have been put into effect by the National Hospice Organization and other hospice model care centers.* Along with the guidelines are objectives which in essence delineate that the program of care is centrally located and administered for the following objectives:

> To serve as the primary unit care, the patient and his family

> To assure effective control of symptoms: physical, psychosocial, spiritual, and emotional

> To assist the patient and family to live usefully, effectively, and as fully as possible

> To assure continuity of care to the bereaved family

> To supplement existing health care services

> To cut down costs of institutional health care.

The hospice, which has been particularly modeled from St. Christopher's Hospice of London, England, also has distinct

---

* A comprehensive list of Hospices in the United States, Canada, and Great Britain is in Cohen, K.P., Hospice: Prescription for Terminal Care. Aspens Systems Corporation, Germantown, Maryland (1979).

characteristics and/or elements which include specific protocols (e.g., criteria for admission, staff support, and supportive services during the bereavement phase of death; a formal
structure which specifies the link between inpatient and in-home
care services; a hospice team; provision of care 24 hours a day,
seven days a week with on-call scheduling of professional team
members; and provision of services regardless of the patient's
ability to pay.

Criteria for admission into the hospice program generally include the following:

1. Willingness of the patient's doctor to continue his association with the patient and/or continue to serve as the primary physician of the patient. (Some centers do have the
   hospice-qualified doctor to direct the program and/or
   serve as the doctor on-call.)
2. Diagnosis of a terminal illness with a lifespan of a few
   weeks to months (3-6 months).
3. That the patient and his family know the diagnosis and prognosis of the illness.
4. That the patient's family, a friend, or neighbor be willing
   to assume responsibility in giving care to the patient.
5. That the patient live within the geographic limits of the
   hospice center. (The boundaries are necessary in order
   to assure a quick and accessible delivery of in-home crisis
   care by the hospice team.)

In summary, hospice care is a family-centered and holistic-
humanistic care that:

1. Alleviates and controls death and dying associated symptoms, particularly physical and intrapsychic pain, experienced by both the patient and his family
2. Diminishes emotional distress and provides means for
   meeting the patient's spiritual needs
3. Promotes measures to resolve interpersonal difficulties
   and socioeconomic problems emanating from the terminal
   illness
4. Provides resources for helping the patient cope with changes
   in his lifestyle and concept of sexuality
5. Eases the psychological impact of the dying process for the
   patient and family to attain peace with the death of a loved
   one.

With due respect to the beneficial effects of hospice care, it
should not serve as a panacea for high-quality and cost-effec-
tive care. There are several implications of the hospice care

concept in terms of ethico-moral issues, health care insur-
ance, legal aspects, legislations, and the current societal beliefs and demands regarding right to health care, the right to
die in dignity, and quality of life. [1,2,5]

The thesis of the hospice movement is supported by the Assumptions and Principles Underlying Standards for Terminal
Illness, which have been identified by the International Work
Group in Death, Dying, and Bereavement.[10] The viability of
this hospice care movement demands consolidated efforts and
commitment among health care givers and advocates, philoso-
phers, theologians, researchers, economists, and health ad-
ministrators and legislators.

HOME CARE SERVICES

An important aspect of a health care delivery system which has
a direct link or is a component of the hospice care movement is
in the in-home care services. The in-home care service is distinct from hospice care in terms of focus and structure. Hospice care may be centrally located in a modern hospice facility that is architecturally tailored to simulate an at-home environment (but with more single and bigger rooms to allow family participation in patient care) or it may be located in an acute-
care facility,[6,12] or it may be in a hospice-based home care
facility.[3] On the other hand, in-home care service may be under the auspices of a certified home health agency.[11] The focus of in-home care service is promotion of the quality of life
of the patient and his family. Thus, a basic requirement for an
in-home care setting is a home that the patient has previously
identified as satisfactory in terms of his lifestyle and level of
functioning. The Coalition for Home Health Services in the State
of New York adopted the philosophy that in-home care become
an integral part of community health care systems.[8] This type
of service should be inclusive of preventive, supportive, and
hospital-type treatment made available to anyone in need of such
a service.[9]

In short, in-home care is conceptualized as a hospital-based
home care, a hospital without walls, and an extension of the
hospital into the community.[4] This type of care is claimed to
have been pioneered by Boston City Hospital in 1780 and was re-
vived in New York City in 1948. An interdisciplinary care is
also provided and referral for services may be self-initiated,
or by inpatient and outpatient services, or through community
organizations.

PARTIAL LIST OF HOSPICES [5,7]

Hillhaven Hospice
5504 East Pima Street
Tucson, AR 85712

Kaiser-Permanente Medical
  Care Program
Hospice Norwolk
12500 South Hoxie Avenue
Norwalk, CA 90650

Hospice of Santa Barbara, Inc.
1525 State Street, Suite 11
Santa Barbara, CA 93101

Penrose Hospital
2215 North Cascade Avenue
Colorado Springs, CO 80907

Hospice Orlando
P.O. Box 8581
Orlando, FL 32806

Highland Park Hospital
718 Glenview Avenue
Highland Park, ILL 60035

Holy Cross Hospital
1500 Forest Glen Road
Silver Spring, MD 20910

Our Lady of Lourdes
  Memorial Hospital
169 Riverside Drive
Binghamton, NY 13905

Hospice of Northern
  Virginia, Inc.
P.O. Box 1590
Arlington, VA 22210

Hospice of Maine, Inc.
32 Thomas Road
Portland, MA 04102

Haven of Northern Virginia,
  Inc.
7300 McWhorter Place
Annandale, VA 22003

Parkwood Community Hospital
7011 Shoup Avenue
Canoga Park, CA 91304

San Diego Hospice
San Diego, CA

Hospice of Marin
Kentfield, CA

Hospice, Inc.
765 Prospect Street
New Haven, CN 06511

Hospice Atlanta, Inc.
1055 McLynn Avenue, N.E.
Atlanta, GA 30306

St. John's Hospital
800 East Carpenter Street
Springfield, ILL 62702

Overlook Hospital
193 Morris Avenue
Summit, NJ 07901

Calvary Hospice
Bronx, NY

Bellin Memorial Hospital
P.O. Box 1700
744 South Webster Avenue
Green Bay, WI 54305

Hospices of Rockland, Inc.
4 Union Road
Spring Valley, NY 10977

REVIEW QUESTIONS

1. Define the hospice care concept.
2. Enumerate the objectives of a hospice care program.
3. Identify the elements or characteristics of a hospice program.
4. What admission criteria are used in the effective operation of a hospice program?
5. Describe the in-home care service as a link to or component of a hospice care movement.
6. What is the focus of in-home care service?
7. What is a necessary requirement that should be met for an in-home care setting?
8. Name at least five hospices in the United States.

REFERENCES

1. Amado, A., et al., Cost of Terminal Care: Home Hospice vs. Hospital. Nursing Outlook, pp. 522-526 (August, 1979).
2. Benoliel, J.Q., Dying is a Family Affair. In: Home Care, Prichard, E.R., et al. (eds.), Columbia University Press, New York, pp. 153-158 (1979).
3. Dunn, M.K., Hospice-Based Home Care Services. In: Home Care, Prichard, E.R., et al. (eds.), Columbia University Press, New York, pp. 153-158 (1979).
4. Eichwald, H., An Organized Home Care Program. In: Home Care, Prichard, E.R., et al. (eds.), Columbia University Press, New York, pp. 148-152 (1979).
5. Markel, W.M. and Sinon, V.B., The Hospice Concept, publication No. 3403-PE. American Cancer Society, New York.
6. Paige, R.L. and Looney, J.F., When the Patient Is Dying: Hospice Care for the Adult. Am. J. Nurs., pp. 1812-1815 (November, 1977).
7. Martinson, I., et al., When the Patient Is Dying: Home Care for the Child. Am. J. Nurs., pp. 1815-1817 (November, 1977).
8. Prichard, E.R., et al. (eds.), Home Care. Columbia University Press, New York (1979).
9. Rossman, I., Home Care of the Cancer Patient. In: Home Care, Prichard, E.R., et al. (eds.), Columbia University Press, New York, pp. 118-119 (1979).
10. The International Work Group in Death, Dying and Bereavement, Assumptions and Principles Underlying Standards for Terminal Care. Am. J. Nurs., pp. 296-297 (February, 1979).

11. Ward, B.J., Hospice Home Care Program. Nursing Outlook, pp. 646-653 (October, 1978).
12. Woodring, S., Hospice Care Project in an Acute-Care General Hospital, 1975-1976. In: Home Care, Prichard, E.R., et al. (eds.), Columbia University Press, New York, pp. 159-164 (1979).

CHAPTER 16
Rehabilitation Oncology

PERSPECTIVES

Rehabilitation nursing is becoming more inclusive of the concept of holistic care and current practices supported by scientific findings in the health field and allied disciplines. Traditional practices such as positioning the patient to prevent bed
sores and contractures are being manipulated to find out if more
definitive and desirable outcomes ensue. Although research by
nurses in the area of rehabilitation is practically nil, the thrust
towards quality assurance and accountability and the increasing
number of doctorally prepared nurses are paving the way to
more scientifically based health care delivery systems. Thus
far, ". . . there is no real evidence that the costly rehabilitation team leads to the most favorable patient outcomes."[7] It is
also suspected that multiple-workers and clients interaction
leads to confusion, dependency or passivity to care, and care
fragmentation. The issues in question are the cost effectiveness, efficiency, and quality of the multidisciplinary team approach to patient care versus the primary care approach. This
issue, as well as other models of care such as the self-care
model, need to be further researched and validated for utility.

Oncology nursing, which is a unique, very challenging specialty,
is a field wherein the science and practice of nursing can be
advanced through more nursing research. To date, the need
for scientific investigation and support of rehabilitation oncology is tremendous. In this chapter, an attempt is made to explore the concept of rehabilitation and its application in the care
of the cancer patient.

REHABILITATION OF THE
PATIENT AND FAMILY

Rehabilitation is considered as tertiary intervention system of
care. This notion should not be literally interpreted as the
process of care which is initiated after the completion of the

primary and secondary systems of care. Rather, it is the process of care delivery aimed at the prevention, maintenance, restorative, and re-educative aspects of patient and family health care.[2,7] It begins from the time of admission to the hospital, continues throughout the course of hospitalization, and extends to the home community setting.[1,3,7]

Specifically, rehabilitation oncology is concerned with the same variables mentioned above. The focus is therefore the same as rehabilitation but the approaches involved in its implementation are quite different. This is apparent in the fact that the approach to the cancer patient as he goes through the loss and grieving process due to a fatal illness necessarily becomes more sensitive to the patient's self-concept and coping mechanisms.

The domain of rehabilitation nursing is that of a holistic man. The range (main elements or variables in this context) are the physical, psychological, social, spiritual, and socioeconomic. Deviations from traditional approaches to the management of these variables in the care of the cancer patient are influenced by the course of the disease and treatment-related factors.[3]

Basic to rehabilitation oncology is the holistic approach which entails rehabilitation of the whole man, augmentation and enhancement of the patient's under-utilized assets and resources, provision of palliative and definitive treatment modalities, promotion of a lifestyle that maximizes the meaningfulness of the person's existence, and provision of assistance in maximizing the patient's assets within the limits of his disabilities and losses.[5,7]

ASSESSMENT OF THE PATIENT

The successful implementation of rehabilitation care of the cancer patient depends to a great extent upon the quality of assessment made at the time of admission to the hospital. It is essential that the assessment process should include the family and patient relationships relative to their losses and assets. The concept of loss may be analogous to the concept of pain. The implications of such concept of pain have already been discussed in Chapter 14. Moreover, objective, concrete losses have psychological, social, spiritual, and socioeconomic correlates. These are unique to the individual and therefore must be evaluated in the assessment process and included in the plan of care for the patient.

The assessment process should focus on important factors that influence patient care outcomes. These factors may be:

1. Disease-related factors
   a. Physical
      (1) Existing disabilities: sensory loss, motor deficits, functional alterations (system-wide aspects), affective and cognitive deficits, and nutritional status
      (2) Potential disabilities: degeneration of body function primarily related to disease or secondary diseases, and age-related factors
   b. Psychological, spiritual, and socioeconomic
      (1) Health practices: health behaviors such as smoking, drug use, sleep patterns, exercise, nutrition, sex habits, and relationships
      (2) Beliefs systems: value patterns, effects or influence of religious meaning and rituals, intrapersonal and interpersonal interactions, coping behaviors, and role of significant others
      (3) Economic resources: primary and secondary financial resources, education, and avocation
   c. Acute disability: pain, fear, imposed immobility, confusion, and disorientation
2. Treatment-related factors
   a. Physical
      (1) Surgery as the primary modality: mutilation of body parts, loss of body parts, functional losses (sensory, motor, affective, cognitive, elimination control, and ingestion of nutrients)
      (2) Multimodal therapy (surgery and adjuvant therapy such as radiation, chemotherapy, and immunotherapy): side effects, toxic effects, focal and systemic sequelae such as nutritional alteration and immunosuppression, direct and indirect effects on the central nervous system, bony structure, and musculature
      (3) Sexuality: See below and Chapter 13
   b. Psychological, spiritual, and socioeconomic
      (1) Rights to care: protection of the patient's rights to treatment and research, and issues relative to cost and benefits of treatment
      (2) Right to quality of life as defined by the patient and family: prolongation of life (assumed when the patient chooses radical treatment), religious-spiritual needs, ethnic-cultural practices
      (3) Sexuality: self-concept, body image changes, sexual meaning attached to body parts (e.g., if the breast is a primary source of erotic stimulation on a patient with mastectomy, then it has a significant impact on the patient), side effects of chemotherapy (e.g., cortisone can cause mood swings and decreased libido,

just as vincristine can cause impotence and increased
or decreased arousal in women) and effects of radiation such as dyspareunia in pelvic irradiation.
(4) Emotional deterioration: withdrawal, regression,
suicide attempts

PLANNING AND INTERVENTION

Active participation and involvement of the patient and his family in the multidisciplinary health care plan is essential. The
patient care objectives are based upon the assessment of the
needs of the patient and family as previously discussed. It
should be noted that the suggested assessment factors are not
exhaustive, and creative approaches to the care of the patient
are encouraged. Another important variable that must be considered in planning care is prognosis of the disease and the objective of treatment modality - curative, palliative or supportive. In any case, the following aspects should be included in
the patient care plan and therapeutic intervention.

1. Specific objectives
   a. Restoration or maintenance of function for quality sur-
      vival
   b. Re-education or modification of roles (family, socie-
      tal, significant others)
   c. Provision of a pain-free, optimum mobility
   d. Resumption or modification of lifestyle
   e. Living with cancer as a holistic person
2. Supports and services
   a. Multidisciplinary team: nurses, social workers, phys-
      ical therapists, psychologists, psychiatrists, vocational
      and placement counselors, religious services, speech
      therapists, inhalation therapists, ancillary workers
   b. Community resources: organizations such as the Ameri-
      can Cancer Society, church-related organizations and
      clubs, Family Association of America (FAA), self-help
      groups such as Friends in Search for Help (FISH),
      Reach to Recovery, Laryngectomy and Ileostomy Asso-
      ciation, etc.
   c. Orthotic and prosthetics: availability and feasibility of
      using either manually or electronically controlled as-
      sistive devices for mutilated and/or lost body organs,
      systems, or en-bloc body parts removal, e.g., trans-
      lumbar amputation
   d. Emotional supports: family relationships, role of sig-
      nificant others, identification of previous coping mech-
      anisms and strengthening them, psychological and

      ego-strengths, crisis intervention team, and religious
      affiliations
e. Vocational re-educative needs: basic skills, constraints
    of disability, employment barriers from job market and
    employers
f. Recreational needs: hobbies, cultural organizational
    affiliations, athletic clubs

SPECIFIC POINTERS TO HOLISTIC CARE

The provision of holistic care can best be achieved if the following factors are included.

Communication Needs

The patient and family must be provided with the necessary information regarding prognosis, treatment, and the implications
of the terminal illness in terms of personal, psychological, social, and financial aspects. This leads to better patient com-
pliance to the rehabilitative regimen. Communication dissonance often occurs in the verbal and nonverbal modes of communicating with the patient and family, especially in the area
of impending death and complications of the disease or treatments. Thus the health care team members should be alert to
contradictory cues. Recognition of the value of silence and/or
therapeutic touch as being more effective than words is very
important. Likewise, respect for the patient's need to reflect
should govern the frequency of interactions with the patient. In
effect, the patient should be allowed to set the pace of the communication process.

Self-Esteem and Body Image

Convey empathetic understanding of the patient's need to use
normal defense mechanisms. These defenses (denial, anger,
bargaining) and the grieving process are initially therapeutic.[2,5,8] Recognize the patient's need for appreciation, respect, and love. Foster patient-family ties and social contact.
Assess the patient's ascription of meanings to specific body
parts. Validate the relative value placed on sexual organs,
face, limbs, and such other qualities as voice for personal and
socioeconomic reasons. Encourage the patient to accentuate
his assets. Avoid showing revulsion to radical effects of therapy, repulsive odor, and cancer site. Consistently be cognizant of the fact that the specific site affected by cancer and its
treatment result in special problems which differ in impact on
every patient. Provide privacy and control over his environment.

Beliefs and Value Systems

Recognize the assumed positive role of religion. Acceptance
of reality and perceptions are influenced by beliefs and value
patterns. As a health care giver, exercise value-clarification
techniques in relating with the patient. Integration of the self
and positive body image should be facilitated. This is particularly important since the patient's behavioral responses ema-
nate significantly from his identity with self and with others.
Be sensitive and alert to the patient's needs for psychotherapy
or crisis intervention. Encourage the use of relaxation techniques.

Patient and Family Education

This aspect of care is focussed on specific needs related to the
disease, the treatment, and the disabilities ensuing from the
disease-treatment response. Performance of daily living at
home and in social settings should be encouraged based upon
the patient's strengths. A structured teaching plan should be
made through collaborative efforts among the multidisciplinary
team, the patient, and his family. Teaching-learning principles should be used. Briefly, as a review, these principles
are: (1) the teaching-learning process begins at the level of the
learner (i.e., level of knowledge, psychomotor skills, affective and sensory abilities); (2) identify, classify, and most of
all, validate the patient's need for learning a new mode of behavior, patterns of living, and vocational/avocational training;
(3) realization that the need to learn, motivation, and the learner's active participation in the learning process are requisites
in the achievement of learning objectives; (4) previous experience, planned-systematic repetition, and positive feedback reinforce and facilitate acquisition and retention of knowledge;
(5) actual, simulated practice such as role playing and return
demonstration concretize what is learned; and (6) for whatever
is learned, periodic and continuous evaluation should be done
by both the teacher and learner.

REHABILITATION OF THE PATIENT
WITH CONTROLLABLE CANCER

Controllable cancers can be managed in terms of cure or palliation. Nonetheless, some kind of chronic needs and/or disabilities can result. Thus, a discussion of the implications of
major radical interventions on body parts relative to rehabilitation care constitute the rest of this chapter.

Continuing rehabilitative care is directed towards use and procurement of assistive devices and resource facilities. Follow-
up care, including home care based services and vocational rehabilitation, are also planned for and initiated at hospital admission if the patient's condition permits. Intertwined with this
process is the timing of the interventions. Chronicity of the rehabilitative process and the disease condition lead to temporal
disruption. Restructuring of time is necessary. Too much time
imposed by the illness and rehabilitative constraints leads to
further physical deterioration, boredom blues, emotional strain,
negative identity, and decreased social skills.[1,6,7] On the
other hand, too little time allowed for patient care management
also has detrimental effects. The patient whose daily life is
enmeshed in treatment-rehabilitation regimens, and whose days
and nights are plagued by symptom control, pain, alimentation
and elimination modifications, and decreased mobility is deprived of time essential for self-reflection and privacy. Moreover, this type of deprival minimizes the necessary time for
meaningful psychic energizer activities. Timing and restructuring of time utilization are therefore crucial in helping to ensure an effective rehabilitative process and positive patient outcomes devoid of unwanted sequelae such as chronic immobility
and debilitating disability. Table 8 will help facilitate a comprehensive understanding of the major aspects of rehabilitation
of the patient with controllable cancer.

REVIEW QUESTIONS

1. Discuss the four major variables within the holistic domain
   of rehabilitation.
2. List the members of the rehabilitation team and define their
   roles and responsibilities.
3. Identify the factors that must be considered during the assessment process which influence patient care outcomes.
4. List four objectives of cancer care rehabilitation.
5. Enumerate supportive/corrective methods for meeting the
   rehabilitation needs of the patient with controllable cancer.

Table 8: Rehabilitation of the Patient with Controllable Cancer

Disease/Treatment Effects	Rehabilitation Needs	Supportive/Corrective Methods
Head and Neck Eye exenteration Orofacial radical excision Glossectomy Radical neck dissection	Preoperative, postoperative teaching regarding prosthesis, its use, and care	Psychological, social, economic needs: counseling, vocational placement, clergy, crisis intervention
	Aesthetic needs	Reconstructive plastic surgery
	Functional related: nerve paralysis, swallowing, masticating, and salivary control, depth perception, phonation, articulation of speech	Maxillofacial prosthesis: eyes, ears, nose, lips, mouth, and palate
		Pedicle flaps or grafts to floor of mouth
	Rotated scapula	Shoulder and arm sling
	Pain and paresis or paralysis	Facial sling
	Accessory nerve and/or trigeminal nerve damage	Nerve graft (using greater auricular nerve for partial replacement of accessory nerve)
	Muscle (arm and shoulder, facial and neck) conditioning and strengthening exercises	Electrical nerve stimulation
		Levator scapula muscle transplant

Table 8 (Cont.)

Disease/Treatment Effects	Rehabilitation Needs	Supportive/Corrective Methods
Larynx Laryngectomy	Speech: phonation, articulation, pitch, intelligibility of artificial larynx, laryngeal transplant, esophageal speech	Speech rehabilitation by professionally trained speech therapist or successfully rehabilitated laryngectomee
	Care of laryngectomy stoma and tube	Laryngeal transplant
		Artificial larynx
	Tube feedings	Facial nerve reconditioning exercises
	Modifying environment to prevent complications	Definitive approach to patient, family, and societal roles, expectations, and occupation
Alimentary and Genitourinary Gastrostomy Pharyngostomy Colostomy Ileostomy	Satiety	Patient and family teaching regarding surgery and its expected outcomes
	Eating patterns and modification	

Ileal-conduit Ileal reservoir Ureterostomy Vesicostomy	Aesthetic needs	Use of ostomy appliances and equipment
	Elimination control	Establishment of elimination control (see Chapters 31, 33)
	Use of ostomy appliances and equipment	Prevention of complications from stoma effects (see Chapters 31, 33)
	Nutritional modifications	
Breast Mastectomy (radical and simple) Lymphatic resection Subcutaneous tissue fibrosis from super-voltage radiation	Maintenance of range of motion	Early routine exercises
	Maintenance of function of affected shoulder and arm	Appropriate prosthesis
	Restoration of external appearance	Nipple preservation and transplant
	Position balance	Audio tapes (preoperatively as needed for teaching)
	Prosthesis	Salt-free diet and/or lympedema sleeves
		Transposition of partially detached omentum beneath chest-wall superficial tissues into axilla and upper arm to control chronic lympedema

Table 8 (Cont.)

Disease/Treatment Effects	Rehabilitation Needs	Supportive/Corrective Methods
Lung Pneumonectomy Lobectomy Thoracotomy effects: splinting of chest, pain, decreased respiratory reserve	Breathing exercises Cardiopulmonary circulation Thoraco/arm/shoulder condi- tioning and maintenance of ROM and function Optimum coughing regimen	Nonvigorous range of motion (ROM) exercises of affected side Manual splinting (pillows or towels for support) Early supervised ambulation Postural drainage Breathing exercises for segmental control of remaining lung Care of thoracotomy tubes and drain- age system (see Chapter 29)
Central Nervous System and Peripheral Nerves Thalamotomy, lobotomy lobectomy Spectrum of personality changes	Maintenance of and/or restora- tion of motor and sensory function Preservation and reconditioning of musculoskeletal structure and func- tion	Special exercises for area-specific disability Galvanic and other nerve stimulation Whirlpool treatment

Spectrum of varying degrees of paralysis and "plegias"	Cognitive and affective sequelae: refocusing or reorienting/re-education	Functional and structural osthotics
Neuropathies		Diathermy treatment
Functional losses and/or uncompensable sensory loss(es)	Safety needs	Reinnervation of viable muscles
		Hot packs or cold packs
Remote effects of cancer: neuromyopathies, pain, muscle wasting		Pain relief with medication; if ineffective, may use hypnosis and other adjuvant techniques
		Substitution of other sensory modalities and/or other patterns of activity
Bone and Soft Tissue		
Amputation of upper extremity	Phantom limb sensation phenomena	Relief of phantom sensations
Interscapulothoracic amputation	Ambulation	Crutch walking
Hemi/total pelvectomy		Early use of prosthesis
Translumbar amputation or maximum hemicorporectomy	Preoperative, operative, and postoperative muscle/stump conditioning exercises	Exercise regimen for maintenance, restoration of structure and function

Table 8 (Cont.)

Disease/Treatment Effects	Rehabilitation Needs	Supportive/Corrective Methods
	Patient and family teaching regarding orthotics and prosthetics	Assistance in self-care and activities of daily living
		Counseling and placement services
	Vocational	Shoulder cap cosmetic prosthesis for clothing support and symmetric appearance

Note: The psychosocial, emotional, spiritual and recreational needs and therapeutic-supportive measures are not included in the above table since these have been discussed earlier in this chapter.

REFERENCES

1. Benson, H., The Relaxation Response. Avon Books, New York (1975).
2. Bouchard, R. and Owens, N.F., Nursing Care of the Cancer Patient. C.V. Mosby Co., St. Louis (1976).
3. Dietz, H.J., Rehabilitation of the Cancer Patient. American Cancer Society, New York (1969).
4. Goesmith, H.S., et al., Omental Transplant in the Control of Chronic Lymphedema. JAMA, 203:1119-1121 (1968).
5. Kellog, C.J. and Sullivan, B.P. (eds.), Current Perspective in Oncologic Nursing. C.V. Mosby Co., St. Louis (1978).
6. McGrory, A., A Well Model Approach to the Care of the Dying Client. McGraw Hill, New York (1978).
7. Murray, R. and Kijek, M.A., Current Perspective in Rehabilitation Nursing. C.V. Mosby Co., St. Louis (1975).
8. Shedd, D.P., et al., The Nurse's Role in Rehabilitation of Cancer Patients With Facial Defects. American Cancer Society, New York (1974).
9. Strauss, A. and Glaser, B., Chronic Illness and the Quality of Life. C.V. Mosby Co., St. Louis (1975).
10. Witkin, M.M., Sex Therapy and Mastectomy. J. Sex Marital Ther., 1:290-303 (1975).

CHAPTER 17
Cancer and Aging

This chapter does not attempt an expository discussion of a multidisciplinary approach to understanding human development in terms of philosophical, anthropological, sociological, psychological, and biological perspectives.[8] Rather, the focus is primarily on what is germane to senescence and cancer as an illness.

The correlates of growing older and senescence are greater wisdom, virtues, social relationships, and spatio-temporal meanings. The cliche, "You are not growing older, only getting better," may not be appropriate and can be devastating to the patient with terminal illness.[6] Likewise, the adage, "Most old people are not all sick or well at the same time," is not necessarily true nor ascribable to the aged cancer patient.[2] Thus the care of the elderly patient with cancer becomes a professional challenge among health care givers. Moreover, statistics indicate that cancer is the second leading cause of death among persons over 55 years of age. Hence, the aging process and the stage of senescence compound and complicate the problems experienced by the patient during his illness and treatment.

To achieve the goals of care of the aging cancer patient, a holistic, multidisciplinary approach that emphasizes coordination and integration of the following responsibilities is essential.

1. Restoring, maintaining, and promoting health and quality of life throughout the health-illness continuum and the dying process.[1,3,8,10]
2. Conscious raising of human potential and the fulfillment of the person's needs for self-actualization.[3]
3. Preventing and alleviating the complications of illness and its therapy.
4. Minimizing the concept of loss imposed by the illness and the aging process which confronts or afflicts both the patient and family members and the givers of health care.[6,7]

GOALS OF CARE FOR THE
AGING CANCER PATIENT

Defining specific goals of care for the aging cancer patient promotes quality care in that each member of the health care team can better understand his role and responsibilities in the care of the patient. These specific goals should also be prioritized and reassessed according to the patient and family members' response. Suggested patient care goals follow.

1. Integrate with patient care the actual losses imposed by aging as they relate to the pathogenesis of cancer, such as:
   a. Immunodeficiency resulting from the aging process (the lowered propensity to produce antibodies results from somatic-cell variations leading to a decreased immune homeostatic mechanism).[12]
   b. Decreased coordination and sensory activity (e.g., sensitivity to pain remains steady up to age 50 and then diminishes differently in different body parts; sensitivity to touch also decreases sharply after age 45,[3] and perceptual ability to sort out, process, and respond to information stimuli decreases with age).[1,8]
   c. Decreased metabolic rate and kidney function, which have direct impact on chemotherapy, immunotherapy, and combined treatment modalities.[2,3,6]
2. Prevent and minimize the hazards of immobility such as hypercalcemia, embolism, osteoporosis, susceptibility to pathological fractures, especially in metastatic bone disease.
3. Incorporate the patient's need for acceptance of changes in body functions and the effects of the cancer and treatment modalities received.[9,10]
4. Recognize a "hope system" which correlates with the dying process and its stages.
5. Facilitate transition from or modification of the patient's premorbid roles and responsibilities.[11]
6. Provide measures for enhancing or maintaining the quality of life, such as the use of appropriate pain relief measures inclusive of pain medication, relaxing exercises, and religious or spiritual activities; socialization that promotes family cohesiveness and support such as in family dinners, card games, in-house movies, and group discussions.[8,9,10]
7. Accommodate the patient's cultural and ethnic practices relative to mode of expression, grooming, pattern of speech, hobbies, food habits and idiosyncrasies, religious rituals and mores, use of humor, and value system.
8. Resolving personal attitudes toward the aged concerning issues on dependency, social worth, political and economic

value, stereotyping of cognitive, affective, and social aspects of the patient's self-concept.[3,4,10] This is particularly important in terms of the recognition of research data that indicates the attainment of a peak level of general intelligence at a certain time in one's life that remains the same into the stage of senescence.[1,5,7,8]

AREAS OF SPECIFIC CONCERN IN THE CARE OF THE AGING CANCER PATIENT

The aging process causes specific concerns relative to physical, psychological, social, sexual, nutritional, and spiritual needs of the elderly patient. These areas of concern are:

1. Physical safety and security.
2. Nutritional history and nutritional needs.
3. Existing and potential psychophysiological disabilities.
4. Interactions of pathological effects of cancer and sensory-motor deficits or losses of aging.
5. Increased risks of surgery and immobility.[11]
6. Dependency versus independence and isolation.
7. Body-image changes.
8. Sexual orientation, sexual dysfunction, and needs.[2,5,7,10]
9. Communication and social skills (age as a cultural barrier).[2,9]
10. Death as the final stage of development.[8]
11. Cultural related "fixated" behaviors.[8]
12. Referral and use of community services and other support systems such as activity groups, reminiscence groups, reality orientation, growth groups, remotivation groups.[11]
13. Transmittal and followup of implementation of the predischarge plan of care.
14. Effects of long-term illness upon the patient and health care givers (e.g., attachment and termination of relationships).

NURSING INTERVENTIONS

Each nursing intervention is goal-directed and goal-specific. The above-mentioned areas of specific concern dictate the specificities of nursing care activities for and with the patient. In effect, patient needs determine the patient care objectives that should be achieved. Health team care is therefore tailored to the patient's actual and potential needs. Guidelines for care relative to the overall effects of cancer, treatments, loss and grieving process, pain, sexuality, nutrition, home care and hospice care, and rehabilitation needs have been discussed in the preceding chapters.

REVIEW QUESTIONS

1. Discuss the correlates of aging.
2. List four (4) nursing responsibilities associated with the holistic care of the aged patient with cancer.
3. Enumerate at least six (6) goals of care of the aged cancer patient.

REFERENCES

1. Butler, R. and Lewis, M., Aging and Mental Health. C.V. Mosby Co., St. Louis (1977).
2. Burnside, I.M., Nursing and the Aged. McGraw Hill Co., New York (1976).
3. Burnside, I.M., et al., Psychosocial Caring Throughout the Life Span. McGraw Hill Co., New York (1979).
4. Christenson, J., Generational Value Differences. Gerontologist, 17:367-374 (1977).
5. Griggs, W., Staying Well While Growing Old: Sex and the Elderly. Am. J. Nurs., 78:1352-1354 (1978).
6. Kellog, C.J. and Sullivan, B.P. (eds.), Current Perspectives in Oncologic Nursing, Vol. 2, C.V. Mosby Co., St. Louis (1978).
7. Larson, R., Thirty Years of Research on the Subjective Well-Being of the Older Americans. J. Gerontol., 32:203-210 (1978).
8. Lugo, J.O. and Hershey, G.L., Human Development: A Multidisciplinary Approach to the Psychology of Individual Growth. McMillan Book Co., New York (1974).
9. Mistler-Lakman, J., Spontaneous Shift in Encoding Dimensions Among Elderly Subjects. J. Gerontol., 32:68-72, (1977).
10. Murray, R.B. and Zentner, J.P., Nursing Assessment and Health Promotion Throughout the Life Span. 2nd ed., Prentice Hall, Englewood Cliffs, NJ (1979).
11. Murray, R.B., et al., The Nursing Process in Later Maturity. Prentice-Hall, Englewood Cliffs, NJ (1980).
12. Roesel, C.E., Immunology: A Self-Instructional Approach. McGraw-Hill Book Co., New York (1978).

PART V
Common Malignancies: Diagnosis and Management

CHAPTER 18
Malignant Tumors of the Bone

Primary malignant tumors of the bone are rare. However, they compose one of the most common types of cancer in children with the highest incidence during childhood and adolescence.

The etiology of primary osteogenic tumors is unknown. Heredity is thought to be a factor in their development. These bone tumors are all sarcomas (osteogenic sarcomas). The term osteogenic sarcoma refers to several varieties of malignant neoplasms of bone cells.[1,7] These tumors present clinical symptoms and radiologic appearances which are almost analogous. Accuracy of diagnosis and optimum therapeutic management of the patient therefore require the combined skills and current knowledge of the pathologist, orthopedist, radiologist, and hematologist. Differential diagnosis involves assessment of some helpful clues which include the age of the patient, site of origin, tumor substance, and characteristics as shown in Table 9.

A unique characteristic of bone neoplasms is their metastatic spread through the hematogenous rather than lymphatic route.[1] These neoplasms tend to metastasize rapidly.

CLINICAL MANIFESTATIONS

1. Local pain, tenderness, swelling
2. Pain is more acute during the night
3. Cachexia
4. General malaise
5. Fever with leukocytosis
6. Impaired mobility of affected parts
7. Anemia, thrombocytopenia
8. Altered immunoglobulin production
9. Pathological fractures
10. Hypercalcemia, hyperuricemia, hypercalciuria

Table 9: Differential Diagnosis of Bone Neoplasms[1,2,5,14]

Tumor-Type	Clues and Characteristics
Osteogenic sarcoma	Tumor substance: osteoid (presence of tumor osteoid establishes the diagnosis)
	Origin: bone-forming
	Cell type: osteoblast
	Bone-digesting: osteoclast
Central Osteogenic	Peaks in second decade with predilection
	Bone affected: metaphysis of long bones (lower end of femur or upper end of tibia or humerus and can extend through the shaft)
Multicentric Carcinomatosis	Affects young children ages 6 to 9. Appears as symmetrical and sclerotic sarcomas of extremities; prognosis for central and multicentric is poor with wild and rapid metastases through the blood stream
Parosteal	Origin: bone surface (periosteum); slow growing
	Prognosis is same as central osteogenic sarcoma when the tumor extends to the medullary cavity
	Clinical symptoms: swelling, pain (more intense at night)
Myeloma (plasmacytoma, plasma cell leukemia)	Origin: marrow
	Cell type: Reticuloendothelial (RE) system
	Most common type of bone neoplasms
	Bone affected: (bones containing red marrow) pelvis, spine, ribs, sternum

Table 9 (Cont.)

Tumor-Type	Clues and Characteristics
Multiple Myeloma	Most common from 50 to 70 years with predilection for males; lytic bone destruction throughout skeleton which can lead to vertebral collapse and cord compression; spreads to liver, lymph nodes, kidney and spleen Clinical manifestations include: fever, pain, malaise, increased sedimentation rate, myelocytic anemia, positive Bence-Jones protein, and increased serum and urine calcium excretion Peripheral neuropathy Pathologic fractures are common Rib involvement shows characteristic "ballooning" 1 to 3 years survival
Extramedullary Myeloma	Affects soft tissues of the nasopharynx, oral cavity, and skin Often painless
Solitary Myeloma	Precedes multiple myeloma Slow growing Arises in same sites as multiple myeloma Prognosis: relatively better if discovered early
Ewing's Sarcoma	Origin: marrow Cell type: reticuloendothelial system Children and young adults (infrequent after age 25) Radiosensitive Bone affected: shaft of long and flat bones Clinical manifestations include: painful, warm erythematous mass, malaise, fever, leukocytosis, increased sedimentation rate Metastasizes rapidly to lungs and other bones Prognosis: grave

Table 9 (Cont.)

Tumor-Type	Clues and Characteristics
Reticulum Cell Sarcoma	Origin: marrow Cell type: reticuloendothelial system Occurrence: 3rd and 4th decade of life; Lodwick's motheaten radiologic appearance Bone affected: medullary cavity of long bones Penetration of cortex produces periosteal reaction Pathological fracture: more frequent than with any other bone tumor 50% 5-year survival
Chondrosarcoma	Origin: cartilage Cell type: chondroblast (forms cartilage) Occurrence: middle or later years of life Half as common as osteogenic sarcoma; slow growing Centrally located tumor expands cortex resulting in marginal sclerosis or endosteal "buttressing" within the shaft of long bones Longest survival
Fibrosarcoma	Origin: fibrous tissue Cell type: fibroblast (forms collagen) Occurrence: rare, affects all ages but frequently middle or later years Bone affected: long or flat bones (pelvis, frequent) involves periosteum, adjacent soft tissues, or medullary cavity; hematogenous spread to lungs, may also spread through lymphatics Prognosis: better than osteogenic sarcoma

Table 9 (Cont.)

Tumor-Type	Clues and Characteristics
Metastatic Cancer	Considered as one of the most common forms of malignant bone tumors. Seeding occurs from primary sites, commonly breast, lung, prostate, thyroid, kidney Bone affected: (mostly red marrow) skull, spine, pelvis, ribs, proximal femur, and humerus Appearance: osteolytic, osteoblastic, or mixed Generalized osteoporosis Vertebral body collapse and rib fractures

DIAGNOSTIC TESTS AND DIAGNOSIS

1. Bone x-ray survey
2. Radioisotope scanning
3. Arteriography (helpful in demonstrating extent of lytic lesions and soft tissue involvement)
4. Biopsy (incisional or aspiration)
5. Laboratory studies which include:
   a. Alkaline phosphatase (increased in Paget's osteosarcoma)
   b. Abnormal albumin-globulin (A/G) ratio
   c. Serum electrophoresis (determines presence of abnormal globulins)
   d. Bence-Jones protein (positive in urine)
   e. Abnormally high serum and urine calcium

TREATMENT MODALITIES

Surgery and extensive radiation therapy serve as the mainstay of therapy.[1] Chemotherapy and immunotherapy as well as combined modalities of treatment have shown some encouraging results. Some studies reveal that patients with sarcoma have circulating antisarcoma antibodies which are localized at the surface of the T cells. These antibodies pertain to the IgM or IgG immunoglobulins.[3] Augmenting and/or stimulating the immune response seems a logical approach and an adjuvant to therapy. As a rule these malignant bone tumors are best managed by a combination of treatment modality, i.e., surgery and radiation postsurgery, radiation and multiple drug therapy, preoperative radiation, surgery and postoperative radiation, and immuno-chemotherapy. Methods of treatment regimen which have been tried specific to tumor-type are shown in Table 10.

Table 10: Treatment Modality Specific to Tumor Type

Tumor Type	Treatment
Osteogenic Sarcoma: Central and Multicentral Osteosarcomatosis	Surgery, radiation, and chemotherapy Radiation: 5000-10000 rads (pre-operatively; 6000-8000 rads (post-operatively
Parosteal	Surgery: interscapulothoracic amputation, hemipelvectomy
Fibrosarcoma	Surgery, radiation, and chemotherapy (resection and bone grafts have been tried on low-grade fibrosarcoma)
Ewing's Sarcoma	Radiation: 5000-6000 rads Multiple drug chemotherapy: cytoxan, adriamycin, and oncovin
Chondrosarcoma	Surgery: hemipelvectomy Radiation: as in Ewing's sarcoma, and radiosulfur
Multiple Myeloma and Metastatic Tumors	Radiation: 1000-4000 rads Radioactive isotope, corticosteroids, and chemotherapy

Surgical interventions include: [4,8,9]

1. Partial limb amputation, e.g., above the knee amputation (a-k amputation)
2. Hemipelvectomy for complete lower extremity amputation
3. Interscapulothoracic amputation for upper extremity
4. Autologous grafting from tibia or ileum after tumor resection. (This method is limited due to the restricted amount of bone which can be resected.)
5. Cadaver bone and cartilage allograft.

Massive resection and allograft transplantation have been tried on some malignant bone tumors such as low-grade chondrosarcoma and fibrosarcoma. The allograft is obtained within six hours after death. Immediate freezing of the bone to decrease its immunogenicity and glycerinization of the cartilage to preserve chondrocyte viability during freezing and thawing is done. As much as possible, the bone size and skeletal configuration should match that of the recipient's. Age range of donors which has been advocated is between 15 and 45 years. Possibility of long-term results of these procedures are still unknown and nonunion and subluxation have occurred. [6,15]

GENERAL PRINCIPLES OF CARE

1. Excruciating bone pain may be alleviated by radiation therapy, steroids, and gamma globulin injections. [13]
2. Decompression of collapsed vertebra is necessary to prevent cord compression.
3. Cord compression may be manifested by paresthesias, neurogenic bladder, paresis, or paralysis.
4. Pathological fractures may be prevented by careful ministering of nursing care, preventing falls, supporting extremities above and below joints, use of braces or bivalved plaster cast.
5. General effects of anemia may be minimized by adequate rest and sleep; high-protein, high-vitamin diet; and folic acid, multivitamin supplements.
6. Thrombocytopenia predisposes to bleeding. Prevent bruising and bleeding by use of a soft tooth brush. Check urine and stools for occult blood.
7. Hypercalcemia causes anorexia, nausea, vomiting, constipation, ileus, abdominal pain, and lethargy. Measures to relieve nausea and vomiting and also prevent constipation should be implemented.
8. Maintain and enforce intake of fluids low in calcium and high in acid ash to ensure good hydration, thereby minimizing formation of kidney stones due to hypercalciuria.
9. Keeping the patient on "NPO" for an extended length of time can precipitate renal failure as a sequela of the hypercalcemia.
10. High doses of radiation to a joint produce fibrosis and/or ulceration of the skin, either of which can lead to possible loss of limb function. Skin care with appropriate application of prescribed ointments will afford relief of the patient's distress.
11. Immunologic response is depressed as a result of various treatment modalities, i.e., radiation or chemotherapy. Protective isolation should be instituted.

12. Postoperative care following hemipelvectomy should include:
    a. Ensure patency of the skin flap catheters (drainage catheters). Maintain general principles of care, continuous suction, and facilitate gravity drainage.
    b. Check and report amount of blood loss. Hemorrhage is a possible complication. Compare vital signs with baseline data to ascertain indications of bleeding.
    c. Watch for skin flap necrosis as well as infection which are likely to occur. Observe sterile technique in caring for drainage and dressings. Note any abnormal odor and color of discharge.
    d. Observe closely for indications of paralytic ileus which may occur as a result of intraperitoneal manipulation of organs during the retroperitoneal dissection. Nasogastric suctioning may be necessary as well as administration of antiflatulent drugs.
13. Steroids may be administered to promote a sense of well-being, anabolism, marrow regeneration, and reduction of hypercalcemia. If steroids are given, monitor the toxic effects of the drug.
14. Body image change and the grieving process associated with loss of body parts and mutilation is another major multidisciplinary concern. Specific approaches are covered in Part IV.

REVIEW QUESTIONS

1. List the general characteristics of malignant bone tumors.
2. Describe the characteristics of multiple myeloma, Ewing's sarcoma, chondrosarcoma, and fibrosarcoma.
3. What are the significant laboratory findings specific to tumor type?
4. Describe the role of the immune system in bone malignancy and its treatment.
5. What type of bone cancer affords the longest survival rate?
6. What are some signs and symptoms of hypercalcemia?
7. How is bone pain due to cancer alleviated?
8. Why are optimum hydration, activity, and ambulation essential in the management of multiple myeloma?
9. List some possible complications of hemipelvectomy.

REFERENCES

1. Rubin, P. and Bakemeier, R. (eds.), Clinical Oncology for Medical Students and Physicians. The University of Rochester School of Medicine and Dentistry and American Cancer Society, New York (1974).

2. Brunner, L. and Suddarth, D., Textbook of Medical-Surgical Nursing. J.B. Lippincott, Co., Philadelphia (1975).

3. Cancer Symposium, 37(4):1788 (April, 1973).

4. Douglas, H., et al., Hemipelvectomy. Surg. Gynecol. Obstet., 138:891-895 (1974).

5. Luckman, J. and Sorensen, K., Medical-Surgical Nursing: A Psychophysiologic Approach. W.B. Saunders Co., Philadelphia (1974).

6. Mankin, H., et al., Massive Resection and Allograft Transplantation in the Treatment of Malignant Bone Tumors. N. Eng. J. Med., 294(4):1245-1247 (June 3, 1976).

7. Marlow, D., Textbook of Pediatric Nursing. W. B. Saunders Co., Philadelphia (1973).

8. Carter, S.K. and Friedman, Osteogenic Sarcoma Treatment Overview and Some Comments on Interpretation of Clinical Trial Data. Cancer Treatm. Rep., 62(2):199-204 (February, 1978).

9. Rao, U., Cheng, A., and Didolkar, M.S., Extraosseous Osteogenic Sarcoma: Clinicopathological Study of Eight Cases and Review of Literature. Cancer, 41(4):1488-1496 (April, 1978).

10. Douglass, H.O. Jr., Osteosarcoma: Survival Gains Resulting From Multidisciplinary Therapy. Progr. Clin. Cancer, 7(83):83-96 (1978).

11. Harrist, T.J., et al., Thorotrast-Associated Sarcoma of Bone: A Case Report and Review of Literature. Cancer, 44(6):2049-2058 (December, 1979).

12. Rosen, G., et al., Primary Osteogenic Sarcoma: The Rationale for Preoperative Chemotherapy and Delayed Surgery. Cancer, 43(6):2163-2177 (June, 1979).

13. Sanerkin, A., Radiotherapy of Chondrosarcoma of Bone. Cancer, 45(11):2769-2777 (June, 1980).

14. Sanerkin, N.G., Definitions of Osteosarcoma, Chondrosarcoma, and Fibrosarcoma of Bone. Cancer, 46(1):178-185 (July, 1980).

15. Pritchard, D.J., Chondrosarcoma: A Clinicopathologic and Statistical Analysis. Cancer, 45(1):149-157 (January, 1980).

CHAPTER 19
Pancreatic Cancer

Primary malignant tumors of the pancreas are relatively rare.
The tumor can arise in any portion of the pancreas but the head
is the most frequent site. Regardless of its location, the natural course of the cancer is that of a rapid and progressively
fatal disease. It affects males three to four times more often
than females, ages 35 to 70, and its peak incidence is in the
sixth and seventh decades.

About 90% of the tumors are adenocarcinomas arising from the
epithelium with two-thirds of them occurring at the head of the
pancreas. Those at the head will compress and invade the ampulla of Vater and common bile duct, thus obstructing biliary
flow. [1]

Islet cell tumors are uncommon, slow growing, and most of them
retain their ability to function, i.e., they continue to secrete
insulin. Removal of the primary tumor will not stop insulin
production by the metastatic tumors elsewhere in the body.
About 10% of the functioning tumors are multiple and 10% of
them are malignant (they metastasize to other organs).

Lymphatic, direct invasion, and hematogenous spread could
cause early perineural spread (thus causing pain), spread to the
lungs, liver, intestines, adrenals, bones, diaphragm, gallbladder, kidneys, heart, mediastinum, heart, ovary, bladder, muscles, skin, and subcutaneous tissue. [2,5,8]

ETIOLOGY

Carcinoma of the pancreas has no known etiology. Scientific
studies on alcoholism, syphilis, chronic pancreatitis and other
carcinogens have no direct relationship with pancreatic cancer.

CLINICAL MANIFESTATIONS

The signs and symptoms are usually of insidious onset except
for a rapid and marked weight loss which is the most common

and typical symptom. Vague, dull, or boring pain which occurs in about 80% of patients may be confined to the midepigastrium or it can be colicky and intermittent, and may radiate to the abdomen, back, chest, or subscapular area. Other symptoms which depend on the type and location of the malignancy include:[1,6,7]

1. Carcinoma of the head and body
   a. Jaundice
   b. Pruritus
   c. Anorexia
   d. Nausea
   e. Vomiting, rapid weight loss
   f. Diarrhea, clay-colored stools
   g. Large, bulky, foul-smelling stools with fat globules (steatorrhea)
   h. Persistent pain made worse by lying down or eating
   i. Pain which may be relieved by sitting or bending forward
   j. Dilated and palpable gallbladder
   k. Signs and symptoms of hyperglycemia, viz., glycosuria; polyuria; thirst; vomiting, hot, dry, flushed skin; Kussmaul breathing; abdominal pain; increased temperature; hypotension
2. Carcinoma of the tail of the pancreas (initial symptoms are usually caused by other organ metastases)
   a. Severe malaise
   b. Weight loss
   c. Palpable abdominal mass.
3. Functioning islet cell tumor (insulinoma)[1,3]
   a. Intermittent attacks of hypoglycemia frequently occurring before breakfast which include:
      (1) Lassitude
      (2) Restlessness
      (3) Weakness
      (4) Fatigue
   b. Signs and symptoms of hyperinsulinism
      (1) Clouding of consciousness
      (2) Confusion
      (3) Staggering
      (4) Convulsions
      (5) Hypothermia
      (6) Frank coma.

DIAGNOSTIC TESTS AND DIAGNOSIS

1. Barium contrast films: Distortion of adjacent organs, widening of duodenal loop, pyloric obstruction seen in tumors at the head of the pancreas.

2. Liver function studies: Indicates extrahepatic biliary obstruction.[1]
3. Laboratory tests: Increased alkaline phosphatase in obstruction of common bile duct, elevated fasting blood glucose, abnormal glucose tolerance test, absence of pancreatic enzymes.
4. Pancreatic scan: May show filling defects; not diagnostic.
5. Selective arteriography: Determines extent of the cancer.
6. Laparotomy and biopsy: Establishes final diagnosis.

THERAPEUTIC MEASURES

Treatment methods for pancreatic carcinoma are merely palliative as most of them have already metastasized widely at the time of diagnosis. A five-year survival is extremely rare, with 90% of the patients dying within one year.

Surgery

Resection is done to relieve obstructive symptoms and for paliation of hyperinsulinism of the islet cell tumor. Some of the surgical procedures which have been done are:

1. Pancreaticoduodenectomy
2. Cholecystojejunostomy
3. Partial pancreatectomy with en bloc resection of the distal stomach, duodenum, and common bile duct (Whipple procedure)
4. Local excision of an insulinoma.

Radiation Therapy

Pancreatic tumors are generally radio-resistant and are located in such a way whereby tumoricidal radiation dose cannot be delivered without risking irradiation of the stomach, liver, intestines, and spinal cord. Split-course radiation of 2000 rads per two weeks alternated with two weeks rest until a total 6000 rads are delivered have shown some beneficial effects in some patients, i.e., 20% five-year-survival in localized, unresectable disease.[4]

Chemotherapy

Successful symptomatic palliation in nonmetastatic adenocarcinomas has been achieved in some cases with the use of mitomycin or 5-fluorouracil.

NURSING IMPLICATIONS

The overall care of the patient includes measures to prevent
and correct hyperglycemia, supportive measures to relieve
symptoms of biliary obstruction, and the maintenance of a satisfactory nutritional state.

Skin Care

Meticulous, frequent, and thorough skin cleansing with cool,
tepid water, lanolin-based soap, or corn starch baths are helpful to relieve pruritus. Instruct patient to refrain from scratch-
ing so as not to irritate skin. Calamine lotion may be applied
to relieve itchiness of the skin.

Dietary

Low-fat diet should be given due to the pancreatic insufficiency.
Medium-chain triglycerides which are well absorbed without
lipolysis would be helpful. Supplementary medications such as
oxandralone (Anavar), vitamin K, and pancreatic tablets such
as pancreozymin, pancreatin (Viokase), and minerals should
be given.

Specific Care If Pancreatitis Is Present

The patient should be closely watched for the effects of kallikrein release (much of it is in the pancreas) into the lymphatics
and plasma. Kallikrein catalyzes kallidin and bradykinin which
are very powerful vasodilators; hence hypotension is always a
possibility.

Specific Care of Patient
With Whipple Surgery

1. Serial checking of physiological parameters such as vital
   signs, blood count, and chemistries should be performed.
2. Gastrointestinal decompression and biliary tube drainage
   should be maintained, ensuring gravity drainage and proper
   functioning of suction apparatus.
3. All intake and output should be carefully measured and recorded.
4. Close observation of any abdominal distention should be
   done since distension may indicate bleeding, leaking of digestive enzymes, or paralytic ileus.
5. Maintenance of parenteral therapy such as IV fluids and
   electrolytes and hyperalimination fluids is very important.

6. Relief of pain postoperatively: adequate analgesics should
    be given postoperatively since in the preoperative period
    an analgesic like morphine sulfate is not given because it
    causes spasm of the sphincter of Oddi which aggravates
    symptoms of biliary/pancreatic obstruction as well as res-
    piratory depression. The pain medication should be given
    before the pain becomes very severe. For unrelenting pain,
    a sympathectomy or a nerve block may be performed and
    every effort should be aimed at increasing the quality of
    life for the patient and his family.

REVIEW QUESTIONS

1. What portion of the pancreas is frequently involved with the
    occurrence of a malignant tumor?
2. List eight signs and symptoms of a pancreatic head tumor.
3. Differentiate hyperglycemia from hypoglycemia, both of
    which can occur in pancreatic carcinoma.
4. Discuss three abnormal laboratory tests associated with
    carcinoma of the pancreas.
5. Describe the surgical, radiotherapy, and chemotherapeutic
    treatment of the patient with pancreatic carcinoma.
6. List specific nursing measures to alleviate pruritus and
    pancreatic enzyme deficiency.
7. Explain why hypotension may occur in pancreatitis.
8. Describe the Whipple procedure and discuss the nursing
    care of the patient who has had this procedure. Specify the
    rationale for each nursing intervention.

REFERENCES

1. Rubin, P. and Bakemeier, R. (eds.), Clinical Oncology for
    Medical Students and Physicians. The University of Roch-
    ester School of Medicine and Dentistry, and American Can-
    cer Society, New York (1974).
2. Bowden, L., Cancer of the Pancreas. CA, 22:275-283
    (September-October, 1972).
3. Clarke, M., et al., Functioning Beta Cell Tumors (Insu-
    linomas) of the Pancreas. Ann. Surg., 175:956 (1972).
4. Haslam, J.B., et al., Radiation Therapy in the Treatment
    of Irresectible Adenocarcinoma of the Pancreas. Cancer,
    32:1341-1345 (1973).
5. Netter, F.H., The Ciba Collection of Medical Illustrations,
    Vol. 4, Endocrine System and Selected Metabolic Diseases.
    Ciba Pharmaceutical Products, New York (1965).
6. Cubilla, A.L. and Fitzgerald, P.J., Pancreas Cancer
    (Nonendocrine): A Review - Part II. Clin. Bull., 8(4):143-
    155 (1978).

7. Cubilla, A.L. and Fitzgerald, P.J., Pancreas Cancer (Nonendocrine): A Review - Part I. Clin Bull., 8(3):91-99 (1978).

8. Cubilla, A.L. and Fitzgerald, P.J., Pancreas Cancer I. Duct Adenocarcinoma, A Clinical-Pathologic Study of 380 Patients. Pathol. Ann., pp. 241-289 (1978).

CHAPTER 20
Thyroid Cancer

Carcinomas of the thyroid generally present as a nodule or a lump in the gland. They are slow-growing with delayed clinical manifestations, low mortality, and morbidity. The patient is usually euthyroid except in the presence of a "functioning" neoplasm which may produce hyperthyroidism. The functioning growth is usually encapsulated, elaborates thyroxine and/or triiodothyronine, and has a variable degree of autonomy from the feedback mechanism of thyroid stimulating hormone released by the pituitary gland.

ETIOLOGY

Factors associated with the development of thyroid carcinoma include radiation effects, prolonged TSH stimulation, chronic nontoxic colloid goiter, follicular adenomas as premalignant and precursor to follicular carcinoma, and genetic predisposition. [6,11,12,13]

GENERAL CLASSIFICATION

Papillary Carcinoma

This is the most common type and accounts for over half of all adults and about two-thirds of childhood thyroid cancers. It affects all ages but occurs more often in young adults, predominantly females, with eight times more predisposition during childbearing age. It is the least aggressive and least malignant type except when it occurs below age 7 and over age 50. The cancer may be small, or may be palpable as a nodule but most often multifocal and bilateral. Metastases is into the regional nodes of the neck, mediastinum, lungs, and other distant organs.

Follicular Carcinoma

This is less common but more aggressive than papillary cancers. It accounts for 20 to 30% of all thyroid cancers, occurs at any age but most commonly between 20 and 50 years. It presents as a small or a large growth, often occurring in clusters containing colloids and, depending on the type, it is often bilateral and tends to recur. Metastasis is also into regional nodes but it readily invades blood vessels and metastasize into the bones, lungs, and liver.

Medullary (Solid) Carcinoma

This is much less common, accounting for only 5% of all thyroid cancers. It affects females more often than males, occurring mostly after age 40. The neoplasm may be small, discrete, or large, hard, irregular, and anaplastic. It grows rapidly and metastasizes into distant organs but regional node involvement is uncommon. The hallmark of this carcinoma is its association with amyloid and calcium deposits throughout the tumor and the production of calcitonin and histaminase. It can elaborate adrenocorticotrophic hormone (ACTH) causing a Cushing syndrome, and the diarrhea which is often associated with the disease is attributed to the production of prostaglandin E_2 and F_2 by the tumor. Nodal and distant metastases into the bones, liver, and kidneys are frequent.

Giant and Spindle Cell Carcinoma

This is the most malignant and deadly of all the thyroid cancers, characterized by a survival rate of about one year. It occurs after age 50, is highly anaplastic and rapidly growing. It never shows any signs of hormonal function, is extremely resistant to radiation, and is almost never curable by surgery. Metastatic involvement of the hypopharynx and esophagus can occur. Tracheal invasion and compression usually cause the patient's death.

CLINICAL MANIFESTATIONS

Signs and symptoms depend on the size and type of carcinoma. The presence of a palpable nodule may be accompanied by pressure symptoms such as hoarseness, dysphagia, dyspnea, and pain. Other symptoms may include:

1. Diarrhea
2. Vocal cord paralysis
3. Heat intolerance
4. Irritability
5. Weight loss and tremors
6. Symptoms of distant metastases.

DIAGNOSTIC TESTS AND DIAGNOSIS

1. Thyroid scan (scanning agents such as 16Se-selenomethionine (16Se) and 99m-technetium (99mTc) are considered superior to radioactive iodine).
2. Needle biopsy (done for cold nodules that appear cystic or that transilluminate).
3. Ultrasonic scan.
4. Chest x-ray, barium swallow.
5. Thyroid angiography.
6. Thyroid function tests. (Except scanning, thyroid function tests are of little value since the patient is usually euthyroid. However, functioning carcinomas may produce hyperthyroidism and therefore can yield abnormal findings.

TREATMENT MODALITIES[1,2,3,5,7]

Surgery

Subtotal thyroidectomy with modified homolateral or bilateral nodal dissection may be performed for papillary and follicular carcinoma. Total thyroidectomy and radical neck nodal excision is done for medullary and anaplastic carcinoma.

Radiation

External radiation has been used for large, inoperable carcinomas and some treatment centers have used megavoltage treatments postoperatively after a total thyroidectomy in lieu of a radical neck dissection. Radioactive iodine has been used to treat local and distant metastases after performance of thyroidectomy.

Thyroid Suppression Therapy

Large doses of exogenous thyroid hormones as adjunctive therapy have been used by some physicians. Simultaneous administration of beta adrenergic blocking agents such as propranolol hydrochloride (Inderal) have increased the patient's tolerance to the treatment regime.

Chemotherapy

Antineoplastic drugs such as doxorubicin HCl (Adriamycin) have been used with some success in treating metastatic thyroid cancer.

NURSING IMPLICATIONS

Nursing care priorities are directed towards alleviating anxiety and discomfort caused by pressure symptoms such as dyspnea and dysphagia, relieving distressing effects of possible thyrotoxicosis, and postoperative nursing care after surgical intervention. The holistic care of the patient who has had radical neck dissection is covered in Chapter 30. In this section, the nursing care of a thyroidectomy patient is emphasized.

Preoperative Care

1. The patient should be in a euthyroid state before surgery is done.
2. Preoperative teaching should include informing the patient of the possibility of hoarseness or aphonia, so that he will not be alarmed and become anxious postoperatively.
3. The patient is also informed of the proper position after surgery and the possibility of having a drainage system.

Postoperative Care

1. Place the patient in a semi-Fowler's or Fowler's position with the head supported on a pillow so that the neck is neither flexed nor hyperextended. Sometimes immobilization may be done by placing the head in between sandbags or with folded blankets placed on each side of the head. Proper positioning of the patient in this manner reduces pain, edema of the suture line, and promotes easier respiration.

2. High humidity oxygen may be given to increase oxygenation and ease breathing.

3. Have available at the bedside a tracheostomy tray in case of emergency procedure to relieve respiratory failure.

4. Observe for signs of anoxia indicated by restlessness or rapid pulse rate.

5. Watch for signs of hemorrhage indicated by pressure symptoms on the trachea and epiglottis such as a choking sensation, difficulty in coughing and swallowing, or tightening of the dressings. The dressings should be checked frequently. Slip a hand underneath the patient's neck and check for any seepage.

6. Observe signs of laryngeal nerve damage. Although hoarseness is expected postoperatively, any increase in it may

indicate laryngeal nerve injury. Crowing respirations or retraction of the tissues of the neck should be noted and reported to the surgeon at once.

7. Monitor the patient for signs of thyrotoxicosis, such as shock, chest pain, palpitation, dyspnea, abdominal pain, diarrhea, fever, somnolence, delirium, and coma. Thyroid storm or thyroid crisis (thyrotoxicosis) is attributed to adrenal insufficiency and release of thyroid hormone into the circulation during surgery. Should this occur, treatment includes administration of steroids, ice packs, or hypothermia to relieve hyperpyrexia. Antipyretics may also be given but aspirin is not recommended because it has synergistic effect with thyroxine. Antithyroid drugs such as methimazole, propylthiouracil, Lugol's solution, or sodium iodide intravenously may be given as necessary. Cardiovascular symptoms may be treated with reserpine, propranolol HCl (Inderal), or digoxin.

8. Watch for tetany as a complication. This can be caused by injury or inadvertent removal of the parathyroid glands during surgery. Observe the patient for occurrence of carpopedal spasm, muscle twitching, vocal cord paralysis, and convulsions. Check serum calcium levels, presence of a positive Chvostek's and/or Trousseau's sign. A Chvostek's sign is elicited by a sharp tapping over the facial nerve anterior to the ear. Twitching of the mouth, nose, and eye indicates a positive reaction. A Trousseau's sign is elicited by occluding the circulation into the arm by using a tourniquet or a blood pressure cuff for approximately 3 minutes. A positive sign is indicated by carpal spasm. Treatment of hypocalcemic tetany is effected with calcium chloride given intravenously and dietary management.

REVIEW QUESTIONS

1. Compare a functioning (hormone-producing) thyroid cancer with a nonfunctioning one.
2. Describe the most common type of thyroid carcinoma.
3. Why does a medullary carcinoma of the thyroid gland cause Cushing's syndrome?
4. What is the most malignant type of thyroid carcinoma?
5. Discuss the care of the patient who is treated with radioactive iodine.
6. How do you check for the Chvostek's sign and Trousseau's sign?
7. Discuss the nursing care of a thyroidectomy patient.

REFERENCES

1. Askar, F.S., A Better Outlook in Thyroid Cancer. Consultant, 12:48 (January, 1972).
2. Becker, K.L., Management of Thyroid Disorders. Postgrad. Med., 53:60 (February, 1973).
3. Brunner, L. and Suddarth, D., Textbook of Medical-Surgical Nursing. J.B. Lippincott Co., Philadelphia (1975).
4. French, R., Guide to Diagnostic Procedures. McGraw Hill Book Co., New York (1975).
5. Shafer, K., et al., Medical-Surgical Nursing. C.V. Mosby Co., St. Louis (1971).
6. Wilson, S.M., et al., Thyroid Carcinoma After Irradiation. Arch. Surg., 100:330-337 (1970).
7. Hellman, D.E., Durie, B.G., et al., Multidisciplinary Management of Carcinoma of the Thyroid. Ariz. Med., 37 (1):19-25 (January, 1980).
8. Sisson, J.C., Bartolo, S.P., et al.: The Dilemma of the Solitary Thyroid Nodule: Resolution Through Decision Analysis. Semin. Nuclear Med., 8(1):59-71 (January, 1980).
9. N Emec, J., Zamrazil, V., et al., Bone Metastases of Thyroid Cancer, Biological Behavior, and Therapeutic Possibilities. Acta Univ. Carol. (Med.), pp. 7-106 (1978).
10. Kimler, S.C. and Muth, W.F., Primary Malignant Teratoma of the Thyroid: Case Report and Literature Review of Cervical Teratomas in Adults. Cancer, 42(1):311-317 (July, 1978).
11. Carney, A.J., et al., C-Cell Disease of the Thyroid Gland in Multiple Endocrine Neoplasia, Type 2b. Cancer, 44(6): 2173-2184 (December, 1979).
12. Getaz, P.E., et al., Anaplastic Carcinoma of the Thyroid Following External Irradiation. Cancer, 3(6):2248-2253 (June, 1979).
13. Holm, E.L., et al., Incidence of Malignant Thyroid Tumors in Humans After Exposure to Diagnostic Doses of Iodine-131. Retrospective Cohost Study. J. N. Cancer Inst., 64(5):1055-1060 (May, 1980).

CHAPTER 21
Cancer of the Adrenal Glands

Malignant neoplasms of the adrenal glands are rare, but when they occur they become widely malignant. The tumor often has already metastasized into the lungs, liver, and the spleen at the time of diagnosis. [5]

Pheochromocytoma, a rarely malignant chromaffin tumor, is mentioned here because about 90% of these tumors occur at the adrenal medulla while the rest occur at the aorta, ovaries, testes, spleen, and bladder. Pheochromocytoma is characterized by malignant and atypical hypertensive crises which are most likely paroxysmal but in some cases can become chronic. About 2% of cases have multiple tumors while about 10% (more so in children) have bilateral medullary tumors. These tumors, like the adrenal medulla, secrete epinephrine while the extramedullary tumors (i.e., chromaffin tissue tumor of the ovaries) secrete mostly norepinephrine, except those that develop in the bladder which can secrete both epinephrine and norepinephrine.

Adrenal cortical tumors are markedly malignant. They occur at all ages, although some authorities claim that they predominantly affect females ages 30 to 40 and especially more so following pregnancy. Others contend that the condition is more prevalent in males. [1] The carcinoma may be nonfunctioning or it may be hormone-producing, thus creating a Cushing's disease or a Cushing's syndrome. [3,4]

ETIOLOGY

Adrenal carcinoma has no known etiology. Factors such as ACTH-producing tumors of the pituitary gland and chronic adrenal hyperplasia have been implicated in the development of carcinoma of the adrenals.

CLINICAL MANIFESTATIONS

Patients with pheochromocytoma present a syndrome associated with atypical hypertensive attack. This consists of:

1. Headache
2. Weakness
3. Nervousness
4. Vomiting
5. Abdominal pain
6. Constipation
7. Sweating
8. Palpitation
9. Angina, pallor, dyspnea
10. Red and puffy cyanotic hands
11. Increased levels of catecholamines, especially in children.

In cortical carcinoma, the patient may manifest symptoms related to the increased levels of cortisone and aldosterone. The symptoms and signs of hyperaldosteronism may include:

1. Moderate hypertension characterized by a rise in systolic pressure which is eventually followed by a diastolic elevation
2. Obesity with the characteristic "buffalo hump"
3. Striae
4. Weakness
5. Polyuria and polydipsia (diabetes)
6. Poor wound healing
7. Hyperacidity
8. Osteoporosis
9. Hirsutism
10. Acne
11. Recess of scalp hair
12. Breast atrophy
13. Rarely, enlarged clitoris
14. Hypokalemic alkalosis
15. Sleeplessness
16. Psychosis.

Some patients may not have the above endocrine syndrome although their carcinoma produces large amount of cortisone. Their signs and symptoms are therefore those of adjacent and distant organ metastases.

DIAGNOSTIC TESTS AND DIAGNOSIS

1. Photoscanning and x-rays, such as retroperitoneal pneumography and adrenal venography, are vital diagnostic tools.

2. 17-Ketosteroids, dehydroepiandrosterone, and 17-hydroxy-corticoids are elevated.
3. Hormonal assay of serum and urinary catecholamines: pheochromocytoma is suspected in the presence of atypical intermittent hypertension which is usually precipitated by stress or by some trigger mechanisms such as changes in position or by the act of micturition.

TREATMENT MODALITIES

Adrenalectomy has produced gradual disappearance of endocrine syndrome and in some cases it caused contralateral adrenal atrophy. Pre- and postoperative radiation have also been used as well as chemotherapeutic palliation of unresectable tumors.[2]

NURSING IMPLICATIONS

Nursing care is based on the individual patient and family needs, but the overall care should include the following measures.

1. Patients with pheochromocytoma should be watched for episodes of acute hypertensive attacks. Prevent and/or minimize stress and other precipitating factors.
2. Accurate timing and complete collection of all urine for catecholamine determination should be done. A 24-hour urine collection is necessary for determination of vanilmandelic acid (VMA) or homovanillic acid (HVA) which are more stable and excreted in larger amounts than the catecholamines (epinephrine and norepinephrine).
3. Proper collection should be made of a single, random voiding or a two-hour urine collection as ordered.
4. The patient should be put on a three-day VMA diet prior to the 24-hour collection for VMA. The diet excludes bananas, tea, coffee, and chocolate.
5. Observation for hyperglycemia reaction as well as hypoglycemia is essential. A rare cortical tumor may produce an insulin-like substance which can cause a drastic fall in blood glucose.
6. The patient who undergoes adrenalectomy is usually given phentolamine hydrochloride (Retigine) to block the vasopressor effects of the adrenal catecholamines during and immediately following surgery. The patient should be checked frequently for fluctuations in blood pressure.
7. Postoperative care of the patient with adrenalectomy includes:
    a. Frequent monitoring of the vital signs.
    b. Maintenance of fluid and electrolytes.

    c. Accurate monitoring of intake and output, especially in the first 48 hours postoperative. If polyuria persists, it should be reported to the physician.

    d. Observation for signs and symptoms of adrenal crisis should be done. This is manifested by weakness, severe abdominal or back pain, hyperpyrexia (which may be followed by hypothermia), hypotension or circulatory collapse, and coma.

8. The patient who is predisposed to adrenal insufficiency due to adrenalectomy, radiotherapy, or chemotherapy should be instructed to carry identification stating his need for hydrocortisone in case of emergency and should also carry with him an injectable preparation such as hydrocortisone sodium succinate. Replacement therapy instructions such as drug dosage and side effects should also be given to the patient and his family.

REVIEW QUESTIONS

1. Discuss the signs and symptoms of pheochromocytoma.
2. Describe the endocrine syndrome which is produced by some adrenal cortical tumors.
3. What foods are excluded in a VMA diet?
4. Why is the drug phentolamine HCl (Regitine) given preoperatively to the patient who is to undergo adrenalectomy?
5. Discuss the postoperative care of the patient with adrenalectomy.
6. List the signs and symptoms of adrenal crisis.
7. What are some of the discharge instructions that should be given to the postadrenalectomy patient and his family?

REFERENCES

1. Rubin, P. and Bakemeier, R. (eds.), Clinical Oncology for Medical Students and Physicians. The University of Rochester School of Medicine and Dentistry, and American Cancer Society, New York (1974).
2. Lubitz, J.A., et al., Mitotane Use in Inoperable Adrenal Cortical Carcinoma. JAMA, 223:1109-1112 (1973).
3. Williams, R.H., Textbook of Endocrinology. W.B. Saunders Co., Philadelphia (1974).
4. Winthrobe, M.M., et al., Harrison's Textbook of Medicine, 7th ed., McGraw Hill Co., New York (1974).
5. Ohman, U., Granberg, P.O., et al., Pheochromocytoma: Critical Review of Experiences with Diagnosis and Treatment. Progr. Clin. Cancer, pp. 135-152 (1978).

CHAPTER 22
Cancer of the Cervix

Cancer of the cervix is the most common cancer of the female reproductive system. Each year, approximately 8000 women in the United States die of this disease. However, it is believed that 75 to 90% of all women with this condition could be saved by early detection, diagnosis, and proper treatment. Cervical cancer has been found to be at least three times more common than cancer of the fundus of the uterus.

ETIOLOGY

Cancer of the cervix is most common between the ages of 30 and 50, rarely occurs before the age of 20, and it is believed that early sexual activity and promiscuity are predisposing factors to this condition. The incidence is also higher in women who are married than in single women regardless of whether or not they have had children. Other factors believed to contribute to the high incidence of cancer of the cervix include low socioeconomic status, increasing parity, and a positive history of venereal disease. For unknown reasons, cancer of the cervix is rare in Jewish women and does not occur in celibate women except for adenocarcinoma. There have been some studies made which indicate that circumcision of the male partner is a factor related to lower incidence. Herpes virus II has recently been linked to cervical cancer. Smegma and deoxyribonucleic acid of spermatozoa have also been considered. To date, there is insufficient evidence to specifically pinpoint the exact cause of the disease, but as research continues the answer to the question of etiologic cause may soon be obtained.

CLINICAL MANIFESTATIONS

In the early phase of cancer of the cervix, it is asymptomatic. There are, however, certain symptoms that may occur in early cervical carcinoma which include:

1. Leukorrhea
2. Irregular vaginal bleeding or spotting
3. Postcoital bleeding
4. Foul vaginal discharge.

When the disease has advanced and has become invasive, then the presenting signs and symptoms are:

1. Pelvic pain
2. Leakage of urine and feces from the vagina
3. Weight loss
4. Anorexia
5. Anemia.

DIAGNOSTIC TESTS AND DIAGNOSIS

Early Detection

Routine Papanicolaou (Pap) smear has been the most important method of detecting any abnormality of the exfoliated cells. For females age 20 to 65 a Pap test every three years at the minimum is recommended; for those under 20, if sexually active, Pap test is done, and after two negative exams it is repeated one year apart. For high-risk women, it should be done more frequently as recommended by the American Cancer Society in 1980.

Several systems are used in classifying cervical smears. Whatever the system may be, it is important to keep in mind as a frame of reference the old classification of cervical smears as follows:

Class 1: Smear normal, no abnormal cells
Class 2: Atypical cells present below the level of cervical neoplasm
Class 3: Smear contains abnormal cells consistent with dysplasia
Class 4: Smear contains abnormal cells consistent with carcinoma in situ
Class 5: Smear contains abnormal cells consistent with invasive carcinoma of squamous cell origin.

If the result of the pap smear is normal, provided there are no symptoms, then there is no need for further consideration until the next routine examination. However, if the smear is questionable, then it should be repeated. If after a repeat pap and the smear persists to be questionable, then further investigative work including biopsy and histological examination should be carried out.

Colposcopy

This should be done when there is an atypical cytologic smear after ruling out and/or treatment of cervicitis and the cytology of atypical cells persists. If after colposcopy there is abnormality seen in visualizing the cervix via the colposcopy, then direct punch biopsy is performed and treatment instituted based on findings. The patient will have to have followup smear and examination for life. If after a colposcopy there is no abnormality seen but the atypical smear cannot be explained and there is no lesion present, then conization is done. If a lesion is present, then biopsy of the lesion is performed and if there is evidence of invasive carcinoma, then metastatic survey and examination for staging is done.

Biopsy

The type and extent of cervical biopsy depends upon any abnormality seen during colposcopy or the results of an abnormal Pap smear. As stated earlier, when the lesion is clearly visible via a colposcope, then one or more punch biopsies may be taken as an office procedure without anesthesia. However, if there is no visible lesion but the Pap smear is suspicious, biopsy excision of an inverted cone of tissue is usually done under general anesthesia in the operating room.

Conization

This is done with a cold knife and not by electrocautery, for the latter may destroy tissue at the cut edge and since the only cancer tissue present may be at this point, the diagnosis may be missed. The incision should be made outside the transformation zone so as to include all potentially neoplastic tissue in the specimen and at least 50% of the canal should be removed, followed by curettage of the remaining endocervical canal.

Conization does not predispose to abortion. Therefore, it should be done in a pregnant woman with a positive cervical smear suggestive of carcinoma. It should be shallower in that it should not extend as far up to the canal as in nonpregnant women.

Schiller Test

This is staining of the cervix with iodine. The normal cervix will take up the stain of the iodine and become brown due to the reaction between the iodine and the glycogen content of normal cells. If the cervix does not take up stain, then there is glycogen depletion which is indicative of abnormality. This test can identify areas for biopsy if no obvious lesion is visualized.

Wedge Biopsy

This has about the same benefits and limitations as does the punch, except that it provides a much cleaner, less traumatized sample wherein some cell layering is evident.

Special Procedures

In addition to the above-mentioned diagnostic tests and procedures for detecting cervical cancer, there are some procedures that should be done for establishing a baseline for future management of the patient.

1. Intravenous pyelogram: This is done for all cases as the most frequent local metastases occur periureterally, and the most common cause of death is due to renal impairment.
2. Cystoscopy: This is done in most invasive cases to rule out bladder involvement.
3. Lymphangiograms: These are used to determine extent of lymph node spread.
4. Special endoscopic procedures as previously discussed, metastatic bone surveys, and liver scans.

TREATMENT MODALITIES

Staging of cervical cancer has been very useful in providing guidelines for determining what modality of treatment should be used. According to the International Classification of Carcinoma of the Cervix, the clinical stages of cervical cancer are:

Stage	O:	Carcinoma in situ, intraepithelial carcinoma.
Stage	I:	Carcinoma confined to the cervix (extension to the corpus should be disregarded).
	Ia:	Microinvasive carcinoma (early stromal invasion).
	Ib:	All other cases of Stage I. Occult cancer should be marked "occ."
Stage	II:	The carcinoma extends beyond the cervix but has not extended to the pelvic wall. The carcinoma involves the vagina, but not the lower third.
Stage	III:	The carcinoma has extended to the pelvic wall. On rectal examination there is no cancer-free space between the tumor and the pelvic wall. The tumor involves the lower third of the vagina. All cases with hydronephrosis or nonfunctioning kidney.
	IIIa:	No extension to the pelvic wall.
	IIIb:	Extension to the pelvic wall and/or hydronephrosis.

Stage IV: The carcinoma has extended beyond the true pelvis or has clinically involved the mucosa of the bladder or rectum. A bullous edema does not classify as Stage IV.

IVa: Spread of the growth to adjacent organs.

IVb: Spread to distant organs.

Another important consideration in determining the management of cancer of the cervix is that of the various degrees of cervical dysplasia.

1. Cervical intraepithelial neoplasia (CIN) grade I, or mild dysplasia: Cervical intraepithelial dysplasia is present when undifferentiated neoplastic cells occupy the lower one-third of the epithelium.
2. CIN grade 2: When two-thirds of the thickened epithelium is involved, it is called moderate dysplasia.
3. CIN grade 3: When the undifferentiated neoplastic cells reach almost to the surface, the lesion is severe dysplasia.
4. Carcinoma in situ: When the entire epithelium is composed of undifferentiated neoplastic cells.

Cervical intraepithelial neoplasia (CIN) form a continuous beginning with mild dysplasia and ending with invasive carcinoma. However, there seems to be general consensus that CIN may have one of three courses, namely, regression, persistence, or progression to carcinoma in situ or invasive carcinoma. Some research findings indicate that roughly three out of every 10 patients who have marked dysplasia, when followed, ultimately develop carcinoma in situ. Other studies indicate a much higher degree of progression.

The treatment of dysplasia depends upon its degree.[8] For mild dysplasia, it could be treated as an outpatient or office procedure with subsequent follow-up examinations with cervical smears. If the lesion is extensive, conization or even hysterectomy may be indicated, particularly if the patient does not wish to have additional children or if infertility is already present due to total obstruction of the fallopian tubes. Follow-up care is essential for the patient after the course of treatment is instituted. Cryotherapy and electrocoagulation have also been used in the treatment of dysplasia.

The treatment modalities for cancer of the cervix include:

1. Surgery (conization, hysterectomy, or radical surgery)
2. Radiation therapy (internal or external radiation)

3. Combination therapy (surgery and radiation)
4. Palliative therapy (symptomatic treatment and perhaps surgery).

The treatment of cervical cancer depends largely on the stage of the patient's cancer upon examination by the physician. It is suggested that a team effort be made to ascertain the best method of treatment to be instituted by a gynecologist, radiation oncologist, and the pathologist. The success of therapy is influenced by the availability of resources needed for effective treatment and follow-up care, the experience and interest of the physicians, the cooperation of the patient, and the commitment of nursing and other health team members. [3,4,5,6]

Preinvasive cancer, Stage O, CIN grade 3 or carcinoma in situ are usually treated with surgery consisting of either conization or hysterectomy. A woman who desires to have more children may be treated with conization provided she is willing to undergo regular follow-up examinations including cervical smears at three-month intervals. If the woman has infertility or does not wish to have additional children, then hysterectomy is the treatment of choice.

Microinvasive carcinoma or stage Ia is treated with radical surgery or radiation therapy. There seems to be a controversy concerning the terminology of microinvasive or superficially invasive in that the term is variously defined as stromal invasion to a depth of 1 mm, 3 to 4 mm, 5 mm, and 9 mm beneath the basement. However, the widely accepted definition of microinvasive is that of stromal invasion with the greatest diameter being 5 mm. Some studies indicate that total abdominal hysterectomy with a wide vaginal cuff is the treatment of choice. According to Nelson, Averette, and some other authorities, until more data are available regarding diagnostic methods, treatment, and long-term follow-up care, stromal invasion by squamous cell carcinoma greater than 1 mm should be classified as frankly invasive cancer stage Ib, and treated by radical surgery or radiotherapy. [2] Stromal invasion less than 1 mm with absence of demonstrable vascular penetration by malignant cells may be classified as stage Ia and treated like stage O carcinoma. The radical surgeries that may be done for stage Ib carcinoma of the cervix are Wertheim abdominal hysterectomy and pelvic lymphadenectomy or Schauta-Amreich vaginal hysterectomy.

Stage Ia, Ib, and stage II cervical carcinoma are treated in most institutions today with radiation therapy. Irradiation consists of internal irradiation of the cervix and upper vaginal area, combined with external irradiation to allow for more even distribution of irradiation to the pelvis and pelvic walls. In more advanced stage I and II disease, the tumor size may be too large to allow effective internal irradiation. In this case, external irradiation is given initially and after the tumor is reduced, then internal irradiation is done. In some cases, due to the extension of the disease, the only possible radiation that can be done is external radiation. If it fails, such as in stage IIb, then pelvic exenteration may have to be done.

The principles of radiation therapy for stage I and II cervical cancers can be summarized as follows:

1. Maximal dose is given to the tumor, with doses to normal tissues maintained within the radiation tolerance of the normal tissue.
2. Combined intrauterine and vaginal internal irradiation is the mainstay of therapy.
3. Supplementary external irradiation is delivered to the parametria and lateral pelvic walls.
4. Due to too large a tumor, the external irradiation may be initiated to reduce the bulk of the tumor, which is then followed by internal irradiation.

Invasive tumors, stages III and IV are primarily treated by radiation. External irradiation is the mainstay of treatment because of the need to deliver a higher dose to the primary tumor and a homogeneous dose to a large-volume tumor. It also reduces the risk of hemorrhage and infection and also restores normal anatomical landmarks in the pelvic cavity. If beneficial effects are achieved, then internal radiation may be done subsequently. In stage III, it may be necessary for the physician to perform a preliminary nephrostomy if renal function is compromised. Statistics indicate that for stage IV carcinoma, there is less than a 5% chance for cure by radiation. In radical surgery of stage IV, a cure rate of 20 to 25% has been effected.

In internal radiation therapy, cesium may be used. In order to prepare the patient for the procedure, it is important for the nurse to know that it can be done either by a "preloading" technique or by the "afterloading" technique. In the former, the applicator used for insertion contains the cesium when the surgeon inserts it into the patient's vagina or cervix in the operating room. In the latter, the empty applicator is implanted in the operating room, then a member of the radiotherapy department puts the cesium into the applicator after the patient has returned to her hospital bed. There are two advantages of the "afterloading" technique. First, it exposes the hospital staff to less radiation, since the insertion is withheld until the patient is in her room, and second, it offers flexibility in the treatment process. After the insertion of the empty applicator, x-rays are taken in the operating room, which show the distance from the applicator thereby minimizing the radiation of the rectum and bladder. In the preloaded technique, there is no flexibility in the position and distance from the radioactive material to the bladder and rectum.

In case of pregnancy, the nurse should be cognizant of the management of the patient with preinvasive cervical cancer and the patient with invasive carcinoma so that she can be supportive to the patient. As stated earlier, the diagnosis of carcinoma in situ is made by a more shallow cone biopsy irrespective of the length of gestation. Once diagnosed as carcinoma stage O, the patient is allowed to continue with her pregnancy and to have vaginal delivery. After delivery, a more definitive treatment is instituted two to three months postpartum as indicated by follow-up examination. If the patient has invasive carcinoma, the pregnancy is usually terminated up to 24 weeks. The subsequent therapy after 24 weeks is determined by the extent of the cancer. The patient who is in the last trimester of pregnancy can be treated by a cesarian section when the fetus is viable. A radical hysterectomy and node dissection may be done during the cesarian section in early cancer or radiation therapy can be administered in the postpartum period.[14]

In palliative therapy, although the approximate recovery rates for various therapeutic intervention in the various stages of cervical cancer are high (95 to 100% in stage O, 70 to 85% in stage I, 65 to 75% in stage IIa, 50 to 65% in stage IIb, 20 to 30% in stage III, and 5 to 10% in stage IV), there are those whose disease progresses beyond the chance for cure and who must therefore be treated with palliation. Surgery plays a limited role in palliation and radiation is used rarely since at this point the maximum tolerated dose has been given to the patient. Hence, symptomatic treatment is given. In terms of chemotherapy, cyclophosphamide (Cytoxan), vincristine, and methotrexate have been used with limited success. The goals of palliative therapy are to make the patient more comfortable through intensive quality nursing care and the use of analgesics as indicated, and to prepare the patient and her family to work through the grieving process.[15,18]

NURSING IMPLICATIONS

In the surgical management of the patient with cancer of the cervix, the nursing care plan should focus on the physical and psychological preparation of the patient preoperatively.[7]

1. Restoration and maintenance of a good nutritional state is essential. Fluid and electrolytes may be administered intravenously with multivitamins. Anemia should be corrected with blood transfusions.
2. Presence of any other medical condition should be evaluated, treated, and/or controlled so as not to present any hazard during the surgical procedure. Diabetes, for example, should be under control to prevent hypoglycemia during surgery and postoperatively.
3. Consent should be signed after the careful explanation of the surgical procedure by the surgeon.
4. No dentures, hairpins, or nail polish should be present when the patient goes to the operating room.
5. All physical preparation of the patient should be done with efficiency in order to convey to the patient a feeling of confidence and trust in the health team.
6. Warm cleansing enemas are given the evening before surgery.
7. Skin preparation involves shaving of the lower half of the abdomen, pubic area, and the perineum.
8. The type of anesthesia that will be used should be explained to the patient by the anesthesiologist.
9. The patient is taught how to do leg exercises, deep breathing and coughing exercises preoperatively.
10. The patient is also informed of what will be expected of her after surgery.

The psychological preparation of the patient is of utmost importance. It should be noted that the patient's husband and/or family should be included in the preoperative teaching in order to promote a better attitude towards the surgical intervention and to enhance group support. Psychological reactions of the patient will vary according to the age and ego strengths as well as self-concept of the patient.

If the patient is premenopausal and her cancer requires hysterectomy, she may react with depression and lowered self-esteem. She may feel that she is no longer a woman or that she may be rejected by her husband. She may have questions about her sexual relationship with her husband after surgery. The nurse can be very therapeutic in this regard when she reassures the patient that the surgery will not interfere with the patient's sexual ability, that she is still a woman, and that the husband will understand the situation. It is important to realize that the nurse should open avenues for communication between the husband, the wife, and herself so that the couple's concerns, especially on the subject of sex, can be discussed. If the patient is pregnant and is allowed to continue with her pregnancy, she should be reassured that everything will be done to promote the welfare of the fetus. The patient should also be informed of the possibility of the need for effecting cesarian section delivery by the last trimester of pregnancy if the situation indicates it.

The principles of care for the patient who is to undergo radiation therapy include the following.

1. For afterloading technique, radioisotope implantation of cesium, the patient is prepared as follows:
    a. Give the patient cleansing enemas and povidine-iodine (Betadine) vaginal douche the evening prior to surgery.
    b. Insert a Foley catheter and connect it to straight drainage to avoid possible displacement of the applicator
    c. Give the patient a bath before she goes to the operating room
2. After insertion of the radioisotope, the patient must remain in bed and lie on her back with the head of the bed elevated 10 to 15 degrees, but her movements must be restricted to prevent dislodgement of the implant.
3. Provide reassurance and observe radiation precautions as already discussed in Chapter 9, Part III.
4. Explain all procedures that have to be done, instructions, in simple, understandable language, and answer the patient's questions.
5. Active range of motion exercises of both arms should be encouraged.
6. Do not give the patient a complete bed bath. Wash face, hands, arms, and chest daily. Do not bathe below the waist. Do not give her a complete back rub.
7. Check the vital signs every four hours. Report any temperature above 100° F.
8. Watch for any rash, skin eruption, vaginal discharge, any excessive vaginal bleeding, abdominal distention, or evidence of dehydration since the patient is prone to dehydration or paralytic ileus.
9. Clear-liquid diet or low-residue diet is usually given to prevent any straining which can cause displacement of the implant. Force fluids to the patient. If the patient is not drinking, report to the physician for possible parenteral fluids.
10. After removal of the implant, the patient should be given a providine-iodine (Betadine) douche and enema (Fleets). She can get out of bed but should be assisted initially until she feels stronger.

11. Discharge instructions that should be given to the patient
    are:
    a. Resume normal activities gradually.
    b. Inquire from her physician when to resume sexual in-
       tercourse. Sometimes it can be resumed in 7 to 10
       days.
    c. Vaginal douche may be done if there is any vaginal dis-
       charge, otherwise it is not necessary.
    d. The patient should avoid direct sunlight on areas ex-
       posed to radiation.
    e. Application of emollient cream on dry skin can be sooth-
       ing.
    f. The patient should notify her physician if she has any
       nausea, vomiting, diarrhea, frequent urination, or in-
       creased temperature.

REVIEW QUESTIONS

1. List some of the etiologic factors associated with cancer of
   the cervix.
2. What are the early signs and symptoms of early cervical
   carcinoma?
3. List the clinical manifestations of advanced cervical cancer.
4. Describe the classification of cervical smears.
5. Enumerate the various diagnostic procedures that may be
   done for detection and diagnosis of cancer of the cervix.
6. Describe the clinical stages of cervical cancer as proposed
   by the International Classification of Carcinoma of the Cervix.
7. List the various types of cervical dysplasia.
8. Name the treatment modalities for cervical cancer.
9. What factors influence success of therapy in cervical cancer?
10. What is the treatment of choice for stage O, stage Ia, Ib,
    and stage II?
11. List the principles of radiation therapy for stage I and II
    cervical cancer.
12. Describe the preloading and afterloading techniques of in-
    ternal radiation therapy.
13. What are the advantages of the afterloading technique?
14. What is the management of a pregnant woman who develops
    cancer of the cervix?
15. Describe the physical and psychological preparation of the
    patient who is to undergo surgical intervention as a mode of
    treatment for cervical cancer.
16. What are some nursing principles to be adhered to in caring
    for a patient who is to have irradiation therapy?

17. List some discharge instructions for the patient who has cancer of the cervix after effective inpatient treatment.

REFERENCES

1. Rudolph, J., Cancer of the Female Genital Tract. In: Clinical Oncology for Medical Students and Physicians - A Multidisciplinary Approach (Rubin, P. and Bakemeier, R., eds.), The University of Rochester School of Medicine and Dentistry, and American Cancer Society, New York, pp. 217-229 (1974).
2. Nelson, J.H., Detection, Diagnostic Evaluation, and Treatment of Dysplasia and Early Carcinoma of the Cervix. CA, pp. 134-150 (May/June, 1975).
3. Brunner, L.S. and Suddarth, D.S., Textbook of Medical-Surgical Nursing. J.B. Lippincott Co., New York, pp. 695-698 (1975).
4. Smith, D.W. and Hanley, C.P., Care of the Adult Patient. J.B. Lippincott Co., New York, pp. 932-947 (1975).
5. Shafer, K., et al., Medical-Surgical Nursing. C.V. Mosby Co., St. Louis, pp. 460, 261 (1971).
6. Peterson, B.H. and Kellog, C.J., Current Practice in Oncologic Nursing. C.V. Mosby Co., St. Louis (1976).
7. Fass, M. and Preston, W. (eds.), Clinical Concepts in Cancer Management - A Self-Instruction. McGraw Hill Book Co., New York, Blakiston Publications (1976).
8. Delgado, G., Stage IB Squamous Cancer of the Cervix: The Choice of Treatment. Ostet. Gynecol. Survey, 33(3):174-183 (March, 1978).
9. Singer, A. and Jordan, J.A., The Management of Premalignant Cervical Disease. Clin. Obstet. Gynecol., 5(3): 629-657 (December, 1978).
10. Jahaveri, G., Microinvasive Carcinoma of the Uterine Cervix. Int. J. Gynecol. Obstet., 16(2):106-114 (1978-1979).
11. Orr, J.D., Cervical Neuroblastoma in Childhood - A Better Prognosis? Clin. Oncol., 4(4):353-358 (December, 1978).
12. Siiteri, P.K., Steroid Hormones and Endometrial Cancer. Cancer Res., 38:4340-4346 (November, 1978).
13. Brewer, J.I., Torok, E.E., et al., Gestational Trophoblastic Disease: Origin of Choriocarcinoma, Invasive Mole, and Some Immunologic Aspects. Adv. Cancer Res., 27: 89-147 (1978).
14. Fennell, R.H. Jr., Microinvasive Carcinoma of the Uterine Cervix. Obstet. Gynecol. Survey, 33(6)406-411 (June, 1978).
15. Jones, W.B., Gestational Trophoblastic Neoplasma, The Role of Chemotherapy and Surgery. Surg. Clin.North Am., 58(1):167-179 (February, 1978).

16. Hajj, S.N. and Herbst, A.L., Evaluation and Management of Diethylstilbestrol-Exposed Offspring. Surg. Clin. North Am., 58(1):87-96 (February, 1978).
17. Van Nagell, J.R. Jr., Donaldson, E.S., and Gay, E.C., Evaluation and Treatment of Patients with Invasive Cervical Cancer. Surg. Clin. North Am., 58(1):67-85 (February, 1978).
18. Van Nagell, J.R., et al., Therapeutic Implications of Patterns of Recurrence in Cancer of the Uterine Cervix. Cancer, 44(6):2354-2361 (December, 1979).
19. Hasumi, K., et al., Microinvasive Carcinoma of the Uterine Cervix. Cancer, 45(5):928-931 (March, 1980).

CHAPTER 23
Ovarian Cancer

While 10 out of every 1000 women in the United States over 40 years old will develop ovarian cancer, only one or two will be cured. [1] The mortality rate of this disease is very high primarily due to its insidious onset and late diagnosis. The highest incidence of ovarian cancer is in the 40 to 60 age group, although it can occur anytime in childhood or adolescence. Ovarian cancer is classified according to cells of origin. Primary epithelial tumors include serous, mucinous, endometrioid, and mesonephric; those of germ cell origin are dysgerminoma, endodermal sinus, embryonal teratoma, and adult teratoma. Sex cord cell tumors are granulosa cell tumor (female) and Sertoli-Leydig cell tumor (male). Germ cells and sex cord tumors comprise gonadoblastoma.

ETIOLOGY

Ovarian cancer has no predilection toward etiologic factors.

CLINICAL MANIFESTATIONS

The degree of symptoms is directly related to the tumor's size, location, degree of malignancy, potential for hormone production, and possible complications such as torsion, rupture, infection, or bleeding. An early sign of ovarian cancer, called the postmenopausal palpable ovary syndrome (PMPO syndrome), is that which is interpreted as a normal sized ovary in the premenopausal woman but represents an ovarian tumor in the postmenopausal woman. [2]

Among the signs and symptoms of ovarian cancer in adults are:

1. Vague abdominal discomfort
2. Dyspepsia
3. Mild digestive disturbances
4. Later, vaginal bleeding in postmenopausal women

222

5. Pain associated with complications, such as intestinal obstruction as the tumor metastasizes to the surface of the bowel.

In children, ovarian neoplasm is manifested primarily by the presence of pain due to a relatively small pelvis and abdominal cavity which causes the neoplasm to stretch the peritoneum and thereby produce pressure symptoms on adjacent structures.

In both adult and pediatric ovarian cancer, a pelvic or abdominal painless mass is most frequently the presenting sign with local pressure and abdominal fullness as additional symptoms. In advanced cases of ovarian cancer, the patient may have ascites, pain, and symptoms resulting from metastatic sites.

DIAGNOSTIC TESTS AND DIAGNOSIS

A complete, systematic evaluation of the patient is mandatory in order to rule out any primary malignancy elsewhere in the body that might have metastasized to the ovary as well as to establish baseline studies for subsequent treatment of the condition.

Among the procedures that may be done are:

1. Careful history and physical examination
2. Pelvic examination and Pap smear
3. Proctosigmoidoscopy as indicated
4. Complete blood count (CBC) and urinalysis
5. SMA-12 (blood chemistries)
6. Chest x-ray
7. Intravenous pyelogram (IVP)
8. Gastrointestinal series
9. Barium enema
10. Paracentesis, laparoscopy, and lymphangiogram (optional)
11. Breast examination and mammography to rule out a primary lesion in the breast
12. Cul-de-sac aspirations and analysis of abnormal cells has been done recently in older women.

The value of pelvic examination in ovarian cancer detection is limited. Only one ovarian cancer in 10,000 examinations of asymptomatic women can be detected. It cannot be palpated until it reaches 15 cm in size. Nonetheless, it is recommended that the examining physician or nurse practitioner should be alert to:

1. A mass in the ovary
2. Relative immobility due to fixation and adhesions
3. Irregularity of the tumor
4. Shotty consistency with increased firmness
5. Tumors in the cul-de-sac described as "a handful of knuckles"
6. Relative insensitivity of the mass
7. Increasing tumor size under observation
8. Bilaterality (70% in ovarian carcinoma versus 5% in benign lesions)
9. An omental cake, nodular hepatomegaly and ascites which are common findings in advanced disease.

Pap smear has been reported to be positive in 40% of patients with advanced ovarian cancer. [1]

TREATMENT MODALITIES

The World Health Organization's histologic typing of ovarian cancer has proved beneficial in the clinical management and subsequent treatment protocols of this condition. This classification is as follows:

1. Serous tumors: adenocarcinoma, papillary adenocarcinoma, and papillary cystadenocarcinoma.
2. Mucinous tumors: adenocarcinoma and cystadenocarcinoma, malignant adenofibroma and cystadenofibroma.
3. Endometriod tumors: adenocarcinoma, adenocanthoma, malignant adenofibroma and cystadenofibroma, endometriod stromal sarcomas, and mesodermal Müllerian mixed tumors, homologous and heterologous.
4. Clear cell (mesonephroid) tumors: malignant carcinoma and adenocarcinoma.
5. Brenner tumors: malignant.
6. Mixed epithelial tumors: malignant.
7. Undifferentiated carcinoma.
8. Unclassified epithelial tumors.

The preferred modality of treatment for ovarian cancer is influenced by the "stage" of the disease. Although the Cancer Committee of the International Federation of Gynecology and Obstetrics (IFGO) has recommended staging of primary ovarian cancer which has been endorsed by the American College of Obstetrics and Gynecology, there are oncologists who feel some inadequacies of such staging. A review of extant literature on the staging of ovarian cancer indicates no major differences. The only noted changes in other proposed stagings are in the addition of a few more items under some of the original staging proposed by the IFGO. The following is a revised staging of ovarian cancer:[1]

Stage   I: Growth limited to the ovaries.

     Ia: Growth limited to one ovary; no ascites.

     (1) No tumor on the external surface; capsule intact.

     (2) Tumor present on the external surface and/or capsule(s) ruptured.
Note: (1) and (2) are additions to the original IFGO staging.

     Ib: Growth limited to both ovaries; no ascites.

     (1) No tumor on the external surface; capsule intact.

     (2) Tumor present on the external surface and/or capsule(s) ruptured.

     Ic: Tumor either Stage Ia or Ib but with ascites (peritoneal effusion which in the opinion of the surgeon is pathologic and/or clearly exceeds normal amounts) or positive peritoneal washings.

Stage II: Growth involving one or both ovaries with pelvic extension.

    IIa: Extension and/or metastases to the uterus and/or tubes.

    IIb: Extension to other pelvic tissues.

    IIc: Tumor either stage IIa or IIb, but with ascites or positive peritoneal washings.
(Note: Stage IIc is an addition to the original IFGO staging.

Stage III: Growth involving one or both ovaries with intraperitoneal metastases outside the pelvis and/or positive retroperitoneal nodes or tumor limited to the true pelvis with histologically proven malignant extension to small bowel or omentum.

Stage IV: Growth involving one or both ovaries with distant metastases. If pleural effusion is present, there must be positive cytology to allot a case to stage IV

Stage IV: Parenchymal liver metastases equals stage IV

Stage V: Special category: unexplored cases which are thought to be ovarian carcinoma. (Surgery, explorative or therapeutic, has not been performed.)

The principles of treatment of ovarian cancer are surgery, radiotherapy, chemotherapy, and combined treatment modalities. Surgery is the primary mode of treatment of ovarian cancer. The surgical intervention performed depends upon the stage of the disease. In general, for women between 40 and 60 years of age who have ovarian cancer of stromal origin and involving epithelial cells, total hysterectomy, bilateral salpingo-oophorectomy, omentectomy, appendectomy, and postoperative irradiation is recommended treatment protocol.[4]

Treatment by stage is as follows:

Stage Ia, Ib, Ic: Total hysterectomy, bilateral salpingo-oophorectomy, omentectomy, appendectomy, and instillation of phosphorus-32 (^{32}PO.

Stage IIa, IIb: Same treatment as above plus external irradiation. Biopsy of any adhesions should also be done to determine the presence or absence of cancer and the extent of the disease.

Stage III: Same as above plus total abdominal irradiation therapy, chemotherapy, or both.

Stage IV: Removal of as much cancer as possible through total abdominal hysterectomy, bilateral salpingo-oophorectomy, appendectomy, and omentectomy. Radiation therapy and chemotherapy with cyclophosphamide (Cytoxan), chlorambucil (Leukeran), and phenylalanine mustard (L-PAM).

It is recommended that patients with advanced ovarian cancer should not undergo extended surgery or pelvic exenteration except in extremely rare instances due to the tremendous trauma the patient has to be subjected to without a reasonable degree of certainty that cure can be effected.

Nonepithelial lesions which comprise 10% of all ovarian tumors and are the most common gynecologic tumor in children and adolescents are best treated with total hysterectomy, bilateral salpingo-oophorectomy, omentectomy, appendectomy, biopsy of para-aortic nodes with postoperative irradiation to the pelvis and para-aortic nodes. However, in a young woman with a unilateral, encapsulated dysgerminoma who wants to maintain childbearing ability, conservative management is indicated since survival rate is high (90%). The treatment for this case is unilateral salpingo-oophorectomy, biopsy of the other ovary and of the para-aortic nodes as well as cytologic examination of pelvic fluid.[3] Follow-up every two to three months for the first three years and then every six months thereafter with chest x-rays is necessary.

Statistics indicate that there is one ovarian cancer per 18,000 pregnancies. Malignancy rate of ovarian tumor in pregnant women is 2 to 5% compared with 18 to 20% in nonpregnant women. The treatment of ovarian cancer in a pregnant woman depends upon the extent of the disease. If low-grade and confined to one ovary, unilateral oophorectomy and bisection of the opposite ovary is done and the pregnancy may be allowed to term. If the cancer has extended beyond the ovary, total hysterectomy and bilateral salpingo-oophorectomy and postoperative irradiation is the mode of treatment. At the term of the pregnancy, cesarian delivery is done for the low-grade ovarian tumor during which time the fallopian tubes and the ovaries are inspected.

NURSING IMPLICATIONS

The principles of physical and psychological care of the patient are the same as in the care of the patient with cervical carcinoma. In addition, the nurse should anticipate the physiological and psychological effects of artificially induced menopause so that she can provide emotional support to the patient. Vasomotor reactions that are likely to be experienced by the patient are hot flashes and excessive perspiration. Headaches, nervousness, heart palpitations, and sleeplessness may also occur. Depression and irritability may permeate the patient's behavior.

The side effects and toxic effects of both chemotherapy and radiotherapy should be closely monitored and the appropriate nursing intervention carried out as previously discussed in Part III, Chapters 7 and 9.

REVIEW QUESTIONS

1. Enumerate the clinical manifestations of cancer of the ovary.
2. Why is there a high mortality rate in ovarian cancer despite major advances in cancer management?
3. Identify the types of ovarian cancer according to cell origin.
4. Discuss the rationale for a complete diagnostic evaluation for the patient with ovarian cancer.
5. Name the various diagnostic procedures that must be done when a patient is suspected of having ovarian cancer.
6. Describe the various stages of ovarian cancer.
7. Identify the various treatment methods according to the stage of the ovarian cancer.
8. What are some of the physiologic and psychological effects of artificially induced menopause?
9. How can the nurse provide emotional support to the patient after a hysterectomy and salpingo-oophorectomy?

REFERENCES

1. Barber, H., et al., Ovarian Cancer. American Cancer Society Professional Education Publication, New York (1975).

2. Rudolph, J., Cancer of the Ovary. In: Clinical Oncology for Medical Students and Physicians - A Multidisciplinary Approach, Rubin, P. and Bakemeier, R., (eds.), The University of Rochester School of Medicine and Dentistry, and American Cancer Society, New York, pp. 237-246 (1974).
3. Kurman, R.J. and Norris, H.J., Germ Cell Tumors of the Ovary. Pathol Ann., 13(1):291-325 (1978).
4. Eastwood, J., Mesonephroid (Clear Cell) Carcinoma of the Ovary and Endometrium: A Comparative Perspective Clinico-Pathological Study and Review of Literature. Cancer, 41(5):1911-1928 (May, 1978).

CHAPTER 24
Breast Cancer

The leading cause of death from cancer in women is carcinoma of the breast, with the highest mortality occurring between the ages of 55 and 74.[1] Excepting melanoma, breast cancer is more unpredictable than other neoplasms due to the hormonal influence on the rate of tumor growth. There are 72 per 100,000 new cases diagnosed each year. At the time of diagnosis, 46% have localized tumor, 42% have regional metastases, and 12% have more extensive metastases. With the public education programs sponsored by the American Cancer Society, about 95% of breast cancers are detected by women themselves through breast self-examination.

Less than 21% of cancers of the breast occur before age 30 and approximately 75% occur in patients over 40 years of age. There is a five-year survival rate of 63% overall; 85% for those with localized lesions, and 53% for those with regional metastases.[1] It is important to note that survival from breast carcinoma depends to a great extent upon early diagnosis, type of cancer present (slow or fast growing), genetic determination, and complete surgical removal of all tissues containing malignant cells before metastases occur.[17]

A great deal of knowledge has been gained about breast cancer through the years in terms of prevalence and highest risk groups. Among those facts which are significant to note are the following:[17]

1. Breast cancer is more left-sided than right-sided.
2. It is more common in the outer than in the inner quadrant.
3. It is more common in women without children. (Mortality rate for women who never had children is 70% higher than for women who have children.)
4. It is more common in women who have not suckled.
5. It is bilateral or breast-successive in 4 to 10% of cases.
6. The male to female ratio is 1:100.
7. There is a five-fold increase among those with familial history of breast cancer.

The high-risk groups of cancer of the breast are:

1. Women over 35 years of age.
2. Women with one or two children.
3. Primigravidas over 25 years of age.
4. Women under age 12 at menarche.
5. Women with 30 years of menses.
6. Women with a history of a relative (mother or sister) with carcinoma of the breast.
7. Women with a history of cystic disease.

ETIOLOGY

Although the cause of cancer is not definitely known, there are certain factors believed to influence the development of breast cancer. The strongest factor being considered is that of genetics. Other factors being explored are hormonal mechanisms (the effect of estrogen in contraceptives has been considered), viral agents, and immunologic processes.

CLINICAL MANIFESTATIONS

Breast cancer has a preclinical stage of 3 to 5 years. The most aggressive breast cancer cell has a doubling time of 22 days. Thus to grow into a 7-cm size tumor (the smallest size which can be felt) the cell must double 30 times, a minimum of 660 days or nearly 2 years of undetected growth. Hence, the only sign in the early stage of the disease is a small palpable mass (lump) which is isolated, movable, and painless. This lump of the breast has been found to occur 50% in the upper-outer quadrant, 20% centrally, 10% in the lower-outer quadrant, and 20% in the medial half of the breast. In the latter stage of the disease, the following clinical manifestations are present:

1. Dimpling of the skin over a hard lump.
2. Puckering of the skin.
3. Changes in the color of the skin over the lesion.
4. Alteration of breast contour.
5. Raising of the nipple.
6. Serous or bloody discharge from the nipple (ulceration).
7. Unusual scaling or inversion of the nipple (signs that the lesion is well established and has invaded surrounding tissue).
8. Fixation of the lump.
9. Pain, erythema (pain is seldom a symptom of early cancer).
10. Nodal axillary masses.

DIAGNOSTIC TESTS AND DIAGNOSIS

There are several procedures used in breast cancer detection and diagnosis. Among these procedures are:

1. Careful breast examination by gentle palpation in different positions. In this examination, check for asymmetry or irregularities; any retraction or distortion of the breast; any axillary lymph node enlargement; thickening, redness or edema of the nipple and areola, color, and texture.[1]
2. Transillumination (A mass that transilluminates is probably cystic unless it is lipomatous or filled with opaque material.)
3. Mammography (A negative result does not rule out malignancy.)
4. Thermography (Neoplastic tissues produce more heat.)
5. Xerography.
6. Excisional biopsy.
7. Aspiration biopsy.
8. Needle localization technique: Dye is inserted with a #22 gauge needle into the suspicious area to provide a marker for the lesion site and a visible tract for the surgeon to follow. After injection of the dye, a mammogram or a xerogram is done.

TREATMENT MODALITIES

Breast surgery, radiotherapy, immunotherapy, hormone therapy, and combination therapy are the treatment modalities used in cancer of the breast.

Breast Surgery

This is the major treatment undertaken. There are several types of surgical procedures done based upon the presenting clinical manifestations, the patient's choice (It is advocated that the surgeon should discuss with the patient the possible alternatives that can be done and allow the patient to think through the advantages and disadvantages of various alternatives before a mutual decision is reached as to what kind of surgery will be done.), the presence or absence of node involvement and metastases, the clinical experience of the surgeon, and availability of resources.

Among the surgical procedures done for cancer of the breast are the following:[18]

1. Radical mastectomy: Removal of the pectoralis major, the pectoralis minor, and the entire breast along with the adjacent lymph nodes is done in an attempt to remove all of the cancer cells from the patient's body.
2. Simple mastectomy: Removal of a breast is done without lymph node dissection.
3. Lumpectomy: Only removal of the tumor is done. Total removal of the breast may not always be necessary. In fact, radical mastectomy has been all but abandoned in England and most of Continental Europe advocates a "lumpectomy" in certain specific early cases.[2] However, most American surgeons do not subscribe to this mode of therapy as they feel there is lack of evidence to support the efficacy of the procedure.
4. Partial mastectomy: The cancer is removed with at least one inch of the healthy tissue surrounding it.
5. Subcutaneous mastectomy: Breast tissue is removed but the skin and nipple are preserved.
6. Modified radical mastectomy: Removal of all of the breast tissue and lymph nodes in the axilla is done but without removing the pectoralis muscles.
7. Extended radical mastectomy: This is done with chest wall resection.
8. Super-radical mastectomy: The sternum is split and the lymph nodes are dissected from the mediastinum.

Studies indicate that there is a higher local recurrence rate in patients who have had partial mastectomy than among those who have had the entire breast removed. It has also been noted that patients with partial mastectomy were subsequently subjected to additional surgery. Hence, most breast surgeons remove the breast and axillary nodes of the patient with noninvasive breast cancer. When the lesion is invasive, less than 1 cm in diameter, and is located in the outer one-half of the breast, the same procedure is used (modified radical mastectomy). If the dominant tumor mass is located in the inner half or in the center of the breast, the internal mammary lymph nodes may be involved. Therefore, they are removed surgically or subjected to postoperative radiation.[14]

Radiotherapy

In women with palpable nodes, simple mastectomy and radiotherapy to the axilla and internal mammary lymph nodes is the mode of treatment. Prophylactic postoperative radiation therapy is done in specific situations, depending on the extent of the disease found at the time of surgery.

Immunotherapy

There have been significant results from immunotherapy in breast cancer. Coley's toxin therapy has produced tumor regression in disseminated cancer of the breast. Local immunotherapy with microbial agents and antigens have also effected tumor regression. The use of BCG vaccine in combination with chemotherapy has prolonged remission and survival in some breast cancer patients. Levamisole, a synthetic immunopotentiating agent, has also resulted in prolongation of disease-free intervals and survival in patients with stage III carcinoma in comparison with those patients treated with conventional surgery and radiotherapy. [3]

Hormone Therapy

The rationale for hormonal therapy is based on the fact that normal function of the mammary gland depends on the action of several stimulating hormones including progesterone, prolactin, somatrophin (the growth hormone), mammogen, and especially estrogen. By altering the hormonal environment of the body, the growth of the primary tumor is inhibited. Thus by chemical ablation of those hormones implicated in mammary carcinogenesis and metastasis, the breast tumor would regress. Recent studies done by Dr. Welsch and co-workers at Michigan State University showed that knocking out prolactin "virtually prevents the appearance" of spontaneous mammary cancers in young mice from a strain that has a high incidence of these tumors. [4] The significance of Dr. Welsh's findings for human cancer of the breast is still to be determined. However, other researchers have found that inhibition of prolactin and estrogen (nafoxidine, an experimental estrogen inhibitor currently being studied in Europe) has effected 34% improvement rate in those patients that were treated with hormone inhibitors.

Combination Therapy

As previously mentioned, surgery may be followed by radiotherapy. Chemotherapy may be given in conjunction with immunotherapy. The decision to use combination therapy depends upon the nature and extent of the disease and the response of the patient to the initial treatment received. [8,13]

An important consideration that the surgeon takes into account in the clinical management of breast cancer is that of staging. The TNM classification for cancer of the breast as mutually agreed upon by the American Joint Committee for Cancer

Staging and End Results Reporting and the International Union
Against Cancer is as follows:

Stage I : Tumor 2 cm or less in its greatest dimension, no fixation to underlying pectoral fascia and/or muscle, no
palpable homolateral nodes, nodes do not contain
growth, and no evidence of metastases.

Stage II : Tumor 2 to 5 cm, skin tethered or dimpled, no pectoral fixation, axillary nodes movable, not significant
or significant, and no metastases.

Stage III: Tumor more than 5 cm with extension to the axillary
nodes, supraclavicular or internal mammary nodes
with fixation, and no evidence of metastases.

Stage IV: Tumor more than 5 cm, node fixation, extension to
the axillary nodes, supraclavicular or internal mammary nodes, and presence of distant metastases.

Treatment of breast cancer by stage may be as follows:

Stage I : Lumpectomy, modified radical mastectomy, radical
mastectomy with or without en-bloc dissection of internal mammary nodes, and postoperative radiation
therapy if the lesion is located retroareolar or in the
medial half of the breast.

Stage II : Radical mastectomy with extensive radiation treatment with maximum tumor dose of 3500 rads, prophylactic castration by oophorectomy or irradiation.

Stage III: Local surgery is contraindicated, extensive irradiation of the primary lesion and the gland fields, extirpation of all possible sources of estrogenic stimulation by castration in the premenopause and up to 10
years postmenopause, and use of corticosteroids.

Stage IV: Surgical ablation (removal of an endocrine organ) such
as in oophorectomy, bilateral adrenalectomy, hypophysectomy; addition of exogenous hormones such as
androgens, estrogens, progesterone, testosterone,
and corticosteroids in large doses. If surgical ablation cannot be done, then adrenal suppression is done
by using high doses of cortisone.

NURSING IMPLICATIONS

The nursing care of the patient with breast carcinoma involves
preoperative care, postoperative care, rehabilitation, care after irradiation, specific principles of care during hormonal
therapy, and care of the patient with inoperable cancer.

Preoperative Care of the Patient
Undergoing Surgical Intervention

1. The patient is initially told by the surgeon if there is a possibility of radical mastectomy. Consent obtained and signed
   by the patient should include consent for radical mastectomy as indicated.

2. Skin preparation includes shaving of the axillary area and
   giving the patient a bath prior to day of surgery.

3. Blood type and cross-match results should be in the patient's chart before going to surgery. Any unusual blood
   type should be communicated to the physician so that efforts can be made to have such blood available before surgery is begun.

4. The nurse should know what the patient was told by the surgeon so that she can provide support and reassurance.

5. The nurse should encourage the patient to verbalize her
   feelings about the surgery, especially as it affects the patient's concept of femininity, body image, and relationship
   with her husband.

6. The nurse should accept the patient's reactions to the diagnosis of cancer, whether it be that of anxiety, anger,
   fear of death, or fear of being mutilated. It is important
   for the nurse to be cognizant of the role of sociocultural
   factors in the patient's perception of her illness. For some
   patients, the affective meaning of the surgery may be just
   a necessary surgical experience, for others, it may mean
   the beginning of a death process.[20,22]

7. If the patient is unable to accept the surgery, inform the
   physician so that postoperative serious sequelae, such as
   depression or inability to recognize and to acknowledge that
   a breast has been removed, may be prevented. A preoperative visit by a recovered mastectomy patient may help
   the patient to accept the need for treatment more readily.[15]

8. If a graft will be needed during the surgical intervention,
   the anterior surface of the patient's thigh is shaved preoperatively for this purpose.

9. Preoperative teaching should include the types of exercises
   that the patient will be expected to do after her surgery.
   This will not only insure more cooperation on the part of

the patient to do the exercises but also reassures the patient that she will come out of the anesthesia, thereby allaying her fear of not waking up again (fear of anesthesia).

10. If the patient has to be transferred to an intensive care unit (ICU) after surgery, she should be told preoperatively so that when she awakens, she will understand the change in her environment. Preferably, the patient should be given a chance to see the ICU and the surgical suite before surgery so that her anxiety may be diminished, since she will have some knowledge of where she will be taken for surgery.

11. The patient should also be informed of what to expect after surgery in terms of having pain (analgesics will be available for her), dressings and dressing changes (including Hemovac drainage), and proper positioning and care of the affected limb.

Postoperative Care of the
Patient With Mastectomy

1. Proper positioning of the patient's affected arm is essential to prevent lymphedema due to venous and lymph stasis. This involves placing one or two pillows under the affected arm to provide support and to elevate the arm so that the hand and elbow are higher than the level of the shoulder. Sometimes the patient's affected arm is bandaged to the body with the elbow bent at right angles, especially if grafting has been done. In this case, the nurse should check any signs of impaired circulation such as swelling, cyanosis of the fingers, coldness, and tingling of the extremity. [19]

2. The care of the drain tube (Hemovac) involves maintenance of negative suction; observation of the color, amount, odor, and consistency of the drainage; and insuring aseptic technique when emptying the Hemovac.

3. If the dressings become saturated, check for any seepage of fluid from the wound by slipping a hand underneath the patient's back. Inform the physician immediately should seepage occur. The nurse should check the dressings every 15 minutes during the immediate postoperative period and then at least three times a day after the first 24 hours postoperation for two to three days. The dressings are not changed until about the 5th to the 9th day postoperation, especially if a graft was done. The drain tube may be taken

out as soon as the amount of drainage is less than 100 cc in a 24-hour period.

4. Prepare the patient for the initial dressing change; talk about it prior to the experience. The patient may react with hysteria, anger, crying, depression, or withdrawal. The nurse should allow for expression of the patient's feelings.

5. Ambulation in the first postoperative day is done with the nurse providing support to the patient by staying on the un-affected side so that if the patient loses balance, the nurse can hold her on the unaffected arm. This would prevent in-jury to the suture line. In ambulating the patient, instruct her to keep her shoulders level and the muscles relaxed. The affected arm is put in a sling for support.

6. Patient teaching should include wound and arm care, pre-vention of infection and lymphedema, and the use of pros-thesis.

7. Encourage the patient to look at the incision prior to dis-charge, but do not insist on it at the first dressing change. To assist the patient to come to grips with her altered body image, try to focus on something positive and specific, such as the signs of wound healing or less swelling which may ease the way towards acceptance of the distorted body im-age. If the patient is hesitant to look at the incision, use general leads such as: "You seem not to be able to look at the incision," which may open the door to a discussion of the patient's feelings. Sometimes the involvement of a rel-ative in dressing change can be very supportive to the pa-tient. Acceptance of the patient by the health team mem-bers and her family for what she is as a person is most es-sential in rehabilitation.

8. Primary nursing can best benefit the patient. When the pa-tient wakes up from anesthesia, it would be very reassur-ing if she sees her primary nurse and if what was done in surgery is explained to her in simple, understandable lan-guage. This is especially important if the patient signed for a "breast biopsy, possible radical mastectomy." The patient needs to know if she still has her breast or not and the extent of the surgery performed. The physician needs to tell the patient what was done and then the nurse can clarify the patient's questions.

Rehabilitation of the
Breast Cancer Patient

The concept of rehabilitation of the breast cancer patient involves a multidisciplinary approach to the care of the patient
as a whole human being within a continuum commencing at the
time of diagnosis and continued through the patient's readaptation to society. The rehabilitation team consists of physicians,
nurses, social workers, long-term mastectomy patient volunteers, the patient, and her family.

Some of the rehabilitative measures that can be done for the patient follow. [10]

1. Assist the patient to express her feelings. The principles
    of care of the patient with fear have been discussed previ-
    ously in Part IV, Chapter 11.

2. Assist the patient to sort out the real from the unreal. Re-
    peated explanation of the diagnosis, treatment, and progno-
    sis may be necessary. Fear of the unknown is very intense
    preoperatively since the patient cannot be sure of the out-
    come of the surgery. Fear of recurrence is experienced
    postoperatively. Honest communication with the patient will
    dispel her fears of the unreal.

3. Refrain from giving false reassurance. Be certain of how
    much the patient has been told about her condition and pro-
    vide emotional support. Be careful in providing reassur-
    ance that pertains to the family relationship such as: "Don't
    worry, I am sure your husband will understand." It is im-
    portant for the nurse to be cognizant of the prior relation-
    ship of the patient with her family, her attitude, and the
    family's attitude towards the surgery. If the family rela-
    tionship is healthy, then it would be helpful to involve the
    family in providing emotional support to the patient.

4. Assist the patient to anticipate the future. The patient
    should be told the length of her physical rehabilitation. She
    should also be informed of the possible effects of her sur-
    gery in terms of mood changes, depression, and the physi-
    ological effects of oophorectomy (if performed).

5. Assist the patient's family to cope with their own feelings
    and to understand the patient. The family needs as much
    support as the patient does. They should be encouraged to
    verbalize their feelings. If the patient is married, the hus-
    band should be included in the patient education program

designed to meet the needs of the patient. A husband who is reassured of the best possible care for his wife can be most supportive to his wife and the rest of the family.

6. Assist the patient to readapt to her lifestyle after surgery. The patient's postoperative exercises are designed to enable her to regain her strength and to restore function. During the first 24 hours postoperation, the patient begins to do exercises with the affected arm in order to stimulate circulation which helps restore function. These exercises include pronation and supination of the hand, opening and closing the hand, flexing and extending of the fingers, bending the wrist forward and backward, brushing teeth, washing the face, combing hair, and squeezing a rubber ball. The nurse should encourage the patient to perform these exercises every day. Additional exercises which may be ordered by the physician for the patient are "climbing the wall" exercise, rope turning, pendulum swinging, hair brushing, and, finally, abduction exercises such as buttoning her dress in the back. If the patient had a graft, the exercises will be gradually increased according to her tolerance and rate of wound healing.

Prior to discharge, the patient may benefit from participation in a Reach to Recovery program, which is sponsored by the American Cancer Society. This program entails visits from a recovered mastectomy patient. The purpose of the visits is to assist the patient in her psychologic and cosmetic needs. The recovered mastectomy patient can share her own feelings and experiences in her readaptation to her lifestyle after her surgery. The types of prosthesis available are discussed with the patient so she can select what she would be most comfortable with.

Since it takes about two to six months for the wound to completely heal, the nurse should give discharge instructions to the patient in terms of what activities she can do to develop her strength further and to promote muscle tone, such as drying her back with a towel, reaching out when making a bed, and gradually resuming her daily work activities. She should be instructed to avoid fatigue, to carry packages on the unaffected side, to examine the remaining breast regularly, and to check with her physician when she can play tennis or golf if these are her major diversional activities.

Care of the Patient
After Irradiation Therapy

The principles of care after irradiation have already been discussed in Part III, Chapter 9.

Specific Principles of Care of the
Patient During Hormonal Therapy

1. Watch for side effects of estrogen therapy, which include nausea, vomiting, pigmentation of remaining nipple and areola, uterine bleeding, stress incontinence, sodium retention manifested by presence of edema, and hyperglycemic reactions.

2. Watch for side effects of androgen therapy, such as fluid retention manifested by weight gain, virilization (deeper voice, coarsening of the skin), hirsutism (appearance of hair on the face and rest of the body), and increased libido.

3. If the patient has edema, give a low sodium diet, diuretics as ordered by the physician, and weigh the patient daily.

4. Observe for signs and symptoms of hypercalcemia as a result of estrogen therapy, which include insomnia, lethargy, anorexia, nausea, vomiting, and eventually coma and vascular collapse if not treated. To prevent hypercalcemia give copious fluids to the patient.

5. If surgical ablation was done to effect change in the hormonal environment of the patient's body, the nurse should be cognizant of the effects of adrenalectomy and hypophysectomy in order to anticipate the needs of the patient. For instance, the patient will need replacement cortisone therapy for the rest of her life. Hence, the nurse should instruct the patient on the importance of taking her cortisone medication regularly as ordered since any lapse in replacement therapy may cause the patient to go into adrenal crisis. This is manifested by decrease in blood pressure, elevation of temperature, nausea, vomiting, diarrhea, abdominal pain, and weakness. There may also be mood changes as cortisone therapy is being regulated. Thus the patient and her family should realize the importance of accepting the patient's behavior of depression, anger, irritability, or elation.

6. The nurse should be aware of the toxic manifestations of corticosteroid therapy, viz., gastrointestinal bleeding,

congestive heart failure due to sodium and fluid retention,
diabetes mellitus, osteoporosis, increased susceptibility
to infection, hypokalemia, and hypertension.

7. The nurse should inform the patient that her requirement
    for steroid can be increased during stressful situations
    such as illness or injury which may cause the patient to
    have adrenal insufficiency. The manifestations of adrenal
    insufficiency are similar to adrenal crisis and the patient
    should be told to contact her physician if she experiences
    these symptoms. [13]

8. The nurse should realize the importance of careful assess-
    ment and observation of the patient after a hypophysectomy
    for signs and symptoms of diabetes insipidus manifested
    initially by excessive urinary output (polyuria) and exces-
    sive thirst (polydipsia). If the polyuria persists, electro-
    lyte imbalance may occur. Therefore, the nurse should
    report to the physician when polyuria persists so that the
    patient may be given pitressin tannate in oil or posterior
    pituitary powder as snuff.

Care of the Patient with
Inoperable Breast Carcinoma

When the metastasis has become so widespread that radical
mastectomy is contraindicated, then palliative treatment is the
goal of therapy. The nurse can play a vital role in the palliative
treatment through various nursing care measures designed to
make the patient more comfortable and to live the remainder of
her life with some meaning and feeling of a sense of control.

1. For the patient with bone metastases, the nurse should han-
    dle the patient gently, especially when turning the patient
    since movement aggravates pain. The nurse should assess
    the efficacy of pain medication so that it can be changed if
    tolerance to the drug develops. If the nursing observation
    validates intractability of the patient's pain, then the physi-
    cian should be informed so that cordotomy may be consid-
    ered as means of relieving the pain.

    The nurse should prevent fractures by instructing the pa-
    tient to be careful in climbing up stairs and to refrain from
    activities that require reaching, twisting, excessive bend-
    ing, or stretching.

2. The patient with chest and soft tissue metastases suffers
    from lesions over her chest, pain on breathing, and

shortness of breath. The nurse can assist the patient to alleviate these discomforts by positioning her in an upright position in bed to ease the breathing and the pain, and by caring for the chest lesions through daily dressing change. To make the patient feel in control of her situation, she should be taught how to change her dressings. The patient's family may also benefit from similar instruction in order to make them feel they are doing something for the patient. If the patient has a problem sleeping due to inability to breathe while lying down, she should be told to sleep in a semi-upright or upright position using several pillows, or may even use a recliner as a bed.[6]

3. When brain metastases is present, the patient may have loss of short-term memory, seizures, visual disturbances, and difficulty in swallowing, eating, talking, and walking. The nurse can provide personalized care of the patient by:[9]
   a. Making herself available to the patient.
   b. Assisting the patient with feedings; it may be necessary to institute tube feedings.
   c. Insuring protection from injury by assisting the patient when ambulating and by having available at the bedside a padded tongue blade, an airway, and suction machine in case the patient goes into seizure.
   d. Talking with the patient slowly so she can better understand.

4. If ascites or pleural effusion occurs, the nurse should anticipate the need for abdominal paracentesis and thoracentesis, respectively. If any of these procedures is to be done, the nurse should instruct the patient on what to do during and after the procedure, provide reassurance to the patient, and have the equipment available for the physician's use.

CANCER OF THE MALE BREAST

The tumor mass found in male breast carcinoma is firm and poorly delimited (with the exception of the colloid variety to carcinoma, which feels soft), as is the female breast tumor.[5] It is much easier to palpate the presence of a palpable mass in males than in females due to the less dense conformation in male breasts. In advanced carcinoma of the male breast, the local signs are the same as for the female. These are ulceration, edema of breast and arm, fixation to chest wall, and presence of metastatic nodules.

The prognosis of male breast carcinoma is more ominous than female breast cancer because (1) the male breast tissue is small and therefore the cancer cells readily reach the lymphatics (60% to 80% of males presenting with breast cancer have axillary metastases) and (2) the appearance of a palpable mass in the male may be considered as a form of benign gynecomastia until fixation and discharge occur, which would then alert the physician that the cancer is already advanced.

In early operable cancer of the male breast, radical mastectomy with axillary node dissection and skin grafting yields a five-year survival rate.

COSMETIC RECONSTRUCTION IN BREAST CANCER PATIENTS

In some studies, it has been found that offering the patient the chance for reconstruction of the breast before the surgery is performed can provide comfort to the patient. It has also been suggested that the patient should be allowed to have a simple breast reconstruction postoperatively.[23] Others have cited silicone implants as means of effecting "astounding" psychological improvement. Notwithstanding the positive effects of reconstructive surgery, its applicability depends to a large extent upon the patient's prognosis.

REVIEW QUESTIONS

1. What is the leading cause of death from cancer in women?
2. What is the overall survival rate of breast cancer?
3. List four factors that influence the prognosis of breast carcinoma.
4. In what part of the breast does cancer occur most?
5. Name the seven high-risk groups for cancer of the breast.
6. Identify some of the etiologic factors believed to cause cancer of the breast.
7. How long can breast cancer remain undetected by palpation?
8. What is the only sign of early breast carcinoma?
9. Enumerate some of the observations that should be noted during a careful breast examination.
10. List the diagnostic tests that may be done in breast cancer detection and diagnosis.
11. Define:
    a. Radical mastectomy
    b. Simple mastectomy
    c. Lumpectomy
    d. Partial mastectomy
    e. Subcutaneous mastectomy
    f. Modified radical mastectomy.

12. List four immunotherapeutic methods used in the treatment of breast cancer.
13. What is the rationale for hormonal therapy in breast cancer?
14. Describe the four clinical stages of cancer according to the TNM classification.
15. What stage of cancer would best be treated with surgical ablation?
16. In what stage of cancer would local surgery be contraindicated?
17. Define rehabilitation.
18. When does rehabilitation of the breast cancer patient begin?.
19. Enumerate six rehabilitation measures which can be done for a patient with breast cancer.
20. What are the side effects of irradiation therapy?
21. What discharge instructions should the nurse give to the patient who has had a radical mastectomy?
22. What are the side effects of estrogen therapy? What are the side effects of androgen therapy?
23. List the signs and symptoms of hypercalcemia.
24. Name the clinical manifestations of adrenal crisis (adrenal insufficiency).
25. List the toxic effects of corticosteroid therapy.
26. What is a complication of hypophysectomy?
27. What drug is used to treat polyuria resulting from hypophysectomy?
28. What type of treatment would be given to a patient with inoperable cancer of the breast?
29. Enumerate nursing care principles in the care of a patient with
    a. Bone metastases
    b. Chest and soft tissue metastases
    c. Brain metastases

30. Why is the prognosis of male breast cancer more ominous than that of female carcinoma?
31. What are the effects of cosmetic reconstructive surgery of the breast after a radical mastectomy?

REFERENCES

1. Oschner, A., Diseases of the Breast. Nursing Digest, IV(2):5-7 (March/April, 1976).
2. Spingarn, N.D., Breast Cancer: New Choices. Nursing Digest, pp. 33-36 (January/February, 1976).
3. Rojas, A.F., Feierstein, J.N., et al., Levamisole in Advanced Human Cancer. Lancet, 1:211-215 (1976).

4. Hope in Breast Cancer Hormone Therapy. Med. World News, p. 80 (May 10, 1974).
5. Fass, M. and Preston, W. (eds.), Clinical Concepts in Cancer Management - A Self Instruction. McGraw Hill Books, Blakiston Publishing Co., New York (1976).
6. Gribbons, C. and Aliapoulios, M., Treatment for Advanced Carcinoma. Am. J. Nurs., pp. 678-682 (April, 1972).
7. Harrell, H.C., To Lose a Breast. Am. J. Nurs., pp. 676-677 (April, 1972).
8. Gutterman, J., Blumenschein, G., et al., Immunotherapy for Breast Cancer. Breast, 2(2):29-33 (April-June, 1976).
9. McCorkle, M.R., Coping with Physical Symptoms in Metastatic Breast Cancer. Am. J. Nurs., pp. 1034-1038 (June, 1973).
10. Rehabilitation of the Breast Cancer Patient. American Cancer Society, New York (1971).
11. Cancer of the Breast: A Report on Research. American Cancer Society, No. 0385 (1971).
12. Egan, J., Sayler, C., and Goodman, M., A Technique for Localizing Occult Breast Lesions. CA, 26(1):32-37 (January/February, 1976).
13. Rubens, R.D., Breast Cancer: Chemotherapy and Management of Special Problems. Nursing Times, pp. 1334-1336 (August 21, 1975).
14. Rubens, R.D., Management of Advanced Breast Cancer. Nursing Times, pp. 1287-1289 (August 14, 1975).
15. Roberts, J., Mastectomy - A Patient's Point of View. Nursing Times, pp. 1290-1291 (August 14, 1975).
16. Goldsmith, H.S., Milk-Rejection, Sign of Breast Cancer. Nursing Digest, pp. 37-38 (January/February, 1976).
17. Savlov, E., Breast Cancer. In: Clinical Oncology for Medical Students and Physicians, American Cancer Society, pp. 129-149 (1974).
18. Smith, D. and Germain, C., Care of the Adult Patient. J.B. Lippincott Co., New York, pp. 974-984 (1975).
19. Shafer, K., et al., Medical-Surgical Nursing. C.V. Mosby Co., St. Louis, pp. 734-745 (1971).
20. Asken, M., Psychoemotional Aspect of Mastectomy: A Review of Recent Literature. Am. J. Psychiatry, 132(1): 56-59 (January, 1975).
21. Rubin, P. (ed.), Cancer of the Breast. Current Concepts in Cancer Multidisciplinary Views. American Cancer Society, No. 3007.04 (1974).
22. Akehurst, A.C., Post-Mastectomy Morale. Lancet, 2: 181-182 (1972).
23. Snyderman, R.K. and Guthrie, R.H., Reconstruction of the Female Breast Following Radical Mastectomy. Plast. Reconstr. Surg., 47:565-567 (1971).

24. Wastell, C., Axillary Lymph Nodes in Breast Cancer. Surg. Ann., 10:123-133 (1978).

25. Hortobagyi, G.N., Gutterman, J.U., et al., Immunotherapy and Chemoimmunotherapy for Human Breast Cancer. In: Immunotherapy of Human Cancer, Raven Press, New York, pp. 321-345 (1978).

26. Bonadonna, G., Valagussa, P., et al., Are Surgical Adjuvant Trials Altering the Course of Breast Cancer? Semin. Oncol., 5(4):450-464 (December, 1978).

27. Carbone, P.P. and Davis, T.E., Medical Treatment for Advanced Breast Cancer. Semin. Oncol., 5(4):417-427 (December, 1978).

28. Harris, J.R., Levene, M.B., et al., The Role of Radiation Therapy in the Primary Treatment of Carcinoma of the Breast. Semin. Oncol., 5(4):403-416 (December, 1978).

29. Veronesi, U., Value of Limited Surgery for Breast Cancer. Semin. Oncol., 5(4):395-402 (December, 1978).

30. Rilke, F., Andreola, S., et al., The Importance of Pathology in Prognosis and Management of Breast Cancer. Semin. Oncol., 5(4):360-372 (December, 1978).

31. Hughes, L.E. and Forbes, J.F., Early Breast Cancer: Part II. Management. Br. J. Surg., 65(11):764-772 (November, 1978).

32. Roswit, B. and Edlis, H., Carcinoma of the Male Breast: A Thirty-Year Experience and Literature Review. Int. J. Radiat. Oncol. Biol. Phys., 4(7-8):711-716 (July-August, 1978).

33. Urban, J.A., Management of Operable Breast Cancer: The Surgeon's View. Cancer, 42(4):2066-2077 (October, 1978).

34. Piro, A.J. and Hellman, S., Effect of Primary Treatment Modality on the Metastatic Pattern of Mammary Carcinoma. Cancer Treatm. Rep., 62(9):1275-1280 (September, 1978).

35. Hubay, C.A., Barry, F.M., and Marr, C.C., Pregnancy and Breast Cancer. Surg. Clin. North Am., 57(4):819-831 (August, 1978).

36. Fisher, B., Redmond, C., and Fisher, E.R., Clinical Trials and the Surgical Treatment of Breast Cancer. Surg. Clin. North Am., 58(4):723-736 (August, 1978).

37. Fisher, E.R., The Pathologist's Role in the Diagnosis and Treatment of Invasive Breast Cancer. Surg. Clin. North Am., 58(4):705-721 (August, 1978).

38. Barna, B.P. and Deodhar, S.D., Immunology, Tumor Markers, and Breast Cancer. Surg. Clin. North Am., 58(4):693-704 (August, 1978).

39. Cooperman, A.M. and Esselstyn, C.B., Jr., Breast Cancer: An Overview. Surg. Clin. North Am., 58(4):659-666 (August, 1978).

40. Haagensen, C.D., Lane, N., et al., Lobular Neoplasia (So-Called Lobular Carcinoma in Situ) of the Breast. Cancer, 42(2):737-769 (August, 1978).

41. Nenci, I., Beccati, M.D., and Pagnini, C.A., Estrogen Receptors and Post-Receptor Markers in Human Breast Cancer: A Reappraisal. Tumor I, 64(2):161-174 (April, 1978).

42. Aisner, J., Specialty Rounds. Management of Disseminated Carcinoma of the Breast. Am. J. Med. Sci., 275 (1):5-16 (January-February, 1978).

43. Rossi, A. and Bonadonna, G., Surgical Adjuvant Chemotherapy in Breast Cancer with Positive Axillary Lymph Nodes. Antibiot. Chemother., 24:229-242 (1978).

44. Heuson, J.C., Leclercq, G., and Mattheiem, W.H., Present Indication for Endocrine Therapy and Chemotherapy in Advanced Breast Cancer. Antibiot. Chemother., 24:189-204 (1978).

45. Woo, K.B., Waalkes, T.P., et al., A Quantitative Approach to Determining Disease Response During Therapy Using Multiple Biologic Markers: Application to Carcinoma of the Breast. Cancer, 41(5):1685-1703 (May, 1978).

46. Cooper, R., et al., Adjuvant Chemotherapy of Breast Cancer. Cancer, 44(3):793-798 (September, 1979).

47. Hagemeister, F.B., Causes of Death in Breast Cancer: A Clinicopathologic Study. Cancer, 46(1):162-167 (July, 1980).

48. Gautherie, M. and Gross, C.M., Breast Thermography and Cancer Risk Prediction. Cancer, 45(1):51-63 (January, 1980).

49. Hall, D.C., et al., Improved Detection of Human Breast Lesions Following Experimental Training. Cancer, 46(2): 408-414 (July, 1980).

50. Manni, A., Transphenoidal Hypophysectomy in Breast Cancer - Evidence for an Individual Role of Pituitary and Gonadal Hormones in Supporting Tumor Growth. Cancer, 44(6):2330-2337 (December, 1979).

51. Moskowitz, M., Breast Cancer: How Can We Reduce Mortality? Consultant, 19(9):47-60 (September, 1979).

52. Plotkin, D., Ten Questions Physicians Often Ask . . . About Managing Mastectomy Patients. Consultant, 19(3): 49-60 (March, 1979).

53. Sheikh, K.M., et al., Ductular Carcinoma of the Breast, Serum Antibodies to Tumor-Associated Antigens. Cancer, 44(6):2088-2089 (December, 1979).

54. Sober, A.J. and Fitzpatrick, F., Melanoma: Be Ready for It. Consultant, 19(9):23-31 (September, 1979).

55. Nemoto, T., et al., Management and Survival of Female Breast Cancer: Results of a National Survey by the

American College of Surgeons. Cancer, 45(12):2917-2924 (June, 1980).

56. Stabile, R.J., Reconstructive Breast Surgery Following Mastectomy and Adjunctive Radiation Therapy. Cancer, 45(11):2738-2743 (June, 1980).

57. See-Lasley, K. and Ignoffo, R., Manual of Oncology Therapeutics. C.V. Mosby Co., St. Louis, pp. 171-178 (1981).

CHAPTER 25
Prostatic Carcinoma

Cancer of the prostate is the most common cancer in elderly males and is the third most frequent cause of cancer death in males. The median age of those afflicted with the disease is 70, with increasing incidence after 50. Carcinoma of the prostate is most predominant among blacks, while the least affected are the Chinese and Japanese. Almost all (97%) prostatic cancers are adenocarcinomas. About 75% of the neoplasms are located in the posterior and medial lobes of the prostate which make them very accessible to digital rectal examination. Since most of the neoplasms are located in the posterior lobe, urinary symptoms tend to occur late. Although most of the tumors grow slowly and are asymptomatic for many years, a few of them are highly malignant and progress rapidly with widespread osseous metastases into the vertebrae, ribs, sacrum, pelvis, and other proximal bones. The osseous spread is attributed to the communication of the plexus of the veins of the prostate gland with the vesical vein plexus, deep dorsal veins of the penis, and internal iliac veins which directly communicate with the vertebral venous plexus.

ETIOLOGY

There is no known cause of prostatic cancer, although hormonal relationships have been established.

CLINICAL MANIFESTATIONS

Early symptoms of prostatic cancer are related to its position at the bladder neck. The symptoms which are associated with prostatic carcinoma include unexplained cystitis, difficulty starting urination, dribbling, increasing frequency, dysuria, and urine retention. These result from bladder-neck obstruction by the neoplastic growth. Later signs and symptoms of a more advanced disease are hard, irregular, and nodular gland, a complete urine retention, deep-seated rectal pain, bone pain, hematuria, and anemia.[2,5]

DIAGNOSTIC TESTS AND DIAGNOSIS

1. Rectal examination: Nodular gland can be felt.
2. Biopsy
   a. Needle aspiration
   b. Open biopsy: open perineal, transrectal, and trans-urethral.
3. Chemical Tests
   a. Serum acid phosphatase (SAP): This is useful in assessing status of the disease before and after therapy. If the SAP level is elevated before treatment and then returns to normal after therapy, it indicates that the therapy was effective. Most often SAP levels increase with onset of relapse. SAP is frequently elevated in prostatic carcinoma and almost never increased in benign prostatic hypertrophy (BPH). It is well to note that SAP levels are also increased by other diseases such as breast carcinoma, osteogenic sarcoma, multiple myeloma, thrombocytopenia, thromboembolic disease, and prostatic infarcts and rectal trauma, e.g., rectal examination.
   b. Alkaline phosphatase: Levels are increased with bone metastases.
4. Bone survey and bone scan: These are done to evaluate the extent of metastatic spread.

STAGING AND TREATMENT

Treatment and prognosis, like other malignant neoplastic growths, are dependent on the stage of the disease. In prostatic carcinoma, stage A refers to a well-differentiated, small, occult lesion in situ. Stage B, the tumor may be still small or large but is confined to the gland. In stage C, the prostatic capsule is invaded, there is partial invasion of the areolar tissue around the base of the seminal vesicles, lymph node involvement and SAP levels are elevated. In stage D, osseous metastases and other extrapelvic involvement have occurred.[2,5]

THERAPEUTIC AND PALLIATIVE MEASURES

Radical Prostatectomy

Radical prostatectomy is the treatment of choice which may be a perineal, retropubic or trans-sacral route. The retropubic approach is favored. This treatment is utilized for stages A and B and for patients who are less than 70 years old and have good prognosis with no evidence of metastases. The prostate gland, seminal vesicles, and cuff of the bladder neck are extirpated.

Complications include incontinence (5 to 15%), impotence (50 to 90%), and increased fibrinolysins which can cause uncontrolled bleeding.[1,3,7]

Radiation

Radiation has been successfully utilized. Interstitial implantation (i.e., gold-198 or [198]Au) plus prostatectomy have shown favorable effects in lessening urinary symptoms and decreasing recurrences. Supervoltage irradiation with a tumor dose of 3000 to 3500 rads has been used to irradiate the prostate and pelvic lymph nodes. This therapy is also utilized in stages A and B and in relieving bone pain from osseous metastases. The advantage of this therapy is preservation of continence, and potency is usually maintained.[4]

Orchiectomy and/or Estrogen Therapy

Orchiectomy and/or Estrogen Therapy have been employed when surgery or radiation treatment cannot be used. This mode of treatment has caused regression in the size of the prostate and bone metastases have disappeared in widespread metastatic disease. Diethylstilbestrol is most widely used. The most common side effect of therapy is gynecomastia which can be prevented by prechemotherapy radiation. Cardiovascular problems, sodium retention, edema, nausea, and vomiting are other side effects. Cyproterone acetate (antiandrogen) has also been used in advanced cases.

Adrenalectomy and Hypophysectomy

Adrenalectomy and hypophysectomy have been tried for ablation of metastatic disease. It has been postulated that the malignant prostate responds to hormonal stimulation or castration just like that of a normal prostate gland. Excisional hypophysectomy and irradiation with radioactive yttrium-90 (^{90}Y) have caused some patients to experience appreciable subjective and objective changes in the progress of the disease.[6,7]

Systemic Administration
of Sodium Phosphate

Systemic administration by intravenous route of sodium phosphate (^{32}P) has been tried in widespread osseous metastases with some objective and symptomatic improvement, especially with the adjuvant use of testosterone.[6]

NURSING IMPLICATIONS

The patient who has had a radical prostatectomy should be monitored for possible hemorrhage due to fibrinolysins. The patient is usually given aminocaproic acid which inhibits plasmin and plasminogen activators, thereby averting uncontrolled bleeding.

Urinary incontinence, a likely sequela of surgery, can eventually be overcome by continued perineal exercises. The exercise which entails contracting the perineal, gluteal, and abdominal muscles can be initiated 24 to 48 hours, postoperatively. Use of absorbent drainage pads with T binder, aseptic dressing changes, open wound care and sitz baths after an abdominoperineal resection is discussed in Part V, Chapter 31.

The suprapubic drain may remain in place longer than 48 hours. Possible urine leakage around the catheter and from the insertion site after its removal necessitates meticulous skin care. Due care is taken to maintain suprapubic (S-P) tube patency and to prevent inadvertent removal.

The urethral catheter is left in place for a much longer period. Closed drainage system is maintained and adequate hydration and optimum activity are encouraged to help minimize infection. Periodic culture of urine and any drainage from the wound are instituted by the nurse as needed.

The threat of an imminent and permanent impotence should have been explored with the patient prior to performance of a radical prostatectomy. Continued emotional support should be given and utilization of family support systems should be encouraged.

REVIEW QUESTIONS

1. What is the most common cancer in elderly males aged 50-70?
2. Why do urinary symptoms tend to occur late in the presence of prostatic cancer?
3. Explain why osseous spread readily occurs in prostatic carcinoma.
4. List six signs and symptoms of advanced carcinoma of the prostate.
5. What is the significance of elevated serum acid phosphatase in cancer of the prostate?
6. Give three complications of radical prostatectomy.
7. Discuss the need for orchiectomy and/or estrogen therapy in prostatic cancer.

8. Why is aminocaproic acid used after a prostatectomy?
9. How can urinary incontinence be alleviated after a radical prostatectomy?
10. Explain why impotence is likely to occur after a radical perineal prostatectomy.

REFERENCES

1. American Cancer Society, Current Concepts in Cancer, Multidisciplinary Views. Cancer of the Urogenital Tract: Part II, (Prostate and Testes) (September, 1974).
2. Brunner, L. and Suddarth, D., Textbook of Medical-Surgical Nursing. J.B. Lippincott Co., Philadelphia, pp. 663-667 (1975).
3. Derrick, F.C., Cancer of the Prostate and Other Prostatic Problems. Postgrad. Med., pp. 123-126 (October, 1973).
4. Hazra, T.A., The Role of Radiotherapy for Prostatic Carcinoma. Geriatrics, pp. 62-64 (December, 1973).
5. Rosenblum, R., Practical Guide to the Diagnosis of Carcinoma of the Prostate. Hosp. Med., pp. 31-35 (January, 1976).
6. Frank, I., Cancer of the Prostate. In: Clinical Oncology for Medical Students and Physicians. Rubin, P. and Bakemeier, R., (eds.), The University of Rochester School of Medicine and Dentistry, and American Cancer Society, New York, pp. 275-279 (1974).
7. Catalona, W.J. and Scott, W.W., Carcinoma of the Prostate: A Review. J. Urol., 119(1):1-8 (January, 1978).

CHAPTER 26
Testicular Cancer

Carcinoma of the testes, which is extremely rare in nonwhites, accounts for 1% of all cancers in men and 12% of all cancer deaths in males between the ages of 15 and 34. In children and infants, testicular neoplasms are categorized into: (1) teratomas (mostly benign), (2) embryonal carcinoma of infantile testis (orchioblastoma), and (3) gonadal stromal tumors (3% behave in malignant fashion). While secondary testicular cancers do occur, they are very rare and are mostly of pulmonary and prostatic origin. Right-sided involvement is over 50% and about 1%, usually appearing asynchronously, occur bilaterally. The tumors are often complex and therefore are not completely understood. Most common classification of testicular malignancy includes those of germinal origin, which are seminomas, embryonal carcinomas, teratocarcinomas, choriocarcinomas, and mixed tumors which are of high percentage. These germinal neoplasms tend to spread rapidly via the lymphatics, usually in sequential fashion (iliac and abdominal para-aortic nodes, mediastinal and left cervical nodes). Hematologic spread (early spread is characteristic of choriocarcinoma) is to the lungs, liver, and kidneys.[3,6,7]

ETIOLOGY

There is no known etiology, although genetic factors have been implicated due to the relatively high incidence of testicular malignancy in twins, in brothers, other members of the same family, and the subsequent involvement of the other testis in patients who developed a testicular carcinoma.

Cryptorchid testes (ectopid testes) or previously atrophic testes are also more prone to malignancy. Some factors associated with the increased incidence of malignancy in the ectopic testes are interference with blood supply, gonadal dysgenesis, endocrine disturbances, and an elevated temperature.

CLINICAL MANIFESTATIONS

1. Testicular carcinomas have no early symptoms that are characteristic of the tumor.
2. Usually the tumor presents as a painless, firm, smooth mass.
3. Gynecomastia and nipple tenderness may be present.
4. Metastatic symptoms include left-sided hydrocele and left renal vein compression from involved para-aortic nodes.

DIAGNOSTIC TESTS AND DIAGNOSIS

1. Transillumination is positive in the differential diagnosis of a hydrocele or a spermatocele.
2. Gonadotrophins are elevated, thereby giving a positive Aschheim-Zondek test. An increased serum gonadotrophin is a very specific indicator of tumor activity.
3. 17-Ketosteroids and estrogens are increased.
4. Tumor cells may be found in the semen.
5. Serum alpha fetoproteins, though not specific for testicular tumor, may be increased.
6. Intravenous pyelogram (IVP) may reveal ureteral deviation.
7. Lymphangiogram (24 hours post IVP) should be done, which may be supplemented by venacavography.
8. Testicular biopsy in situ (aspiration) is absolutely contra-indicated.

TREATMENT MODALITIES

The method of treatment for carcinoma of the testes is often controversial, with the exception of treating a primary tumor whereby an orchiectomy with ligation of the spermatic cord at the inguinal ring is the treatment of choice. The modalities of treatment which may be instituted are:[2,3,4,5]

1. Orchiectomy (removal of testicle) and retroperitoneal node dissection (lymphadenectomy) and postoperative radiation of lymphatic channels.
2. External radiation using supervoltage technique (usually cobalt) as treatment of choice for seminomas. Other authorities include with this mode of treatment irradiation of the mediastinal and supraclavicular areas. Lymphadenectomy and chemotherapy may follow if radiation is unsuccessful.
3. Orchiectomy and retroperitoneal lymphadenectomy are done for embryonal carcinomas and teratocarcinomas.
4. Orchiectomy and radical lymphadenectomy combined with chemotherapy are done for choriocarcinoma.

5. Chemotherapy, combined with pre- and postoperative radiation are done for disseminated carcinomas.

NURSING IMPLICATIONS

The unique nursing concern in this type of malignancy is its target population. With young males in their early prime of sexuality, development, and procurement of life goals, the challenges of helping them live their lives to their utmost potential and fulfillment in a relatively smooth and positive way cannot be overemphasized. The threat of cancer, the rigors of radiation and chemotherapy, and the uncertainty of the effects of the disease on one's lifestyle are ever-present realities. With orchiectomy (some surgeons do not remove the scrotum because there is a possibility of scrotal implantation) and local radiation treatment, impotency and sterility should not be a problem unless bilateral involvement has occurred, in which case sterility would be a sequela. Hormonal depletion and loss of seminal fluid on ejaculation can occur. Testosterone is necessary for normal sexual behavior and occurrence of erection, development of accessory sex organs, and sexual characteristics. The nurse should explain to the patient prior to therapy that measures will be instituted to retard or arrest the possible ill effects of the treatment he will receive. Synthetic hormones (testosterone proprionate or testosterone acetate) should be given to augment the deficit and prosthetic devices are always a possibility for the unique needs of the individual patient.[1,2]

REVIEW QUESTIONS

1. What is the target population of testicular cancer?
2. Why is transillumination helpful in diagnosing testicular tumors?
3. Explain why genetic factors are attributed to the development of testicular cancer.
4. What are the factors associated with the increased incidence of malignancy in an ectopic (cryptorchid) testes?
5. Discuss three modes of therapy for germinal cancers of the testes.
6. Give three functions of testosterone.

REFERENCES

1. Bergersen, B., Pharmacology in Nursing. C.V. Mosby Co., St. Louis (1976).
2. Grabstald, H., Testicular Cancer. No. 3377, American Cancer Society, New York (June, 1975).

3. Frank, I., Testis Cancer. In: Clinical Oncology for Medical Students and Physicians. Rubin, P. and Bakemeier, R., (eds.), The University of Rochester School of Medicine and Dentistry, and American Cancer Society, New York, pp. 275-279 (1974).

4. Katz, M.E., Grosbach, A.B., et al., Testicular Germ Cell Tumors: Diagnosis, Management, and the Potential for Cure. Cancer Clin. Trials, 1(4):247-271 (Winter, 1978.

5. Javadpour, N. and Bergman, S., Recent Advances in Testicular Cancer. Curr. Probl. Surg., 15(2):1-64 (February, 1978).

6. Raney, R.B., Jr., Hays, D.M., et al., Paratesticular Rhabdomyosarcoma in Childhood. Cancer, 42(2):729-736 (August, 1978).

7. Aristizabal, S., Davis, J.R., et al., Bilateral Primary Germ Cell Testicular Tumors: Report of Four Cases and Review of the Literature. Cancer, 42(2):591-597 (August, 1978).

CHAPTER 27
Leukemias and Related Nursing Care Principles

Leukemia is a fatal disease of the blood-forming tissues characterized by an abnormal proliferation and maturation of any of the cellular elements of the blood (granulocytes, lymphocytes, monocytes) that affect the bone marrow, spleen, liver, lymph nodes, and the blood components. There are several types of leukemia which occur at varying degrees in children, adults, and at all ages. Acute lymphocytic leukemia (ALL) is a disease which attacks mainly children and young adults; acute myelogenous leukemia (AML) occurs with similar frequency at all ages; chronic myelogenous leukemia (CML) affects those in middle and late life; and chronic lymphocytic leukemia (CLL) is a disease of the aged. Other types of acute leukemia which affect children and young adults include acute monocytic leukemia (AM_OL), acute myelomonocytic leukemia (AMM_OL), and stem cell or undifferentiated leukemia (AUL).

ETIOLOGY

Epidemiologic studies reveal certain evidence that links environmental, genetic, viral, and immunologic factors to the causation of leukemia. Nevertheless, only a very limited number of cases can be identified which indicate that these causative factors have definitely played a role in the occurrence of the disease. Hence, it is still widely acknowledged that the specific cause of leukemia is unknown.

Some of the environmental factors believed to play a role in the causation of leukemia include the following.

1. Ionizing radiation: Patients exposed to massive radiation doses have been found to develop leukemia.[1,2]
2. Chemicals and drugs: Benzene exposure has apparently been associated with subsequent development of leukemia.[3] Other drugs which also have been observed to have a direct role in the subsequent occurrence of leukemia are phenylbutazone,[4] arsenic,[5] and chloramphenicol.[6]

3. Marrow hypoplasia: The marked reduction in hematopoietic cells in the marrow is believed to be a predisposing factor to the development of leukemia.
4. Environmental interactions: This involves the interaction of factors in the environment that tend to increase the incidence of leukemia, which to date have not been fully explored and identified.

In the genetic theory, it is believed that there is an inherited predisposition to leukemia. This is based on the findings of increased rate of occurrence of leukemia in Down's syndrome (mongolism), Fanconi's anemia, Bloom's syndrome, and in Klinefelter's syndrome. There has been a reported increase in the frequency of leukemia in siblings, which further supports the genetic theory of leukemia causation.

Studies have indicated increasing evidence of the role of viruses in animal leukemia.[8] Hence, there is reason to believe that viruses can cause leukemia in humans.[9] Through electron microscopy, certain viruses have been identified in human leukemic cells.[10] On the other hand, immune deficiency has been proposed as a predisposing factor in the development of neoplasia. Several lines of evidence also suggest that the progression of tumors may be related to host immune capabilities.[11]

DIAGNOSIS AND DIAGNOSTIC TESTS

1. Laboratory findings: Normochromic and normocytic anemia and thrombocytopenia are present in nearly all cases of leukemia. Presence of hyperuricemia and myeloblasts in the peripheral blood, and a low, normal, or elevated to marked degree of white cell count.
2. Histochemistry: This is useful in differentiating the type of leukemia present. The differential diagnosis of the type of leukemia has been based on the activity of the enzyme muramidase. This enzyme is present only in cytoplasmic granules. Since lymphocytes (blasts) do not have granules, the muramidase levels are reduced in lymphocytic types of leukemia but are markedly elevated in acute and chronic myelocytic forms. The myelocytes tend to have weak or absent staining with periodic acid-Schiff stain.[12]
3. Bone marrow aspiration or biopsy: These will show an increase in leukemic blasts, often marked; normal precursors are significantly reduced in numbers.

CLINICAL MANIFESTATIONS

All of the various types of leukemia share any combination of the following signs and symptoms:

1. Easy fatigability and malaise.
2. Pallor due to the anemia resulting from crowding of bone marrow with leukemic blasts and decreased formation of megakaryocytes and erythroid precursors.
3. Bleeding due to decreased platelets; the patient may have epistaxis; bleeding gums; petechiae; gastrointestinal, retinal, and intracranial hemorrhage; and ecchymosis.
4. Enlarged liver, spleen, cervical, and axillary lymph nodes may be seen due to leukemia cell infiltration, as these circulate in the bloodstream.
5. Anorexia, weight loss, and irregular fever may be seen due to increased basal metabolic rate.
6. Increased susceptibility to infection may occur due to decreased white blood cells.
7. Meningeal leukemia may result due to infiltration of the central nervous system with the leukemic cells.
8. Signs of respiratory infection such as fever and chills may be present.
9. Pain over long bones and sternum may occur due to the leukemic cells infiltrating the bone marrow.

TREATMENT MODALITIES

The clinical management of leukemia depends upon the type of leukemia involved and the goal(s) of treatment.

Acute Lymphocytic Leukemia (ALL)

This type of leukemia is most common among children between 3 and 4 years; boys are slightly more affected than girls except in the first year. About 80% of children with leukemia have acute lymphocytic leukemia and there are about 2000 to 3000 new cases diagnosed each year. The initial treatment plans for acute lymphocytic leukemia are:[42]

1. Remission induction therapy
2. Consolidation therapy
3. Maintenance therapy.

Remission induction therapy: This may be initiated by chemotherapy using the POMP protocol (prednisolone, vincristine, Oncovin, methotrexate, and mercaptopurine) for five days followed by a 5- to 10-day rest period to allow for bone marrow

recovery. These drugs kill the leukemic cells selectively without damaging the bone marrow precursors of normal red and
white blood cells and platelets. If the child responds to treatment, remission occurs as early as two weeks and generally
no later than six weeks. If it fails, another protocol is tried.
According to Lichtman and Klemperer, initial therapy with vincristine and prednisone leads to a complete remission in 85%
to 90% of children with ALL.[13] Remission is achieved when
blood and bone marrow studies show no evidence of leukemic
cells. L-asparaginase may be given daily intravenously to kill
leukemic cells by preventing them from incorporating an amino
acid essential for protein synthesis. (Normal cells make their
own.)

Consolidation therapy: The initial treatment regimen may be
continued or modified.

Maintenance therapy: Depending on blood and bone marrow findings, the patient is placed on remission maintenance treatment,
generally one course per month for an indefinite period or until
the patient shows signs of relapse. The use of cytarabine (Cytosar) and thioguanine therapy every 12 hours for about 10 days
has been effective. These drugs stop the leukemic cells in the
cell-division stage from synthesizing DNA. Repeated therapy
with these drugs kills over 99% of the leukemic lymphocytes.[32]

Other modalities used in the treatment of ALL include chemotherapy and radiotherapy, immunotherapy, and marrow transplant.[44]

Chemotherapy and radiotherapy: In case of recurrence of the
disease in other parts of the body like the gonads, thymus, and
central nervous system, the use of systemic chemotherapy appears to be inadequate. When meningeal leukemia occurs, intrathecal methotrexate during the first five to eight weeks after
diagnosis with or without cranial irradiation has proved an effective mode of therapy. Carmustine (BiCNU) can cross the
blood-brain barrier and kill leukemia cells that may stay out of
the reach of other drugs in the central nervous system. It is
given alone or with x-ray irradiation.[43]

Immunotherapy: This is generally instituted after six to eight
months of intensive chemotherapy.[40] The procedure for BCG
vaccination regimen and irradiation has been dealt with in Part
III, Chapters 8 and 9, respectively.

Marrow transplant: A patient with ALL can be a candidate for
marrow transplant if he either has not achieved remission or
has relapsed after remission.[37,39]

Prognosis: Children two to eight years of age have the best long-term survival. Those over eight years do not fare as well for some unclear reasons. If the white cell count stays less than 25,000, there is a five-year survival; if it is markedly increased, the survival is two to three years.

Acute Myelogenous Leukemia (AML)

This is seen with almost the same frequency in all ages, although the frequency is increased somewhat in those over 40 years of age. [46]

The principles of treatment of AML rest on two important premises:

1. That two competing clones are present in the bone marrow: a leukemic, and a normal or nearly normal clone.
2. That profound suppression of the leukemic marrow cell population is required in AML to allow the opportunity for a return of normal hematopoiesis. [13]

In view of the need to effect profound suppression, intensive chemotherapy is the treatment of choice. This will be done during the first two months after diagnosis. Remission is achieved in about 50% of patients when the karyotype of mitotic cells is normal, which suggests replacement by a normal or near normal clone. Combined chemotherapy of at least two drugs is maintained for at least two to three years if still in remission and then treatment may be discontinued. Some regimen of drug therapy may be maintained indefinitely if tolerated by the patient. The drugs used in combination are cytarabine, which inhibits biosynthesis of DNA, and thioguanine. [48]

Bone marrow transplant: This may be done for a patient with AML whose prognosis is poor or has relapsed from remission.

Supportive care therapy: The intensive chemotherapy reduces blood cells to very low levels incompatible with life. Hence, supportive measures are undertaken to combat the ill effects of intensive chemotherapy as follows: [31]

1. Platelet transfusions of specialized cell fractions from the blood are made so that when the patient cannot make his own normal marrow cells function, the cells can be replaced.
2. White cell transfusion, reverse isolation techniques, and use of protected environments as well as prophylactic gut-cleansing antibiotics to reduce infection risks during

periods of severe granulocytosis have not yet added greatly to overall results of treatment and are still being studied. Nevertheless, it is important to note that the major cause of death in acute leukemia is infection. Therefore, it is necessary to protect the patient from possible sources of microorganisms.

Prognosis: The median survival of untreated patients with AML is about two months. Intensive chemotherapy has increased the median survival rate to about 13 months.[14]

Chronic Lymphocytic Leukemia (CLL)

This type of leukemia is of slow onset and no symptoms are felt until the patient seeks medical check up for some unrelated medical problem during which time routine laboratory findings would reveal very high concentration of lymphocytes in the circulation, bone marrow, lymph nodes, liver and spleen. CLL is rarely seen in adults less than 35 years of age and increases in frequency with succeeding years. It is more prevalent in males than females and of all the leukemias, familial clustering is most notable, especially in siblings.

Patients with CLL who are symptom-free do not require treatment. Those who have active illness, in whom anemia, thrombocytopenia, hypermetabolism, and splenomegaly are present need treatment in order to reduce the lymphocyte mass in the bone marrow and tissues. Chemotherapy with alkylating agents, especially chlorambucil or cyclophosphamide, is often used. Sometimes splenectomy is beneficial if the patient has hypersplenism. If lymph node masses begin to cause discomfort and disfigurement, local x-ray irradiation is used until it can no longer control the nodes or until systemic reactions of fever, sweating, fatigue, anorexia, and weight loss occur.

Prognosis: The median survival rate of individuals with CLL is approximately seven years after diagnosis. Thus, vigorous therapy has not been necessary. Nonetheless, the possibility of a normal clone of lymphocytes being restored after intensive chemotherapy has paved the way for the development of clinical trials to test this possibility.

Chronic Myelogenous Leukemia (CML)

CML is uncommon before 20 years and increases in frequency with each succeeding decade; it is slightly more predominant in males than females. The onset is insidious and some patients may be discovered as having the disease during a routine medical checkup.

Initial treatment of CML is aimed at relief of fever, sweating, easy fatigability, malaise, reduction of excessive leukocytosis, and arrest of progressive anemia. Chemotherapy with busulfan (Myleran), an alkylating agent given orally, is the modality of treatment. The dosage is based on weekly white cell counts. The goal is to reduce the white cell count from as high as 200,000/mm3 to 20,000 to 5000. Drops below 5000/mm3 are avoided because of possible bone marrow damage and to protect the kidneys from the uric acid resulting from drug-induced cell destruction. Allopurinol is given with plenty of fluids to control hyperuricemia, uricosuria, and renal shutdown. Maintenance therapy with busulfan has no special benefits and increases the risk of the patient developing side effects. Although a patient with CML may be well for awhile, eventually he will enter an accelerated phase of the disease, a blast crisis marked by sudden spurts of immature myeloblasts, and will respond poorly to busulfan. The prognosis at this period is grave and survival is not long, maybe weeks or a few months.

Prognosis: CML's median survival rate is about 3.5 years. The use of busulfan has prolonged survival only slightly but has made the chronic phase less of a morbid experience.[13] In most patients, they are well for several years.

NURSING IMPLICATIONS

The nursing care of the patient with leukemia entails an empathetic and compassionate approach with a great deal of commitment to utilize the best of all available professional skills to provide the most beneficial treatment for the patient. Because of the intricacies of the various modalities of treatment used, the nurse has a vital role in the multidisciplinary approach to patient care. From the time of the patient's diagnosis to the initiation of treatment plans during the maintenance treatment up to the terminal phase of the illness, the nurse will face a tremendous challenge to her professional skills.

Awareness and recognition of the patient's and/or the family's reactions to the diagnosis is essential for the nurse to be able to provide appropriate intervention. As previously discussed in Part IV, Chapter 11, the patient's initial reaction is that of shock or disbelief. But for the child with leukemia, the psychological reaction varies according to the age of the child. The preschool leukemic is mostly concerned with separation anxiety from his parents and of the unfamiliarity and strangeness of a new environment in the hospital. The preteen school age child will have similar concerns plus the ability to comprehend correctly or incorrectly any information he is told or hears. The teenager will be more concerned with the effects of the disease on his lifestyle, activities, and independence from his parents, his dreams for the future, and the reactions of others to his illness.[15]

The principles of nursing intervention during this period should be focused on the following.

1. Honest communication with the patient and the family.
2. Encouragement of questioning and respect for the psychological defenses exemplified including denial, anger, and hysteria.
3. Discussion of the fears of the patient and the family.
4. Referring the concerns of the patient and the family to the appropriate professional who can best handle the situation, such as a social worker or a minister.
5. Establishing rapport with the parents of the child so that parental overprotectiveness and its effects can be explored more easily.
6. Discussion of the possible side effects of various tests and treatment modalities so that the patient and family can better participate in the overall treatment plan within a cooperative and supportive framework. There are occasions when knowledge of the ill effects of therapy can produce anxiety and some hesitancy on the patient or family. The nurse can best deal with this problem by maintaining open lines of communication with them.

The goal of psychosocial intervention is to assist the patient and his family in their adjustment to the illness, hopefully towards acceptance of the disease and its effects on the family constellation lifestyle and relationships. In order to achieve this, the nurse should be sensitive to the following needs of the patient and family:

1. Need for support and assistance in coping with the need to modify family schedule of activities, such as altering vacation plans on account of the patient's illness.
2. Need for support in coping with guilt feelings associated with the occurrence of the illness.
3. Need for understanding and compassion in their emotional outbursts and loss of control of the situation. Denial may have to be tolerated if it helps the family go on with their daily life activities.
4. In the leukemic child, the parents need guidance in how to share the diagnosis with the siblings and how the siblings can be part of the health team's efforts to care for the child.
5. Need for group support among family members themselves.

During the initiation of treatment plans and in the treatment process, the nursing responsibilities are primarily in the preparation of the patient for the treatment, both physically and emotionally, and making careful assessment and observation of the patient's reactions to the treatment he receives.

When intensive chemotherapy is used, the patient and family are told before treatment of the possible side effects of the drugs as discussed in Part III, Chapter 7. For the leukemic child, it is especially important to emphasize the possible physical changes of loss of hair, personality changes (irritability and nightmares), water retention causing edema of the face and extremities, decreased energy, nausea, vomiting, skin rash, mouth ulcers, decreased attention spans, weight loss, and infection so that the parents can be better prepared to cope with these changes. The purpose of reverse isolation should be explained to the parents so that they can help the nursing staff in allaying the child's anxiety when seeing people wearing masks and gowns, which can be very frightening at first. It is the responsibility of the nurse to monitor closely any untoward effects of therapy. If a patient is given intravenous chemotherapy for instance, the nurse should (a) prevent extravasation in order to prevent necrosis of tissue, (b) apply hot packs to extremities to dilate the veins and thereby facilitate intravenous infusion, and (c) observe for the proper rate of infusion and any toxic effects. The nurse should watch for any bronchial spasm if the patient is given L-asparaginase. It is important to note that when drugs which can cause bronchial spasm are administered, they should be given in the presence of a physician and the vital signs should be monitored every 15 minutes.

When irradiation is given to the patient, its toxic effects should be watched closely. In bone marrow transplant, the principles of care include the following:[16,47]

1. Preparation for marrow transplant
   a. Before marrow infusion, the patient's marrow cells and all his leukemic cells must be killed by massive chemotherapy and total body irradiation.
   b. The patient is hydrated with one liter of IV 5% dextrose in water four hours before each dose of cyclophosphamide (Cytoxan) intravenously and every four hours thereafter.
   c. Furosemide (Lasix) is given IV one hour and six hours after each cyclophosphamide (Cytoxan) treatment in order to effect diuresis. The patient is also asked to urinate every three to four hours. The urine pH is maintained at 7 by intravenous administration of sodium

bicarbonate and oral acetazolamide (Diamox) tablets. Allopurinol is given orally to prevent buildup of uric acid deposits.

d. The patient's weight and serum creatinine phosphokinase levels are monitored and daily EKG is done to detect any cardiomyopathy.

e. In the operating room, under general anesthesia, the donor undergoes marrow extraction from the iliac crests by multiple needle aspiration of 400 to 700 cc. This is then filtered, heparinized, and mixed with culture media for infusion.

f. After irradiation, the nurse should watch for side effects of radiation therapy such as nausea, vomiting, alopecia, diarrhea, fever, and severe parotitis (puffy red face). There may be erythema 48 to 72 hours later. Hyperpigmentation may occur in two to three weeks (sun-tanned appearance). Severe mucositis may occur, which is very painful. If it does occur, the patient is kept NPO and hyperalimentation fluids are given to maintain the nutritional state of the patient.

g. A central venous pressure is inserted several days prior to marrow transplant to monitor fluids given and any volume overload during treatment.

h. The patient is washed with a hexachlorophene antibacterial cleanser (pHisoHex), undergoes total body irradiation, is put in an isolation or protected environment and the marrow infusion is given intravenously.

i. During the infusion and afterwards, the patient is watched for volume overload, allergic reaction, and signs and symptoms of pulmonary emboli.

2. Care of the Patient After Marrow Transplant
   a. Strict sterile reverse isolation is maintained.
   b. Vigorous antibiotic therapy is given using cephalothin IV, carbenicillin, and gentamycin as ordered. Nystatin tablets as mouthwash and gentamycin elixir are given to sterilize the gastrointestinal mucosa.
   c. Antibiotic creams are applied to every body orifice and skin folds four times a day.
   d. A hexachlorophene (pHisoHex) bath and shampoo are given twice daily.
   e. Culture of the room is done weekly; the patient's skin and orifices are cultured three times a week.
   f. Furniture and equipment are washed daily.
   g. All foods served to the patient are sterilized.
   h. A daily complete blood count is done (WBC, RBC, platelets, and absolute granulocyte counts). The lowest WBC is expected to occur seven to nine days post-transplant

and then gradually increases as the new marrow begins to function.

i. Daily blood and platelet transfusion is given to protect the patient against hemorrhage and infection for about 25 days. Before any blood is transfused, it is irradiated with 1500 rads to destroy lymphocytes that might cause graft-versus-host reaction.[26]

j. Bone marrow biopsies and aspirations are done once a week for the first four weeks to insure graft "take" and to check any signs of leukemia relapse.

k. Careful observations should be made of any of the following complications which can occur after transplant:[23]

(1) Rejection: This rarely occurs with proper immunosuppression.

(2) Leukemic relapse: This is due to leukemic cells being resistant to cyclophosphamide (Cytoxan) therapy and irradiation prior to transplant, the development of a leukemic growth pattern by the engrafted marrow, or a virus which may cause leukemia change in the engrafted marrow.

(3) Graft-versus-host reaction (GVHR): This is manifested when the lymphocytes (from the donor's graft) infiltrate the host's body and release a lymphokinin that injures and kills host cells by direct contact. The signs and symptoms of GVHR are (1) generalized rash, often in the palms and soles of the feet which become bullous followed by generalized erythema; (2) nausea, vomiting, diarrhea, and abdominal pain; and (3) changes in the liver enzymes and bilirubin levels, and enlarged liver.

The treatment of GVHR includes: (1) intravenous methotrexate on the 3rd, 6th, and 11th day after marrow transplant, then every week for 100 days to overcome methotrexate toxicity; and (2) ATG (antihuman thymocyte globulin) is given to combat GVHR if severe liver and intestinal involvement develop.[25]

There are certain specific nursing care principles in the care of a pediatric leukemia patient which the nurse should adhere to as follows:[17,18,19,22]

1. Gentle handling of the patient to minimize the risk of pain or fracture.

2. Use of primary care nursing.

3. Hand washing of both patient and nurse, especially after bladder and bowel elimination to control infection source.

4. Keep the nails short and clean to protect the patient from injury and thereby prevent foci of infection.
5. Check any skin lesions and report findings to the physician.
6. Frequent mouth care - use of soft toothbrush, rinses, and inspection of any ulceration should be done. If lesions are present, warm sodium bicarbonate or diluted hydrogen peroxide oral rinses are given to the patient. Lidocaine HCl (Xylocaine) ointment may be applied to the mucosal lining of the mouth for comfort. Soft foods and cool drinks should be given rather than a regular diet. The latter has a soothing effect.
7. Avoid any contact with anyone who has had a communicable disease.
8. Medications are given with fruits, ice cream, or soft drinks to make them more palatable.
9. To prevent constipation, give plenty of fluids and fruits, except apples and bananas which tend to be constipating. If unsuccessful, stool softeners such as dioctyl sodium sulfosuccinate (Colace) may be given as prescribed by the physician. Laxatives or enemas are not routinely used.
10. Oral or axillary temperatures are taken, but not rectal to prevent any rectal fissures. Report any temperature of 101°F. Acetaminophen (Tylenol) is usually ordered for any fever, since aspirin interferes with platelet function.
11. Check the urine amount and color, note any frequency or urgency of urination which may indicate urinary tract infection.
12. Therapeutic lotion and bath oil (Alpha Keri) are applied to skin to combat dryness.
13. Watch for any fungal overgrowth such as Candida infections of the mouth, esophagus, genital, and anal areas. Oral Candida infection is indicated by a dark, furry coating or a white patchy coating on the tongue. Treatment for this condition is oral nystatin. In the care of genital or anal candidiasis, nistatin tablets (Mycostatin) or nystatin-neomycin sulphate-gramicidin-triamcinolone acitonide (Mycalog) ointment is used.
14. Involve the parents in the care of the child but assist them to strike a balance between time spent with the child in the hospital and their own lives at home and at work.
15. Institute a program for parents, nurses, hematologists, and other health team members to meet together and discuss the disease, treatment plans, and any areas of concern as well as pent-up feelings. In some institutions, a hematology clinic is made available for this purpose.

In the terminal phase of leukemia, the nursing care is aimed at primarily preparing the patient and the family for the imminent death and providing comfort and reassurance that the patient has lived a meaningful life. The various measures that can be helpful for the dying patient have already been discussed in Chapter 12, Part IV.

Knowledge of the causes of death in adults with leukemia certainly enhances the nurse's appreciation of the need to carefully observe the patient for any signs of infection, toxic effects of therapy, and the patient's coping mechanisms.

REVIEW QUESTIONS

1. What is leukemia?
2. Enumerate the different types of leukemia.
3. Identify some factors believed to cause leukemia.
4. Which diagnostic test is conclusive of leukemia?
5. What enzyme activity would provide a means of differential diagnosis of the type of leukemia present?
6. Enumerate some of the clinical manifestations of leukemia.
7. What are the goals of initial treatment plans of ALL?
8. Define remission.
9. How soon would remission occur after induction therapy of ALL?
10. What drugs are used in the treatment of meningeal leukemia?
11. List the signs and symptoms of meningeal leukemia.
12. What is the prognosis of ALL, AML, CML, and CLL?
13. List the two important premises upon which the principles of treatment of AML are based.
14. What supportive care measures are usually given to a patient with AML?
15. Which type of leukemia is usually asymptomatic and may be discovered during a routine regular physical examination?
16. What drug is used to combat hyperuricemia?
17. What characterizes a blast crisis?
18. Describe the nursing approach to a patient with newly diagnosed leukemia.
19. What is the goal of psychosocial intervention at the time of diagnosis? What is the goal during the course of the disease? What is the goal at the terminal phase of leukemia?
20. List the needs of the patient and family that the nurse should meet in caring for the patient with leukemia.
21. Describe the role of the nurse in intensive chemotherapy, irradiation, and bone marrow transplant.
22. What are some specific nursing care principles to be adhered to when caring for a child with leukemia?
23. How do the adult, preschool, and preteen age pediatric react to the diagnosis of leukemia?

24. Name the complications of bone marrow transplant.
25. Define GVHR. What nursing observations would indicate occurrence of GVHR?
26. Describe the treatment of GVHR.
27. Describe the care of the patient before a marrow transplant and after the marrow transplant.
28. In the terminal phase of leukemia, what are the major goals of nursing intervention?
29. What is the major cause of death in adults with leukemia?

REFERENCES

1. Van Pelt, A. and Cogden, C.C., Radiation Leukemia in Guinea Pigs. Radiat. Res., 52:68 (1972).
2. Vigliani, E.C. and Saita, G., Benzene and Leukemia. N. Eng. J. Med., 271:812 (1964).
3. Ryser, H.J., Chemical Carcinogens. N. Eng. J. Med., 285:271 (1971).
4. Leavesley, G.M. and Stenhouse, N.S., Phenylbutazone and Leukemia. Med. J. Australia, 22:963 (1971).
5. Kjeldsberg, C.R. and Ward, H.P., Leukemia in Arsenic Poisoning. Ann. Intern. Med., 77:935 (1969).
6. Brauer, J.J. and Dameshek, W., Hypoplastic Anemia and Myeloblastic Leukemia Following Chloramphenicol Therapy. N. Eng. J. Med., 277:1003 (1967).
7. Miller, R.W., Genetics of Leukemia: Epidemiologic Aspects. Hum. Genet., 13:100 (1968).
8. Kinkaid, R., Cancer Viruses in Animals. Science, 169: 828 (1970).
9. Bryan, W.R., Maloney, J.B., et al., Viral Etiology of Leukemia. Ann. Intern. Med., 62:376 (1965).
10. Porter, G.H. III, Dalton, A.J., et al., Association of Electrondense Particles with Human Acute Leukemia. J. Nat. Cancer Inst., 33:547 (1964).
11. Ellman, L., Green, I., and Martin, W.J., Histocompatibility Genes, Immune Responsiveness, and Leukemia. Lancet, 2:1104 (1970).
12. Hayhoe, F.G. and Cowley, J.C., Acute Leukemia: Cellular Morphology, Cytochemistry, and Fine Structure. Clin. Hematol., 1(1), W.B. Saunders Co., London (1972).
13. Lichtman, M. and Klemperer, M., The Leukemias. In: Clinical Oncology: A Multidisciplinary Approach, Rubin, P. and Bakemeier, R. (eds.), The University of Rochester School of Medicine and Dentistry, and American Cancer Society, New York, p. 472 (1974).
14. Gunz, F.W., Levi, J.A., and Vincent, P.C., The Outlook for the Adult with Acute Leukemia. Med. J. Australia, 2:403 (1972).

15. Leventhal, B. and Hersch, S., Modern Treatment of Childhood Leukemia: The Patient and His Family. Nursing Digest, III(4):12-15 (July/August, 1975).

16. Walker, P., Bone Marrow Transplant: A Second Chance for Life. Nursing 77, 7(1):24-25 (January, 1977).

17. Martinson, I., The Child With Leukemia. Am. J. Nurs., pp. 1120-1122 (July, 1976).

18. Silver, H., et al., Handbook of Pediatrics. 8th ed., Lange Medical Publ., Palo Alto, CA (1969).

19. Isler, C., Care of the Pediatric Patient with Leukemia. RN Magazine, pp. 14-19 (February, 1972).

20. Rodman, M.J., Drug Therapy Today. RN Magazine, pp. 30-34 (February, 1972).

21. Desotell, S., A Brighter Future for Leukemic Patients. Nursing 77, 7(1):19-23 (January, 1977).

22. Foley, G. and McCarthy, M.A., The Child with Leukemia - The Disease and Its Treatment. Am. J. Nurs., p. 1108 (July, 1976).

23. Santos, G.W., Tutschka, P.J., et al., Bone Marrow Transplantation in Malignancy. Curr. Probl. Cancer, 4(6):3-22 (December, 1979).

24. Graze, P.R. and Gale, R.P., Autotransplantation for Leukemia and Solid Tumors. Transplant. Proceed., 10(1):177-184 (March, 1978).

25. Clarkson, B.D., Current Concepts of Leukemia and Results of Recent Treatment Programs. Transplant. Proceed., 10(1):157-162 (March, 1978).

26. Schiffer, C.A., Aisner, J., et al., Platelet Transfusion Therapy for Patients with Leukemia. Progr. Clin. and Biol. Res., 28(267-279 (1978).

27. Jacobs, P., The Transplantation of Bone Marrow. Cent. Afr. J. Med., 24(Suppl. 9):33-42 (September, 1978).

28. Barton, J.C. and Conrad, M.E., Current Status of Blastic Transformation in Chronic Myelogenous Leukemia. Am. J. Hematol., 4(3):281-291 (1978).

29. Turner, A. and Kjeldsberg, C.R., Hairy Cell Leukemia: A Review. Medicine (Baltimore), 57(6):477-499 (November, 1978).

30. Golomb, H.M., Hairy Cell Leukemia: An Unusual Lymphoproliferative Disease: A Study of 24 Patients. Cancer, 42(Suppl. 2):946-956 (August, 1978).

31. Levine, A.S. and Deisseroth, A.B., Recent Developments in the Supportive Therapy of Acute Myelogenous Leukemia. Cancer, 42(Suppl. 21):854-864 (August, 1978).

32. Frei, E. and Sallan, S.E., Acute Lymphoblastic Leukemia: Treatment. Cancer, 42(Suppl. 2):828-838 (August, 1978).

33. Linman, J.W. and Bagby, G.C. Jr., The Preleukemic
Syndrome (Hemopoietic Dysplasia). Cancer, 42(Suppl. 2):
854-864 (August, 1978).

34. Groopman, J. and Ellman, L., Acute Promyelocytic Leukemia. Am. J. Hematol., 7(4):395-408 (1978).

35. Brouet, J.C. and Seligmann, M., The Immunological
Classification of Acute Lymphoblastic Leukemias. Cancer, 42(Suppl. 2):817-827 (August, 1978).

36. D'angio, G.J., Complications of Treatment Encountered in
Lymphoma-Leukemia Long-Term Survivors. Cancer, 42
(Suppl. 2):1015-1025 (August, 1978).

37. Thomas, E.D., Buckner, C.D., et al., Marrow Transplantation in the Treatment of Acute Leukemia. Adv. Cancer Res., 27:269-279 (1978).

38. Arlin, Z.A., Fried, J., et al., Therapeutic Role of Cell
Kinetics in Acute Leukemia. Clin. Hematol., 7(2):339-
362 (June, 1978).

39. Sanders, J.E. and Thomas, E.D., Bone Marrow Transplantation for Acute Leukemia. Clin. Hematol., 7(2):295-
311 (June, 1978).

40. Alexander, P. and Powles, R., Immunotherapy of Human
Acute Leukemia. Clin. Hematol., 7(2):275-294 (June,
1978).

41. Wiernik, P.H., Treatment of Acute Leukemia in Adults.
Clin. Hematol., 7(2):259-273 (June, 1978).

42. Mauer, A.M., Treatment of Acute Leukemia in Children.
Clin. Hematol. 7(2):245-258 (June, 1978).

43. George, S.L., Design and Evaluation of Leukemia Trials.
Clin. Hematol., 7(2):227-243 (June, 1978).

44. Lusher, J.M. and Ravindranath, Y., Acute Lymphoid Leukemia. Pediat. Ann., 7(7):466-482 (July, 1978).

45. Bodey, G.P. and Rodriguez, V., Approaches to the Treatment of Acute Leukemia and Lymphoma in Adults. Semin.
Hematol., 15(3):221-261 (July, 1978).

46. Reiffers, J., Acute Myeloblastic Leukemia in Elderly Patients: Treatment Prognostic Results in 22 Cases. Cancer,
45(11):2816-2820 (June, 1980).

47. Garrett, T.J., Bone Marrow Transplantation in the Therapy of Adult T-Cell Acute Lymphoblastic Leukemia. Cancer, 45(8):2006-2008 (April, 1980).

48. Keating, M.J., Factors Related to Length of Complete Remission in Adult Acute Leukemia. Cancer, 45(8):2017-
2029 (April, 1980).

CHAPTER 28
Carcinoma of the Liver

Primary liver cancers are infrequent in the United States, although secondary, metastatic liver carcinomas are frequent, occurring in about 50% of late cancers. Epidemiological studies reveal that Orientals have the highest incidence of the disease and that the average age of patients who develop liver carcinoma is between 60 and 70 with 6 to 10 times more occurrences in males.[1]

The primary neoplasms are adenocarcinomas which arise from either the hepatic (liver) cells or the bile ducts. The right lobe, which is larger than the left lobe by about a factor of six is more frequently involved in the development of the disease. The tumor may be either single or multiple; it may be small or large enough to replace the entire lobe. The mode of spread is through the sinusoids, the portal vein, and the lymphatics. Regional lymph node extension and distant metastases into the lungs, brain, and bones may at times give the first clinical symptoms of the disease.[9,13,14]

ETIOLOGY

Factors associated with liver cancer are prolonged, postnecrotic cirrhosis, hemochromatosis, and intestinal parasites, e.g., schistosomiasis.

CLINICAL MANIFESTATIONS

Signs and symptoms of liver carcinoma are not pathognomonic of the disease. The symptoms depend largely on the extent of the disease, the degree of hepatocellular damage, and functional failure. In general, the patient may manifest the following:

1. Weight loss (initially)
2. Increased in weight due to ascites and extracellular fluid retention
3. General weakness

4. Cachexia
5. Anemia
6. Abdominal fullness and pain which may radiate to the back
7. Fever
8. Obstructive jaundice
9. Abnormal liver function tests
10. Splenomegaly
11. Hepatomegaly with palpable tumor nodules
12. Presence of a bruit or venous hum over the liver.

DIAGNOSTIC TESTS AND DIAGNOSIS [6,7,8,9]

1. Alkaline phosphatase and Bromsulphalein excretion tests are elevated.
2. Splenoportal venography
3. Liver scan using $99mTc$ colloid or radioactive colloid gold would reveal "cold-filling defects" in the area of neoplasm.
4. Serum immunoelectrophoresis can be done for the detection of alpha-fetoproteins which may be present in about 75% of cases with primary liver carcinoma.[6]
5. Biopsy by needle aspiration or by exploratory laparotomy.

TREATMENT MODALITIES

Surgery

Surgery is done for nonmetastatic, solitary, and localized cancer. A subtotal hepatectomy or a lobectomy may be done. Some sources claim that 90% resection of the liver is possible because of the liver's great capacity to regenerate.

Chemotherapy

Chemotherapy may consist of methotrexate, 5-fluorouracil and other drugs administered either systemically or by intra-arterial hepatic perfusion. This treatment method has caused tumor regression and prolonged survival in some patients. A few cases of 7-year survival and a 1% 5-year survival rate have been reported by some authorities.[11,12,15]

Radiation Therapy

Radiation therapy may be used as adjunctive treatment or for palliation of symptoms. Liver carcinomas are radioresistant and by virtue of their location, tumoricidal radiation dose is restricted to as low as 3000 rads.

NURSING IMPLICATIONS

The care of the patient includes the principles of care related
to chemotherapy and surgical resection of vital organs of the
body. Emphasis for this particular type of malignancy is on
supportive care prior to, during, and after administration of a
specific therapy. Focusing on the basis of symptomatology, the
care of the patient may be summarized as shown in Table 11.

Table 11: Patient Care in Carcinoma of the Liver [2,3,4]

Patient Problem	Nursing Management
Discomfort and pain	Proper position of patient in a semi-Fowler's or Fowler's position to ease breathing
	Frequent change of position to mobilize and improve cardiopulmonary function
Edema	Fluid and sodium restriction in diet
	Daily weights
	Accurate intake and output measurements
Ascites	Measurement of abdominal girth or circumference
Pruritus	Meticulous skin care using lanolin-base soap, corn-starch bathing
	Patient instructed not to scratch to prevent injury to the skin
Decreased proteins and coagulation factor which result from hepatic failure	Prevent injury and bruising; periodically check platelet levels
	Check for "liver flap" by asking the patient to dorsiflex his hand while the arm is supported; tremor or clenching of the finger means a positive finding

Table 11 (Cont.)

Patient Problem	Nursing Management
Anemia	Monitor laboratory hemoglobin and hematocrit
	Give patient foods high in iron; supplementary vitamins and iron medication may be given as ordered
	Provide adequate rest and sleep
Feminization in males and masculinization in females	Provide emotional support on altered body image
Portal hypertension which can cause congestive cardiac failure, renal failure, gastrointestinal bleeding, esophageal varices, and pericarditis[5]	Give cardiac glycosides as ordered
	Diuretic therapy should be maintained
	Check vital signs at least four times a day
	Observe for any bleeding, i.e., test for occult blood in stools (hematest)
Encephalopathy and hepatic coma due to toxicity of ammonia on brain cells with resultant hypoxia	Administer drugs such as steroid, glutamic acid, large doses of L-dopa, vitamin E, lactulose, and antibiotics
Patient can have pre-coma convulsions	Check patient for confusion, drowsiness, agitation, presence of coarse or flapping tremors (asterixis)
	Asterixis is checked by having patient hold the BP bulb. The degree of asterixis will be reflected in the BP manometer
	EEG may be done which can reveal slow waves with increased amplitude
	Check for the presence of fetor hepaticus which is characterized by an acetone and/or "old wine" odor

Table 11 (Cont.)

Patient Problem	Nursing Management
	Protein-free diet or a diet restricted to 20 to 40 g protein to rest the liver cells
	To treat hepatic coma, intestinal antibiotics such as neomycin will lessen bacterial action. Anticipate side effects of the drug such as diarrhea and vitamin K deficiency, which can cause bleeding
	Minimize factors that precipitate hepatic coma, such as infection, bleeding, protein diet, and drugs (morphine sulphate, barbiturates, and other opiates)

REVIEW QUESTIONS

1. List some etiologic factors associated with liver cancer.
2. Enumerate some of the signs and symptoms of cancer of the liver.
3. Discuss the diagnostic tests done for liver carcinoma.
4. What is the treatment of choice for nonmetastatic liver cancer?
5. List the drugs that may be used for treatment of liver carcinoma.
6. Discuss the nursing management of the following problems that can occur due to cancer of the liver:
   a. Discomfort and pain
   b. Edema
   c. Ascites
   d. Pruritus
   e. Decreased proteins and coagulation factor
   f. Anemia
   g. Feminization/masculinization
   h. Portal hypertension
   i. Encephalopathy
   j. Hepatic coma.

REFERENCES

1. Rubin, P. and Bakemeier, R. (eds.), Clinical Oncology for Medical Students and Physicians. The University of Rochester School of Medicine and Dentistry, and American Cancer Society, New York (1974).
2. Clinical Ascites, An Etiologic Approach to Management. Hospital Practice, pp. 67-72 (August, 1973).
3. Conn, H.D., Current Diagnosis and Treatment of Hepatic Coma. Hospital Practice, p. 65 (February, 1973).
4. Hayter, J., Impaired Liver Function and Related Nursing Care. Am. J. Nurs., p. 2374 (November, 1968).
5. Mikkelsen, W.P., Portal Hyptertension: Clinical Assessment. Hosp. Med., pp. 56-90 (November, 1973).
6. Netter, F.H., The Ciba Collection of Medical Illustrations, Vol. 3, Digestive System, Part III, Liver, Biliary Tract, and Pancreas. Ciba Pharmaceutical Products, New York (1957).
7. Netter, F.H., The Ciba Collection of Medical Illustrations, Vol. 4, Endocrine System and Selected Metabolic Diseases. Ciba Pharmaceutical Products, New York (1965).
8. Sanders, T.P., Liver Scanning. Postgrad. Med., pp. 191-195 (January, 1973).
9. Horrie, A., et al., Ultrastructural Comparison of Hepatoblastoma and Hepatocellular Carcinoma. Cancer, 44(6): 2184-2193 (December, 1979).
10. Lai, C.L., Histologic Prognostic Indicators on Hepatocellular Carcinoma. Cancer, 44(5):1677-1683 (November, 1979).
11. Petrek, J.A. and Minton, J.P., Treatment of Hepatic Metastases by Percutaneous-Arterial Infusion. Cancer, 43 (6):2182-2188 (June, 1979).
12. Lee, Y.T. and Irwin, L., Hepatic Artery Ligation and Adriamycin Infusion Chemotherapy for Hepatoma. Cancer, 41(4):249-255 (April, 1978).
13. Srouji, M.N., Chatten, J., et al., Mesenchymal Hemartoma of the Liver in Infants. Cancer, 42(5):2483-2489 (November, 1978).
14. Grieco, M.B. and Miscall, B.G., Giant Hemangiomas of the Liver. Surg. Gynecol. Obstet., 147(5):783-787 (November, 1978).
15. Pettavel, J. and Morgenthaler, F., Protracted Arterial Chemotherapy of Liver Tumors: An Experience of 107 Cases Over a 12-Year Period. Progr. Clin. Cancer, 7: 217-233 (1978).

16. Lee, Y.T., Nonsystemic Treatment of Metastatic Tumors of the Liver - A Review. Med. Pediatr. Oncol., 4(3):185-203 (1978).
17. Terblanche, J., Liver Tumors Associated with the Use of Contraceptive Pills. S. African Med. J., 53(12):439-442 (March, 1978).

CHAPTER 29
Lung Carcinoma

Carcinoma of the lung is the number one cause of cancer deaths in men. It affects males four times more than females. The average age of those afflicted is 60, with about 1% under 30 and 30% over 70 years. Approximately 5% of all patients will survive for five years and 20% will live over one year. There is a high morbidity and mortality rate; the average length of survival after diagnosis is only 6 to 9 months.[1]

The most common types of lung cancer are squamous cell or epidermoid carcinoma (60%) followed by undifferentiated carcinomas (30%) and adenocarcinomas (10%). The majority of lung cancers arise from the major bronchi rather than the peripheral areas of the lung. The right lung is affected more often than the left lung and more than 50% of all lung cancers occur in the upper lobe. The mode of spread is generally by extension into the bronchi, pulmonary blood vessels, pleura, thoracic wall, diaphragm, and the pericardium. Compression and invasion of the brachial plexus, the vagus, the phrenic, and the recurrent laryngeal nerves can occur. The squamous carcinomas, well-differentiated carcinomas, adenocarcinomas, and large anaplastic tumors tend to invade locally and metastasize widely into distant organs. Small cell anaplastic (oat cell) carcinomas are the most rapidly spreading tumors, such that when diagnosed they are considered inoperable. Common lymphatic spread is to the hilar, mediastinal, and paratracheal nodes and during relapse, retrograde spread into the epigastric region occurs.

Distant metastases involve virtually every organ in the body. The first one affected is the brain due to the venous vertebral intercommunication between the lung and the brain. Other major organs for metastatic spread are the liver, the skeleton, the adrenals, and less commonly the opposite lung.[2,14,15]

ETIOLOGY

Environmental factors have been implicated more than heredity and individual characteristics. There is a higher incidence of lung cancer in urban than in rural areas. Epidemiological studies have shown no difference in social settings but occupational hazards such as coal mining are directly implicated in lung cancer. Cigarette smoking is a well-known factor in the development of lung carcinoma. Other factors, which are correlated with the individual's predisposition, are chronic lung infections and diseases (such as bronchitis, tuberculosis, and bronchiectasis) and other carcinogens like coal tars and asbestos.

CLINICAL MANIFESTATIONS

Signs and symptoms of lung cancer depend largely on the extent of the disease and its location. For example, a tumor in the main bronchus can readily cause bronchial obstruction, hence an atelectasis. As previously stated, the disease often masquerades as other respiratory tract diseases. The most common alerting signs include:

1. Change in pulmonary status such as cough that becomes chronic.
2. Occurrence of unilateral wheezing.
3. Dry cough that becomes productive.
4. Presence of mucoid, rust-streaked, or purulent sputum.
5. Hemoptysis.
6. Obstructive pneumonitis and chest pain.
7. Atelectasis.

Other symptoms that are indicative of advanced carcinoma of the lungs are:

1. Vocal cord paralysis
2. Hemorrhagic pleural effusion
3. Shoulder and arm pain due to compression of the brachial plexus by an apical or superior sulcus tumor.

It is important to note that various extrapulmonary manifestations of a metastatic lung cancer may antedate the signs and symptoms of the primary disease. For convenience, these extrapulmonary manifestations are grouped according to specific organ function derangement as follows:[1,2]

1. Central Nervous System: Loss of memory, personality changes, faulty speech, progressive dementia.[15]

2. Metabolic: Wasting of the host with severe weakness, hypersecretion of adrenal cortex (mostly associated with oat cell carcinoma); electrolyte imbalance due to increased ACTH and ADH, hypercalcemia, and hypophosphatemia; Cushing's and carcinoid syndrome; hypercalcemia due to ectopic PTH.
3. Neuromuscular: Peripheral neuropathy with sensory or mixed sensory-motor defects; cortical or cerebellar degeneration with ataxia, vertigo, nystagmus, intention tremor, carcinomatous myopathy with muscle weakness and wasting, particularly of the trunk and limb girdle; polymyositis with or without dermatomyositis.
4. Dermatological: Acanthosis nigricans; nonspecific dermatoses; ichthyosis; erythema gyratum repens.
5. Hematological: Anemia (nonspecific macrocytic, normochromic); erythrocytosis; fibrinolytic purpura.
6. Vascular: Migratory thrombophlebitis; recurrent thrombophlebitis; nonbacterial endocarditis characterized by fibrin plaque deposits on heart valves; arterial embolization from detached fibrin plaques.
7. Skeletal: Clubbing of fingers (most frequent); rheumatoid arthritis (may precede other clinical manifestations of lung cancer); pulmonary hypertrophic osteoarthropathy.

DIAGNOSIS AND DIAGNOSTIC TESTS

Careful, thorough assessment of history and physical examination are crucial in establishing a diagnosis. Generally, lung cancer is asymptomatic in its early stage and the clinical manifestations mimic those of any other upper-respiratory infection. Stereoscopic chest x-rays or x-rays of the anterior/posterior, lateral, oblique, and apical lordotic (taken on both inspiration and expiration) are of utmost importance since most lung cancers are centrally located. Other diagnostic tests that may be done are as follows:[1]

1. Bronchoscopy and bronchography.
2. Sputum cytology (Papanicolaou technique).
3. Bronchial brush biopsy.
4. Percutaneous needle biopsy under videoscope (used for peripheral nodular lesions; has the risk of seeding needle tract and/or causing a pneumothorax).
5. Mediastinoscopy to examine nodes around the trachea and mediastinal node dissection (presence of contralateral node involvement indicates inoperability).
6. Radioisotope venacavogram to determine pulmonary blood flow.

7. Scalene node biopsy: This is done as a method to determine operability. Once scalene node biopsy is positive, most physicians consider it as a contraindication to surgery. (The node location is important to remember. The right scalene nodes drain the right lung and left-lower lobe while the left scalene nodes drain the lingual and left-upper lobe.)

8. Lung scan does not have any value to diagnosis as it does not differentiate cancer from a lung infarct or pneumonitis.

TREATMENT MODALITIES [1,10,11,12]

1. Surgery: Surgical resection is the treatment of choice for localized, excisable lesion. A lobectomy or a pneumonectomy (removal of the entire lung and adjacent nodal dissection) may be performed based on the extent of the disease and the functional capacity of the patient. Surgery is contraindicated as a palliative measure or in the presence of extrathoracic metastases. [18]

2. Radiotherapy: Supervoltage radiation is used to deliver higher depth dose and to achieve fewer side effects and skin reactions. Irradiation is used for palliation of inoperable cancers and for patients who refuse surgery. A tumoricidal dose of 4500 to 6000 rads can cause a radiation pneumonectomy. Irradiation of localized; asymptomatic intrapulmonary lesions have also been tried with some success. Bronchogenic stump recurrences are treated with radiotherapy. [4,16]

3. Preoperative radiation: Use of preoperative radiation is restricted to apical or superior sulcus tumors.

4. Atmospheric and hyperbaric oxygen breathing during radiation treatment have been tried with no substantial benefits.

5. Enhancing radiosensitivity with chemotherapeutic agents has been also tried but has been, thus far, unrewarding. Some of the chemotherapeutic drugs used to enhance radiosensitivity include: vitamin K, 5-fluorouracil, dactinomycin, hydroxurea, nitrogen mustard, and procarbazine (Matulane). Immunotherapy has also been used. [13,17]

6. Intrapleural instillation of radioactive gold, phosphorus, or nitrogen mustard are utilized for treating pleural effusion.

7. Chemotherapy with alkylating agents has been used for palliation of symptoms of metastatic disease. A small percentage of patients achieve beneficial effects which last for a period of two to three months.

8. Radiotherapy and/or rhizotomy (resection of nerve roots) have been tried for pain relief in Pancoast tumor, and Horner's syndrome.

9. Combined preoperative and postoperative radiation has also been used.

NURSING IMPLICATIONS

Resection of part or all of the lung subjects the patient to the complications of surgery. The patient should be closely monitored for complications (which occur in 20% of all patients) such as pulmonary embolism, empyema, pulmonary edema, bronchopleural fistula, cardiac arrhythmias, cor pulmonale, and incisional chest pain which can persist for several months after surgery. [7]

Acute pulmonary edema is more likely to follow a pneumonectomy due to drastic reduction in the pulmonary circuit and increased permeability of the capillaries induced by hypoxia. Emergency treatment with alternating tourniquet on extremities, morphine sulphate intravenously to decrease the patient's anxiety and pain, rapidly-acting diuretics also given intravenously, and/or a phlebotomy must be instituted.

Chest tube drainage attached to a water seal with or without suction is used in the patient who has had a lobectomy. Make certain that optimum gravity drainage is maintained by avoiding kinks on extension tubing (by taping a tongue blade on tube proximal to any connection), looping the tubing on the side of the bed while providing leeway to prevent detachment of tubing from the chest tube or undue tugging when the patient turns to his side. Maintain the prescribed negative pressure, usually at 20 cm of water. Too high a suction can produce tension pneumothorax. Refill water on suction control chamber of a Pleurevac setup and sufficient bubbling of the water-seal chamber reservoir should be maintained. Observe for oscillation of water inside air vent tubing. The water should oscillate when the patient takes a deep breath or coughs. Oscillation will stop when the lung is fully expanded or when the chest tube is obstructed. Continuous air bubbling in water-seal bottle not attached to suction indicates air leak. Check for exact locus. If appropriate, apply a clamp on the chest tube as close to its insertion as possible. Careful assessment of the patient's respiratory status is necessary in cases of air leak, disconnected chest tube, or disrupted water-seal drainage setup. Immediate clamping of the chest tube will prevent atmospheric air entry into the pleural cavity. However, if pneumothorax, hemothorax, or massive pleural effusion have occurred, the disconnected chest tube need not be clamped right away to allow the escape of air and fluid. Reestablishment of the closed-chest drainage system should follow. [6,8]

Prevent obstruction of the tubing. If "milking" the chest tube is necessary, the process is facilitated by placing petroleym jelly (Vaseline) on the finger used for milking or stripping the tube.

One hand should be used to hold and firmly immobilize the tube close to its insertion and "milk" towards the drainage away from the patient. When the patient is turned to the operated side, prevent compression of the tubes by placing rolled hand towels along each side of the tubes.

Placing the patient preferably on his unoperated side in a semi-Fowler's or Fowler's position would facilitate breathing and gravity drainage. This would also promote expansion of the affected lung. Deep breathing and coughing deeply at the end of expiration, four to eight times every hour will also increase oxygenation. Giving the prescribed analgesic or firm splinting of the incision with towel or soft pillow placed anteroposteriorly on the affected chest should prevent the patient from chest splinting due to pain during the breathing and coughing exercises. Perform arm and shoulder range of motion exercises to prevent shoulder ankylosis, promote circulation, and decrease pain.

Chest x-rays should be done daily to assess tube placement and efficacy. Accurate, hourly (or more frequently as needed) notation of the patient's overall condition and quantity and characteristics of chest drainage should be done. A creamy, milky, or yellowish chest drainage may mean a chylous fistula. Notify the physician and continue monitoring the patient.

Supportive care of the patient receiving chemotherapy has been discussed in preceeding chapters. Similarly, the nursing care of the patient receiving irradiation has been explored earlier in Part III, Chapter 9. Additionally, for irradiation in lung carcinoma, specific supportive care is planned for possible occurrence of tracheitis, esophagitis, radiation myelitis, or vocal cord paralysis.

REVIEW QUESTIONS

1. What is the number one killer of men who die of malignant disease?
2. Explain why lung cancer has a fatal outcome.
3. What are the predisposing factors to development of lung carcinoma?
4. Explain why brain metastases readily occur in carcinoma of the lung.
5. List three vital nerves which can be invaded by carcinoma of the lung.
6. Give five diagnostic procedures for diagnosing lung cancer.
7. What are the manifestations of lung carcinoma?

8. Give at least two clinical manifestations of the following extrapulmonary metastatic diseases: CNS, neuromuscular, skeletal, metabolic, hematologic, vascular, and dermatologic.
9. Discuss the role of surgical resection, chemotherapy, and radiotherapy in treating lung cancer.
10. What are the complications of a lobectomy/pneumonectomy?
11. Explain why acute pulmonary edema can occur after a pneumonectomy.

REFERENCES

1. Rubin, P. and Bakemeier, R. (eds.), Clinical Oncology for Medical Students and Physicians. The University of Rochester School of Medicine and Dentistry and American Cancer Society, New York (1974).
2. American Cancer Society, Current Concepts in Cancer: Multidisciplinary Views, Bronchogenic Carcinoma, New York (April, 1975).
3. Liddle, H.V. and Thomas, J.M., AB-1o3 (NSC-37096) in the Treatment of Bronchogenic Carcinoma. Cancer Chemother. Rep., 39:61-65 (July, 1964).
4. Carter, S.K., New Drugs on the Horizon of Bronchogenic Carcinoma. Cancer, 30:1402-1409 (1972).
5. Guttman, R., Results of Radiation Therapy in Patients with Inoperable Carcinoma of the Lung. Am. J. Roentgen., 93:99-103 (January, 1965).
6. Kersten, L., Chest Tube Drainage Systems: Indications and Principles of Operation. Heart and Lung, II:97-107 (January-February, 1974).
7. Luckman, J. and Sorensen, H.C., Medical-Surgical Nursing. A Psychophysiologic Approach. W.B. Saunders, Philadelphia (1974).
8. Morgan, C.V. and Orcutt, T.W., The Care and Feeding of Chest Tubes. Am. J. Nurs., pp. 305-308 (February, 1972).
9. Har, T. and Takita, H., Depression of T-Lymphocyte Response by Non-T Suppressor Cells in Lung Cancer Patients. Cancer, 44(6):2090-2098 (December, 1979).
10. Vogh, S., et al., MACC Chemotherapy for Adenocarcinoma and Epidermoid Carcinoma of the Lung. Cancer, 44 (5):864-868 (September, 1979).
11. Weiss, R.B., Small-Cell Carcinoma of the Lung: Therapeutic Management. Ann. Intern. Med., 88(4):522-531 (April, 1978).
12. Zubrod, C.G. and Selawry, O., The Treatment of Lung Cancer. Adv. Intern. Med., 23:451-467 (1978).

13. McKneally, M.F., Nonspecific Immunotherapy for Lung Cancer. In: Immunotherapy of Human Cancer, Raven Press, New York (1978).
14. Greco, F.A., Einhorn, L.H., et al., Small Cell Lung Cancer: Progress and Perspectives. Semin. Oncol., 5 (3):323-335 (September, 1978).
15. Bunn, P.A. Jr., Nugent, J.L., and Matthews, M.J., Central Nervous System Metastases in Small Cell Bronchogenic Carcinoma. Semin. Oncol., 5(3):288-298 (September, 1978).
16. Seydel, H.G., Creech, R.H., et al., Radiation Therapy in Small Cell Lung Cancer. Semin. Oncol., 5(3):288-298 (September, 1978).
17. Forbes, J.T., Greco, F.A., et al., Immunologic Aspects of Small Cell Carcinoma. Semin. Oncol., 5(3):263-271 (September, 1978).
18. Van Dongen, J.A. and Van Slooten, E.A., The Surgical Treatment of Pulmonary Metastases. Cancer Treatm. Rev., 5(1):29-48 (March, 1978).

CHAPTER 30
Head and Neck Tumors

About 95% of head and neck cancers originate in the mucosal linings and are thus epithelial in nature, the largest number of the lesions being squamous cell epithelioma. The remaining 5% are adenocarcinomas, mixed tumors, and rarely, sarcomas.

Head and neck tumors altogether account for 3% of cancers in the United States and most often affect men over 50 years of age. Most of these tumors do not look like cancers (innocent looking) initially as they usually present as thickening, minute ulcers, or areas of slight irritation.[4]

Cancers of the head and neck are believed to arise de novo or in areas where there is chronic irritation such as leukoplakia (chalky, white, thickened patches on the tongue or buccal mucosa) or hyperkeratosis. As the cancers grow, the innocent-looking ulcers become elevated fungating masses or ulcerations in areas of thickened tissue. These tumors spread by direct extension, lymphatic invasion and dissemination, and ultimately, distant metastases.[1]

Perineural lymphatics are involved very often and neck cancers and neck node involvement are very common. Remote metastases to distant organs from the clavicle are relatively uncommon.

The symptoms of head and neck cancers depend upon the type of lesion, its location, and extent of its spread.

1. Cancers of the nose and paranasal sinuses often cause a bloody discharge, pain in the teeth or face, and/or mass in the nasal fossa. Early signs which should be taken seriously include presence of mass and subsequent obstruction of breathing, and feelings of pressure, local pain, and paresthesia in the paranasal sinus.
2. Cancer of the nasopharynx is usually manifested by neurological impairments, deafness, dyspnea, and/or enlarged neck nodes.

289

3. Cancer of the oropharynx is often asymptomatic. With the growth of the lesion, there may be dysphagia and occasional pain. Enlargement of lymph nodes due to metastases is common.

CANCER OF THE LIP

The tumor usually occurs on the lower lip as a fissure or a painless, indurated ulcer with raised edges. Lip cancer metastasizes to the regional lymph nodes infrequently and then usually only in the late stage of the disease when the growth of the lesion has been controlled. Hence, the rate of cure is high. Lip lesions account for about 15% of all head and neck tumors, rarely occur in blacks and those below 40 years of age. Its incidence increases with each succeeding decade.

Etiology

The cause is unknown but the following are believed to be predisposing factors:

1. Prolonged exposure to the sun and wind (actinic radiation).
2. Constant irritation from the warm stem of a pipe (pipe smoking).
3. Chronic leukoplakia.
4. Syphilis.

Clinical Manifestations

Painless ulceration which persists for more than two weeks is indicative of lip cancer.

Diagnostic Tests and Diagnosis

1. Biopsy: A negative biopsy should be repeated.
2. Bidigital examination of submental and submaxillary triangles for evidence of metastases.

Treatment Modalities

The treatment can either be surgery or radiotherapy, depending upon the extent and size of the tumor. The general principles considered before the treatment of choice is selected and implemented are as follows:

1. For a small lesion (less than 1 cm in size), either surgery or radiotherapy is done. The chance for cure is about the same in either case (90%).

2. For lesions more than 1 cm in size but less than half of one lip, surgical excision and reconstruction or irradiation are used.
3. For extensive tumors which involve the entire lip, irradiation is the treatment of choice since it gives better cosmetic effects.
4. A big (4 cm or more in size), noninvasive, superficial carcinoma is better treated by irradiation because this method will cure just as well as surgery plus do a better cosmetic job.
5. Palpable lymph nodes may be present but often are due to inflammatory reactions. A limited observation period of six to eight weeks is justified before any decision is made to perform a neck dissection and suprathyroid dissection.

Results and Prognosis

1. There is a five-year survival rate in about 90% of uncomplicated lesions.
2. Delayed neck dissection still offers a high cure rate.
3. There may be local recurrences and, rarely, distant metastases.

Nursing Implications

1. Patient education is recommended on the importance of seeking medical attention if there is an ulcer that does not heal in two to three weeks.
2. Make the patient aware of the etiologic factors associated with cancer of the lip to prevent occurrence of the disease.
3. The principles of care of the patient who undergoes surgery, radiotherapy, and chemotherapy have been discussed in Part III. To assist the patient cope with his fears, the principles discussed in Part IV, Chapter 11 are essentially the same.

CANCER OF THE TONGUE

Cancer of the tongue accounts for a smaller incidence than does cancer of the lip. When all cancers of all sites are considered, tongue cancer accounts for a small percentage (about 1 to 2%) of new cancer cases each year. It is important to note that tongue cancer, like lip cancer, occurs mostly in males; the sex ratio being 4 to 1. The highest incidence of the disease is in the sixth and seventh decades. The risk of having the disease increases with age.

Etiology

There is no specific cause of cancer of the tongue. However, several factors have been implicated:

1. Use of all forms of tobacco is probably the most significant.
2. Cigarette smoking.
3. Chewing betel nut.
4. Alcohol intake. (The long-term heavy drinker has three or four times the chance of getting tongue cancer as an abstainer or an occasional drinker.)[13]

Clinical Manifestations

About three-fourths of all tongue cancers occur in the anterior two-thirds, and about 40% of these patients will have neck metastases on first examination; while about one-fourth of all tongue cancers occur in the base, and about 70% of these patients will have neck metastases when first seen.[1] Tongue cancers metastasize much earlier and more readily than lip lesions, thus long-term prognosis is considerably poorer.

The lesions of the anterior two-thirds usually have the following characteristics:

1. They begin with premalignant changes of leukoplakia with or without surface inflammation or erosion.
2. The patient complains of feeling "something funny" on the tongue.
3. Localized pain is present in the late stage of the disease.
4. Ulceration and bleeding of the enlarged tumor occur, thereby worsening the pain.
5. Decreased mobility of the tongue, especially if the lesion infiltrates the muscle and the floor of the mouth or jaws, can occur.
6. About 40% will have enlarged metastatic cervical nodes, submaxillary, and digastric nodes.

Diagnostic Tests and Diagnosis

1. Biopsy is essential, especially at the edges of the lesion.
2. Culture to determine any presence of superimposed infection.
3. Exfoliative cytology and biopsy are recommended.
4. X-ray studies should be done of mandible and chest.

Treatment Modalities

1. A small primary lesion is treated satisfactorily with irradiation or surgery.
2. Some authorities believe that combined (en bloc) resection of the tumor, floor of the mouth, mandible, and contents of the lateral neck yields the best curative results if used in all cases. This is not used routinely, however, due to:
   a. Inability of the patient to tolerate the procedure or to adjust to it, primarily due to age.
   b. The fact there are cancers that are small enough to be treated with limited resection.
   c. The patient may not want to have such an extensive surgery.
   d. Some authorities advocate irradiation to the primary lesion as the treatment of choice.
3. Small (2 cm or less) lesions on the free margin of the tongue may be treated with partial glossectomy.
4. Larger lesions (over 2 cm) may be treated with irradiation to the primary lesion plus a neck dissection for the metastases.
5. Lesions at the base of the tongue (often fairly large, about 2 cm) may be treated the same way as larger lesions. In larger lesions, laryngectomy may have to be done also.
6. If irradiation therapy is to be used, the following should be taken into consideration:
   a. External therapy alone is rarely adequate to shrink the lesion and should, therefore, be supplemented by radium implants into the tongue.
   b. Needle implants or some other kind of irradiation requires skillful management, since it takes about 8 to 10 days to achieve the desired effects of radiotherapy.

Nursing Implications

The care of the patient with cancer of the tongue depends greatly on the needs of the patient as a result of the chosen modality of treatment. The care of the glossectomy patient includes:

1. Preparation of the patient for partial glossectomy or total glossectomy should include not only the psychosocial aspects as discussed in Part IV, but also telling the patient and his family about the changes that will occur after surgery and the methods that will be used to assist the patient to communicate with others.
2. Provision of a magic slate, a pencil and paper, or a tiny blackboard with chalk will enable the patient with hemiglossectomy or total glossectomy to communicate.

3. Oral feedings will not be possible for some time postoperatively so the patient will have to be maintained on parenteral fluids.

4. Suctioning should be done frequently postoperatively to insure decreased secretions resulting from difficulty in swallowing saliva or expectorating secretions. A gauze wick may be used to direct saliva into an emesis basis. Sometimes a dental suction device may be used to carry away saliva as it accumulates.

5. Mouth care as ordered may include the use of sterile water, a mild alkaline mouthwash, hydrogen peroxide, or a solution of sodium bicarbonate. Sterile equipment and aseptic technique should be used in carrying out the procedure to minimize the risk of postoperative infection. A catheter may be used for this purpose by placing it along the side of the mouth between the cheek and the teeth and then injecting the irrigating solution with gentle pressure. Drain the remaining fluids into an emesis basin or suction the patient.

6. After initial parenteral therapy, the patient may be fed through a nasogastric catheter or a soft catheter that is passed into the throat and beyond the operative site. Liquid food, 200 to 400 cc, may be given every three to four hours. The patient should be watched closely after a liquid diet for any nausea or vomiting.

7. Watch for any diarrhea due to the liquid diet and then report to the physician if it persists. The dietician may be consulted in order to provide a nutritive diet that will minimize occurrence of untoward effects.

8. Speech training may be instituted if the patient has speech difficulties.

If the patient is treated with needles or molds containing radium or other radioactive substance, he should be given specific instructions as follows:

1. Talking with the needles in place will be difficult.

2. If an intraoral mold is used, the patient will be unable to talk.

3. The patient should know that abrupt movement or change of position may dislodge the radium implant. Therefore, the patient should not attempt to do any of these without assistance from the nurse. If the patient has discomfort in the mouth he must report it immediately and not attempt to change the position of the mold or radium.

In addition to the principles of care during radiotherapy which have been discussed in Part III, Chapter 9, the following nursing measures should be undertaken for the patient with irradiation of the tongue:

1. Allowing the patient to lie down for brief periods may help alleviate his discomfort. Administration of sedatives as ordered will also be helpful.
2. Supporting the chin with a sling will promote comfort.
3. Have available suction equipment at the bedside in case of choking or bleeding.
4. Observe for sloughing off of tissues which can cause a fetid odor.
5. Give meticulous mouth hygiene, such as mouth irrigation with one-half teaspoon sodium chloride and one-half teaspoon of sodium bicarbonate to a quart of water as a gargle. Gargling may be repeated as often as every four to six hours. Hydrogen peroxide or Dobell's solution may be used in case of sloughing off of tissues. A solution of 15 drops of common chloride household bleach in a glass of water helps to control mouth odors and is relatively acceptable to many patients.

CANCER OF THE MOUTH

Cancers of the mouth account for 15% of all oral cavity lesions. The average age of onset of the disease is 60 years.

Etiology

There is no known specific cause of cancer of the mouth. The etiologic factors previously discussed in cancer of the tongue have also been implicated in cancer of the mouth. [13]

Clinical Manifestations

Mouth cancer usually presents as an infiltrative lesion with a fissure-like ulceration. Spread is rapid and it involves the contralateral side and the mandible. About 50% of cases present with adenopathy (submaxillary) that is frequently bilateral.

Diagnostic Tests and Diagnosis

1. Direct examination with bimanual palpation
2. Biopsy
3. Radiographs of mandible and chest

Treatment Modalities

The principles of treatment are essentially the same as in cancer of the tongue. However, with involvement of the mandible, it is recommended that the treatment of choice would best be that of combined resection of the floor of mouth, a partial mandibulectomy, and an en bloc neck dissection.[10,12]

Due to high occurrence of early lymph node metastases, an elective neck dissection is to be given serious consideration as a modality of treatment. In an elective neck dissection, the nodes may not be palpable but possible microscopic foci are removed.

Nursing Implications

The nursing care of the patient with cancer of the mouth is very much like that of the patient with glossectomy and interstitial irradiation of the tongue. Additionally, there are other factors that should be considered, especially for the patient with inoperable cancer of the mouth.

Although surgery and radiation are the mainstay of therapy for cancer of the mouth, when the cancer becomes inoperable, irradiation may be the only choice of treatment. Surgery may be considered as a means of palliation of symptoms, but the primary treatment is that of irradiation.

The prevention of the complications that occur after irradiation of the mouth is a definite nursing responsibility. Among the problems encountered as a result of radiotherapy to the mouth are:

1. Mucositis
2. **Xerostomia**
3. Dental decay
4. Trismus.

Mucositis is an inflammation of a mucous membrane. In head and neck patients, this is a result of the radiation to the intraoral membrane. The severity of mucositis depends upon the dose, fractionation, volume of tissue irradiation, and the type of radiation.

Nursing Management

1. Give the patient frequent oral irrigations with a warm solution of hydrogen peroxide and normal saline. This will

cleanse the oral tissues, minimize local pain, and lubricate membranes.
2. Irrigate every four hours and after meals.
3. Instruct the patient to minimize or eliminate smoking or alcohol intake.
4. Clean dentures with soap and water after meals or soak them in a denture cleaner. Preferably, the patient may have to refrain from wearing the dentures to prevent further irritation of the gums. Should this be done, the nurse should provide emotional support to the patient since it is sometimes a considerable concern of the patient to be without his teeth.

Xerostomia, or dryness of the mouth, is unpleasant and occurs about one or two weeks after irradiation has begun. Diminished saliva interferes with eating, swallowing, and talking. Give the patient a great deal of fluids and administer a saliva substitute such as carboxymethylcellulose and sorbitol with a pH of 7.2 via spray. The patient may be instructed how to spray his mouth whenever he needs it. The effect of this chemical is to dissolve the viscous mucus and makes the mucosa slippery. The effects last for one or two hours.

There is a higher incidence of dental decay as a result of irradiation therapy. The radiation decay first occurs at the junction of the clinical crowns of the teeth and the gingival margin.[2] It is believed that dryness of the mouth and the altered pH of the scanty saliva are major causes of dental caries.

The practice of tooth extraction prior to irradiation has been abandoned at most institutes and hospitals since the advent of more advanced methods of prevention and improved restorative materials. The successful management of the patient's problem of preventing dental decay depends upon a concentrated effort on the part of the patient, nursing, and dental personnel.

1. Use of the Bass technique insures cleaning the surfaces most vulnerable to decay. This technique involves the use of a soft small brush placed at an approximate angle of 45 degrees between the gingiva and the teeth. The lingual surfaces of upper and lower anterior teeth are cleaned with either the tip or the heel of the brush. The suggested type of brush to be used are Right Kind, Oral B Sulcus brush, and Pycopay Softex. A toothpaste with a high fluoride content should be used. Interproximal areas should be cleaned with dental-floss, toothpicks, interproximal brushes, or even pipe cleaners.[2]

2. Topical application of fluoride on the teeth after thorough brushing has been effective in controlling dental caries.

Trismus, an inability to open the mouth fully, is often seen in en bloc resection and radiotherapy. This makes it difficult to do mouth care. However, an effort should be made to use catheters to irrigate the mouth as described earlier.

For the patient with radical neck dissection, the nursing care involves the preoperative care, postoperative care, and the care of a patient with tracheostomy. [2,3,5,6,7,8,9]

Preoperative Care of the Radical Neck Dissection Patient

1. Inform the patient of the possibility of a tracheostomy, its purpose, how it will be taken care of, and how it will affect his ability to communicate.
2. Provide reassurance that the surgery will not make him less acceptable to others.
3. Understand the meaning of his illness to him and his family, know his support systems, values, and self-concept.
4. Support healthy coping mechanisms; do not break any coping mechanism unless another mechanism can be effectively substituted.
5. Make the patient feel the caring, supportive, and accepting attitude which he needs.
6. Other principles of care have been discussed in other chapters where surgical intervention is the mode of treatment.

Postoperative Care of the Radical Neck Dissection Patient

1. Maintenance of a patent airway (tracheostomy tube), nasogastric tube suction, and drainage system is very important.
2. Prevent complications such as wound infection, airway obstruction, carotid blowout, chylous fistula, decreased venous return causing edema of face and neck with "purplish" color of the face, and increased cerebrospinal fluid.
3. Frequent observations are required to detect onset of any of the above-mentioned complications and to prevent them from occurring as much as possible.

Nursing Management

1. Airway obstruction: Observe for any wheezing, stridor, retraction, or respiratory difficulty. Suction the patient every hour initially or more frequently as indicated.

2. Infection: Maintain close monitor on temperature and use aseptic technique in tracheostomy care and suctioning.
3. Carotid blowout: Apply direct pressure over the area stat. Preventive measures such as keeping the suture line intact, free from infection, and maintaining the drainage system are very essential. Normal drainage is 240 to 300 cc in the first 24 hours which then becomes scant and serous. If drainage is a lot less than normal, check the drainage system as it may not be working. The accumulation of fluid under the skin flaps can cause infection and necrosis of tissue which may cause carotid blowout.
4. Chylous fistula: This may result from injury to the thoracic duct during surgery or due to injury or necrosis of tissue postoperatively. Institute preventive measures as in carotid blowout. Observe for the type of drainage, such as milky drainage after feeding which may indicate fistula. The fistula may heal spontaneously or it may require surgical suturing.
5. Involve the patient and the family in subsequent self-care, including care of the tracheostomy. This will enhance the rehabilitation of the patient.
6. In positioning the patient, place him in a **Fowler's** position to ease breathing and promote drainage. This also decreases venous pressure on the skin flap.
7. Give the patient means of communication such as a magic slate, **flash cards**, or pencil and paper.
8. Care of the skin flaps includes application of bacitracin twice daily as ordered using aseptic technique.
9. Anticipate the removal of the catheter drainage setup about 4 to 5 days postoperation so the patient can be informed and prepared. The sutures may be removed about 5 to 10 days postoperation depending on the amount of drainage, absence of any complications, and rate of healing of the patient.

CANCER OF THE LARYNX

Cancer of the larynx emanates from the epithelial coverings of the structures comprising the larynx, i.e., the epiglottis, aryepiglottic folds, and true and false vocal cords. Ninety-five percent of all tumors of the larynx occur in males, they are rare in blacks, and the peak incidence is in the fifth to sixth decades of life.

Etiology

1. Chronic alcoholism.
2. Excessive use of tobacco.

Clinical Manifestations

1. Hoarseness that persists for more than one week.
2. Dyspnea when lesion is advanced.
3. Dysphagia in very extensive lesions.
4. Small lesions are painless, advanced lesions cause sore throat.
5. Unexplained unilateral adenopathy.

Diagnostic Tests and Diagnosis

1. Indirect laryngoscopy is essential in all cases of hoarseness.
2. Direct laryngoscopy is required for more accurate visualization.
3. Biopsy is essential before any treatment is instituted.
4. Diagnostic x-ray studies such as laryngeal tomography, laryngogram, and chest film are recommended.

Treatment Modalities

Depending on the size and extent of the tumor, the procedures that may be done are:

1. Horizontal partial laryngectomy may be used when the lesion is small and confined to the epiglottis. It is preferred, however, that radiation be done in this case. For radiation failures, then supraglottic laryngectomy may be done.
2. If the lesion is larger and extends beyond the epiglottis to the aryepiglottic folds and false cords, surgery alone (supraglottic laryngectomy) or combined therapy (surgery and radiation) procedures produce best results.
3. If the lesion is small and confined to the true vocal cord, and if the cord is mobile and not fixed, either radiation or surgery can give equally good results.
4. For larger lesions with extension beyond the true cords and presence of fixation of vocal cords, then total laryngectomy is done.
5. In case of cervical metastases (clinically palpable lymph nodes or microscopic nonpalpable) the patient can be treated by elective neck dissection or radiation therapy.

There are certain complications of radiation therapy, viz., edema and chondritis. On the other hand, total laryngectomy can produce loss of voice and/or permanent tracheostomy. Partial laryngectomy can result in hoarseness and hazard of aspiration.

Nursing Implications

The nursing care of the patient is similar to what has been discussed in the care of the neck dissection patient with tracheostomy. Additionally, the patient with partial laryngectomy should be instructed to rest his voice for at least three days postoperatively or until the doctor gives specific approval. The patient should only whisper until healing is complete.

In the total laryngectomy patient, the patient is told preoperatively that he will breathe through a special opening made in his neck for the rest of his life and that he will no longer have normal speech. The emotional support that the patient needs is tremendous and every effort should be made to make him feel receptive of the proposed surgery. A visit from a recovered laryngectomy patient may be very beneficial for the patient preoperatively.

Speech rehabilitation may be started as soon as the tracheostomy tube has been removed. The patient should be informed of available resources such as the International Association of Laryngectomees and the local chapter of the American Cancer Society such as the Lost Cord Club or a New Voice Club. All of these can assist the patient readapt to his new life after total laryngectomy. Esophageal speech may be learned by the patient in about two to three months after surgery. If unsuccessful, a speech aid such as a vibrator or an electronic artificial larynx may be prescribed for him.

Discharge instructions for the patient should include:

1. Care of the tracheostomy, including what activities to avoid, such as swimming.
2. Wearing an identification card which alerts people that he is a partial neck breather or a total neck breather. The former indicates that he mainly breathes through the neck opening. However, there is a connection between the lungs and the nose as well as the mouth. The larynx may or may not be present and a metal or plastic tube may or may not be in the neck opening. The latter indicates that the patient breathes only through the neck opening. There is no connection between the lungs and the nose or mouth.

REVIEW QUESTIONS

1. In what portion of the lip is malignancy likely to occur most?

2. What percentage of all head and neck lesion does cancer of the lip account for?
3. List some of the etiologic factors implicated in lip cancer.
4. Define leukoplakia and hyperkeratosis.
5. What type of therapy would be the best method of treatment for lip cancer? Why is this method preferred?
6. Identify some of the factors that would influence the type of treatment for head and neck cancers.
7. In what portion of the tongue would cancer most likely occur?
8. When would glossectomy or hemiglossectomy be the preferred treatment of choice in cancer of the tongue?
9. Discuss the nursing care of a glossectomy patient.
10. Define an elective neck dissection.
11. Why would elective neck dissection be done in cancer of the mouth?
12. Discuss the complications of irradiation therapy in cancer of the mouth. What is the nursing management of each complication?
13. Describe the Bass technique of preventing dental caries.
14. List the complications of radical neck dissection.
15. What important nursing observations should be made in each of the complications of radical neck dissection?
16. Describe the nursing care of a patient with tracheostomy.
17. Discuss the nursing care of a patient who is to undergo laryngectomy.
18. Describe esophageal speech.
19. How does an electronic larynx work for the aphonic patient?

REFERENCES

1. Fass, M. and Preston, W. (eds.), Clinical Concepts in Cancer Management - A Self-Instruction. McGraw Hill Book Co., Blakiston Publications, New York (1976).
2. Trowbridge, J.T. and Carl, W., Oral Care of the Patient Having Head and Neck Irradiation. Am. J. Nurs., pp. 2146-2148 (December, 1975).
3. Tierney, E.A., Accepting Disfigurement When Death Is the Alternative. Am. J. Nurs., pp. 2149-2150 (December, 1975).
4. Rubin, P. and Bakemeier, R. (eds.), Clinical Oncology for Medical Students and Physicians. The University of Rochester School of Medicine and Dentistry and American Cancer Society, New York (1974).
5. Lawless, C., Helping Patients with Endotracheal and Tracheostomy Tubes Communicate. Am. J. Nurs., pp. 2151-2152 (December, 1975).

6. Ewing, D., Electronic Larynx for Aphonic Patients. Am. J. Nurs., pp. 2153-2156 (December, 1975).

7. Nicholson, E., Personal Notes of a Laryngectomee. Am. J. Nurs., pp. 2157-2158 (December, 1975).

8. American Cancer Society, First Aid for (Neck Breathers) Laryngectomees. New York (July, 1973).

9. McConell, E.A., How To Truly Help the Patient With a Radical Neck Dissection. Nursing 76, pp. 58-65 (November, 1976).

10. Amer, M.H., et al., Factors That Affect Response to Chemotherapy and Survival of Patients With Advanced Head and Neck Cancer. Cancer, 43(6):2202-2206 (June, 1979).

11. Danziger, J., Computerized Tomography in Rhabdomyosarcoma of the Head and Neck. Cancer, 44(2):463-467 (August, 1979).

12. Hanna, D.C. and Clairmont, A.A., Submandibular Gland Tumors. Plast. Reconstr. Surg., 61(2):198-203 (February, 1978).

13. Mashberg, A., Garfinkel, L. and Harris, S., Alcohol as Primary Risk Factor in Oral Squamous Carcinoma. Cancer, 31(3):146-155 (May/June, 1981).

CHAPTER 31
Cancer of the Alimentary Tract

Cancer of the gastrointestinal tract presents a variety of occult to easily detectable clinical manifestations and presenting symptoms which are dependent on the exact locus of the neoplasm. Consequently, therapeutic intervention may or may not be initiated early enough to effect a cure. As a rule, the farther the malignancy is from the cervical esophagus, the better the cure rate and prognosis. Many patients have been successfully cured primarily with surgical intervention for some colorectal malignancies.

CANCER OF THE ESOPHAGUS

Malignant neoplasms of the esophagus affect most commonly the elderly over the age of 60 with a 3:1 ratio of males to females. The cancerous growth is rarely detected with screening procedures unlike that of the "coin" lesion in the lung, which may be discovered during routine chest x-ray. The continuous spread of the disease as well as metastasis through the lymphatic chain and blood stream has already caused an advanced inoperable stage with distant metastases to the lungs, liver, and bone when the patient seeks medical attention. Consequently, cancer of the esophagus is associated with high mortality and morbidity.

The neoplasm usually begins at the surface of the mucosa and is often located at the distal portion (lower third esophagogastric junction) and least often at the upper third (cervical esophagus). Most esophageal cancers are epidermoid squamous cell carcinomas which are more radiosensitive than the adenocarcinomas. Some authorities believe that the only definitive cure is surgery and that radiotherapy and chemotherapy are only adjunctive treatments or they are utilized only for palliation of symptoms.

Etiology

Heredity has been implicated in the development of gastrointestinal cancer, which is believed to be a multifactorial inheritance.

To date, there are no definitive etiologic factors. However, the following are considered to be **predisposing factors:**

1. Smoking
2. High alcohol consumption
3. Plummer-Vinson syndrome (nutritional deficiency)
4. Lye stricture of the esophagus.

Clinical Manifestations

1. Dysphagia accompanied by weight loss
2. Cervical adenopathy
3. Signs of cachexia
4. Sialorrhea
5. Regurgitation
6. Aspiration
7. Laryngeal paralysis
8. Ulceration (hematemesis, hemoptysis)
9. Perforation into the trachea, mediastinum, lung, or pleural sac
10. Radiating pain or pain in the back (usually indicates mediastinal extension).

Diagnostic Tests and Diagnosis

1. Barium swallow and cineradiography (shows slowed peristalsis, strictures, or filling defects).
2. Exfoliative cytology (esophageal and gastric saline lavage).
3. Fiberoptic esophagoscopy with biopsy.

Patient Management

The goal of therapy is to render the most humane form of treatment possible so that the patient may be able to eat, hopefully until the end of his life, by a careful determination of the most effective treatment modality.

Various methods of treating the patient have been investigated but the outlook is still very grim. Some medical treatment centers have employed the following approaches:1

1. Staging workup, which includes bronchoscopy, chest x-rays, scalene node biopsy, liver and bone scan, mediastinoscopy and mediastinal node biopsy, skeletal survey (rarely done), and pretreatment laparotomy to determine celiac nodes and liver involvement.

2. Utilization of artificial tubes such as the Mousseau Barbin placed endoscopically to bridge the tumor for temporary relief of dysphagia. [1]
3. Radiation therapy for epidermoid squamous cell carcinoma located in the cervical esophagus above the aortic arch.
4. Rotational irradiation of the entire length of the esophagus with 5000 to 6000 rads in four to six weeks.
5. Combined preoperative concentrated radiation (500 rads daily for four to five days) followed by esophagectomy within five to six days for upper- and midthoracic esophageal cancers.
6. Treatment protocol[2]
   a. Stage I and II: Preoperative radiation and/or surgery may be used in selected cases.
   b. Stage III: Gastrostomy, radiation alone, or surgery may be used as palliative procedure.
   c. Stage IV: Gastrostomy or irradiation are contraindicated in the presence of fistula or perforation; judicious use of analgesics for patient's pain is recommended.
7. Postoperative radiation, which is limited to 4500 to 5000 rads due to a higher radiosensitivity of the transplanted colon or stomach, may be employed.
8. Irradiation with chemotherapy (e.g., bleomycin).

Complications of Therapy

1. Radiation
   a. Esophageal perforation, hemorrhage (immediate), and stricture (late)
   b. Pneumonitis, fibrosis of the lung with fatal cor pulmonale
   c. Myelitis of the spinal cord for doses greater than 5000 rads.
2. Surgery
   a. Anastomotic leak
   b. Fistula
   c. Empyema
   d. Pneumonia
   e. Malnutrition.
3. Use of artificial tubes
   a. Tumor erosion from pressure of tube
   b. Dislodgement of tube which may cause perforation into the mediastinum
   c. Blockage of tube.

Surgical Removal and
Reconstruction Procedure[1]

Several surgical interventions have been advocated. The first
thoracic esophagectomy was performed in 1940. By 1942,
esophagogastrectomy and esophagogastrostomy were done,
whereby the stomach was brought up antethoracically to re-
establish gastrointestinal continuity. In 1955 interposition of
the right colon was used to re-establish continuity of the alimentary tract. Since patients with esophageal cancers are extremely debilitated, a three-stage surgical approach is advocated for upper- and midthoracic esophageal cancer.

The three-stage surgical approach is as follows:[1]

Stage 1: Celiotomy with en bloc nodal dissection (lymph nodes
around the celiac axis and paracardia are removed) and a gastrostomy is performed. Gastrostomy feeding is usually initiated three days after surgery. Preoperative radiation is 500
rads daily for four to five days.

Stage 2: Using a right thoracotomy approach, a total thoracic
esophagectomy is performed. The upper (cervical) portion of
the esophagus is pulled up and exteriorized into the neck as an
external esophagostomy. After four to five days this "external" esophagus is connected to the gastrostomy by a rubber
catheter. With this connection, the patient is able to take food
by mouth. (See Figure 7.)

Stage 3: Six to twelve months after the second stage, reconstruction procedure is performed. Esophagogastrostomy is
created by first doing a pyloroplasty and fashioning the stomach into a "roll" which is brought up antethoracically and anastomosing it with the previously exteriorized esophagus. (See
Figure 8.)

Improved and advanced technology have encouraged some surgeons to do a more radical surgery, which involves total esophagectomy with splitting of the diaphragm and resection of the
tail of the pancreas, the spleen, and celiac nodes. Reconstruction of the alimentary tract is achieved by either an esophagogastrostomy or by substernal transplantation of the right colon
anastomosing it to the cervical esophagus and stomach (esoph-
agogastrocolic anastomosis).

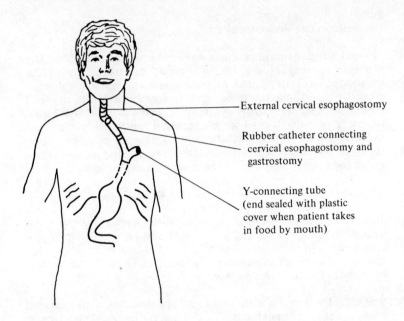

Figure 7: External Cervical Esophagostomy

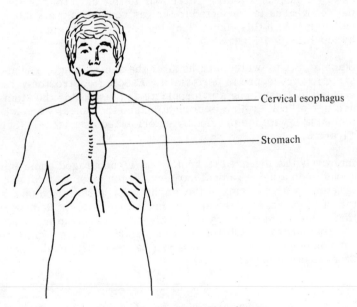

Figure 8: Cervical Esophagus

Nursing Care Implications

1. Prevention of aspiration (presurgical intervention).
2. Monitoring patient for radiation and surgical complications.
3. Care associated with gastrostomy and exteriorized esophagostomy (skin care and prevention of skin breakdown):
   a. Gastrostomy feeding should be given by gravity.
   b. Blenderized food containing adequate nutritive value should be given to the patient.
   c. The usual amount for each meal should be 200 to 500 cc.
   d. Giving the patient something to chew before the feeding stimulates gastric secretions and provides some satisfaction of normal eating.
   e. Provide emotional support to patient and encourage him to participate in his tube feedings until he can be taught how to do it. This lessens the psychological trauma of not being able to eat the normal way.
4. Principles of care related to radiation and chemotherapy should be followed.
5. Principles of care related to the patient who has chest tubes should be followed.
6. Patient-family teaching for home care should be done between three-stage surgical procedures and continued follow-up care.

CANCER OF THE STOMACH

Cancer of the stomach was first clinically identified by Borman in 1926 according to its gross clinical presentation.[1] The most common type is adenocarcinoma (about 97% of them, with over 50% being situated in the pyloric area, 25% along the lesser curvature, 10% each in the cardia and entire stomach, and about 2 to 3% along the greater curvature). The remaining 2 to 3% are sarcomas of which most are lymphomas and leiomyomas. The disease is more prevalent in males, and in the United States and England it is most common among lower socioeconomic groups. It is believed that a 60 to 90% cure may be effected by gastric resection if the cancer is still in situ (localized, early stage). The key to the success of therapy is early detection. Unfortunately, this is very rare due to the insidious onset of the disease and its being asymptomatic until it has reached an advanced stage. Efforts at early detection are aimed at identifying high-risk populations and subjecting them to modern diagnostic tools. Epidemiologic research shows various findings in etiologic factors and incidence. The highest incidences of adenocarcinoma of the stomach are found in Japan, Finland, Chile, and Iceland, with death rates over four times that of the United States white population.

Etiology and Predisposing Factors

There is no definitive etiology of stomach cancer. Some studies indicate that individuals in families predisposed to develop cancer of the gastrointestinal tract carry cells that have developed increased ability to proliferate and that this may be due to combined actions of various genes as well as environmental and other conditions, such as:

1. Nutrition
   a. Deficient intake of vitamins A and C and presence of an antivitamin A in reheated fats and other foods.
   b. High intake of smoked foods (phenol being in all smoked foods, tar, soot).
   c. High intake of talc-treated rice (talc contains fibrous silicates classified as asbestos).
   d. High intake of salted fish, vegetables, and starch.
   e. Deficient intake of fresh fruits and vegetables.

Some authorities believe that lower incidence of gastric cancer is associated with having corn as a staple food in the diet.

2. Pernicious anemia: Associated with high incidence of gastric adenocarcinoma.
3. Chronic gastritis and chronic peptic ulcer.
4. Premalignant lesion: Polyps (villous adenoma), hyperplastic gastrophy, and hiatal hernia. (The last two have more frequent association with malignancy than normal mucosa.

Clinical Manifestations

Since stomach cancer is of insidious onset, the patient may not manifest dramatic symptoms unless the cancer is already far advanced. The patient may only complain of vague abdominal pain (pain is unlike that of the characteristic ulcer pain) which is unresponsive to routine medical remedies. Anorexia and weight loss may or may not be present while achlorhydria and iron deficiency anemia are indicative of malignancy.

Diagnostic Tests and Diagnosis

1. Occult blood determinations in stool.
2. Exfoliative cytology using abrasive balloon or chymotrypsin lavage (highly accurate if positive).
3. Fiberoptic gastroscopy.
4. Upper GI series.
5. Gastric analysis to determine presence or absence of hydrochloric acid in the stomach, either by histamine test or tubeless gastric analysis method.

Treatment Modalities

Gastric adenocarcinomas are not sensitive to irradiation and hardly, if at all, respond to chemotherapy. The high doses of radiation required to effectively treat the neoplasm will be lethal to the highly sensitive GI tract. In some centers, a combination of radiation therapy and chemotherapy have been utilized. One such combination which improved survival more than either modality is the use of 5-fluorouracil and 3500 to 4000 rads loading dose. To date, radiation and chemotherapy are used as adjuvants to surgical intervention.

Surgical intervention remains to be the treatment of choice. Surgery should be performed before metastases beyond the confines of the stomach and adjacent lymphatic pathways have occurred. Historically, surgery of the gastrointestinal tract for treatment of cancer included the following.[10]

1875: First successful gastrostomy.
1879-1880: First attempt by Pean for cancer resection.
1881: Billroth performed the first gastroduodenostomy (Billroth I) while Wolfler performed the first gastroenterostomy
1897: Schlatter performed the first total gastrectomy.
1949: Hunnicutt introduced replacement of the gastric pouch by other viscera and in 1951 Lee employed segments of the colon.

Extremely radical surgeries were performed in the 1950's. The scope of a radical surgery included removal of the entire stomach, spleen, the greater omentum, the body and tail of the pancreas, the hepatic artery up to its junction with the gastroduodenal artery and sometimes the left lobe of the liver. This type of surgery resulted in a high mortality. With the improvement of surgical approaches and postoperative management of the patient, the high mortality rate has improved but the survival rates have not been favorably affected by super-radical procedures. In the presence of hepatic, rectovesicular or rectouterine metastases, ascites, or serosal implants, surgery is done only as a palliation of obstruction, impending perforation, or bleeding. Some of the surgical approaches to gastric resection are shown in Figure 9.

The types of surgery that may be done include:

1. Total gastrectomy: Removal of the entire stomach and duodenum, total gastrohepatic omentum, the greater omentum, the spleen, a cuff of the esophagus, and an en bloc dissection of the splenic, celiac, and pericardial nodes.

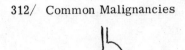

Billroth I
(gastroduodenostomy)

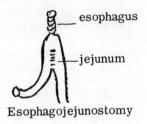

Esophagojejunostomy

Billroth II
(gastroenterostomy)

Esophagojejunostomy Roux-Y
technique

(A) & (B) =
jejunum

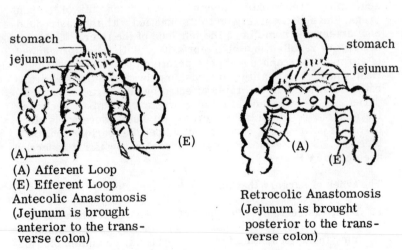

(A) Afferent Loop
(E) Efferent Loop
Antecolic Anastomosis
(Jejunum is brought
 anterior to the trans-
 verse colon)

Retrocolic Anastomosis
(Jejunum is brought
 posterior to the trans-
 verse colon)

Figure 9: Gastric Resections

2. Radical subtotal gastrectomy: Resection of most of the large part of the stomach en bloc with the greater omentum and gastrohepatic omentum with wide regional lymph node resection, splenectomy, and pancreatectomy. If contiguous spread has occurred in the liver and transverse colon, excision of the involved parts may also be performed.

Nursing Implications

The care of the patient after surgical intervention includes the following:

1. Maintenance of fluid and electrolytes.
2. Gastric drainage for at least 48 hours or until gastric residual is less than 200 ml.
3. Patency of gastric drainage tubes should be maintained using an intermittent, low-suction apparatus.
4. Instillation of a buffer or iced isotonic solution via the gastric tube should be done cautiously to prevent anastomotic leakage or injury to the suture line.
5. Enemas should be avoided during the immediate postoperative period since cramping may interfere with healing and/or cause tension on the anastomosis, thereby interrupting suture line integrity.
6. Adjuvant measures which may be given to the patient include antibiotics; vitamins B, C, and E; and anticoagulants as prophylaxis against thromboembolism.
7. Careful monitoring of the patient's condition to ascertain onset of any postoperative complications such as perforation, stomal obstruction, hemorrhage, and infection so that immediate measures may be undertaken to combat the complication. Prevention of the occurrence of the above-mentioned postoperative complications is one of the goals of nursing intervention.
8. Awareness of the possibility of late complications of surgery is essential. Some of these late complications that should be watched for are summarized in Table 12. The nurse should also note that the overall sequelae and prognosis of the patient after surgery depend to a great extent on the degree of malignancy, the kind of surgery done (extent of resection), and the general vitality of the patient.

The therapeutic measures that may be done to combat the various late complications of surgical intervention are also included in Table 12.

Table 12: Complications of Surgery and Related
Therapeutic Measures

Complications	Medical and Surgical Intervention
Afferent loop syndrome (found in patients with long antecolic anastomosis) (See Figure 9.)	Antibiotics (tetracycline 250 mg for two weeks) or other antibiotics; revision of the procedure with short loop or conversion of Billroth II to Billroth I.
Diarrhea (severe) leading to decreased absorption of nutrients (The severe diarrhea is attributed to increased transit time of food, achlorhydria, which predisposes to bacterial overgrowth in the upper GI tract.)	Antispasmodics and sedatives; omission of milk and milk products; bile-absorbing resin; hydrochloric acid and antibiotics; Reversal of an intestinal loop, or interposition of jejunal loop
Weight loss due to vomiting, diarrhea, and/or postgastrectomy syndrome	High caloric diet, especially high in protein and fat; hyperalimentation regimen; frequent small feedings; Surgical construction of gastric pouch; insertion of an antiperistaltic jejunal loop or a by-pass of the gastrojejunostomy
Vomiting associated with afferent loop or dumping syndrome or obstruction	Correction of postgastrectomy syndrome; detour of bile from resected stomach or from esophagus, either by enteroanastomosis or by a Roux-Y procedure; medical intervention usually not satisfactory
Dumping syndrome (due to rapid entry of food into jejunum, hypovolemia due to rapid fluid shift, and hyperglycemia followed by hypoglycemia due to high insulin release)	Frequent small, dry meals; Tolbutamide for functional hypoglycemia; avoid excessive salt and carbohydrates; anticholinergics or antispasmodics, sedatives, and vitamin B-12; resting and/or lying down after meals; avoid psychogenic causes; no fluids during meals and an hour after

Table 12 (Cont.)

Complications	Medical and Surgical Intervention
	meals; interposition of jejunal loop between stomach and duodenum; lysis of adhesions
Anemia: macrocytic and microcytic (vitamin B-12, iron, and folic acid deficiency)	Ferrous sulfate, cyanocobalamin, folic acid; conversion of Billroth II to Billroth I
Osteoporosis and osteomalacia (decreased calcium absorption)	Vitamin D supplement; increase intake of calcium and phosphorus

ILEOCOLONIC AND RECTAL MALIGNANCY

Neoplastic tumors of the small intestine are uncommon. They occur in younger people (slightly more common in men than women) than do malignant tumors of the colon and rectum. Children are practically not affected. The peak incidence is at the fifth and sixth decade of life. About 90% of all the small intestine tumors occur in the ileum, while the most common symptomatic adenocarcinomas are located in the duodenum and jejunum. Besides the metastatic deposits arising from tumors elsewhere in the body, the other primary tumors include leiomyosarcoma, lymphoma, and carcinoid tumors. These tumors infiltrate the mucosa, serosa, mesentery, adjacent lymph nodes and spread by direct extention into other organs. Regardless of the tumor type, the signs and symptoms are intermittent epigastric or periumbilical pain, and, depending on the site (e.g., the duodenum) there may be biliary obstruction, malabsorption, bleeding, and bowel obstruction.

Colorectal neoplasms are considered the second most frequently fatal cancer in the United States. It equally affects men and women, although carcinoma of the colon is more common in women whereas cancer of the rectum is more common in men. Two out of three patients are over 50 years old with cancer appearing earlier in those who have familial polyposis and chronic ulcerative colitis.

Colonic cancers spread into regional lymph nodes in at least 50% of all cases. Most of them spread into the periaortic nodes following the course of mesenteric vessels. Rectal cancer spreads into the perineal and groin nodes rather than retroperitoneally. They also rarely extend longitudinally over 5 cm from the gross tumor. However, attachment to the adjacent abdominal structures such as the small bowel, genitourinary tract, and ovaries is frequent. Distant lymphatic and hematogenic spread to the liver, lungs, bones, and kidneys as well as seeding into the peritoneal cavity can occur.

Various sources indicate different percentages in the distribution of the tumors along the colon and rectum. However, there seems to be general consensus that two-thirds of colorectal neoplasms are within 24 cm of the anal orifice, which make them detectable by digital examination and proctosigmoidoscopy.[35] According to Morton, the distribution of neoplastic tumors is as follows: rectum, 50%; sigmoid, 20%; descending colon, 6%; transverse colon, 8%; and cecum and ascending colon, 16%.[16]

PREDISPOSING FACTORS

1. Multiple polyposis: Mendelian dominant affecting both sexes and has a very high tendency to become malignant. They can occur in all parts of the colon.
2. Gardner syndrome: Hereditary disease which can eventually become malignant.[3,34]
3. Chronic ulcerative colitis: A definite risk factor with a familial tendency.
4. Adenomatous polyps: Approximately 15% become malignant. Controversy still exists as to their being premalignant. They are small, reddish lesions, frequently on a stalk, occurring most frequently in the rectum and sigmoid but can arise in any part of the colon.
5. Villous adenomas: High likelihood of developing invasive cancer. They are soft, spongy lesions with no stalk arising from colonic wall, usually in the sigmoid and rectum. They possess many villous projections on their surface.
6. Diet: Higher incidence of colon cancer is attributed to the lack of unabsorbable cellulose in the diet causing a longer transit time of fecal material through the colon.[33]

Clinical Manifestations

General signs and symptoms include anorexia, nausea, vomiting, weight loss, abdominal cramps and pain, anemia, GI bleeding, perforation, intestinal obstruction, jaundice, hepatomegaly, cachexia, inguinal hernia, an asymptomatic palpable mass, and abdominal distention. The type of symptom depends on the location of the tumor and stage of the disease. Dull pelvic pain is associated with metastasis beyond the local lymph nodes.

The signs and symptoms according to location are:

1. Right colon (cecum, ascending colon, and one-half of transverse colon)
   a. Right lower quadrant pain, intractable anemia, weight loss.
   b. Manifestation of bowel obstruction if tumor is large.
   c. Signs and symptoms of small bowel obstruction (if ileocecal valve is obstructed by tumor) such as anorexia, nausea, vomiting, upper abdominal pain and palpable mass.
2. Left colon (one-half of transverse colon and sigmoid colon).
   a. Change in bowel habits.
   b. Decreased caliber of stools, such as pencil-like appearance.
   c. Mucus and blood in stools.
   d. Feelings of incomplete bowel evacuation.
   e. Signs of bowel obstruction, such as constipation, lower abdominal crampy pains and distention.
3. Rectum
   a. Rectal bleeding.
   b. Prolapse of tumor through the anus.
   c. Sense of incomplete evacuation.
   d. Tenesmus and pain (pain is a late feature).

Diagnostic Tests and Diagnosis

1. Rectal examination: One-half of all colon cancers can be detected this way.
2. Sigmoidoscopy: Two out of three colorectal tumors can be seen and biopsied.
3. Fiberoptic endoscopy: Visualization of the right colon can be accomplished by gas insufflation. Biopsy forceps and polypectomy snares can be passed to remove the polyps and tissue for histological examination.
4. Barium enema and air contrast: Especially helpful in diagnosing tumors of the cecum.
5. Silicone foam enema: The expelled silicone cast may show indentations imprinted by tumors, or polyps and cells for histology may also be recovered from surface of the silicone.

Carcinoembryonic antigens (CEA) have been identified as tumor markers but are nonspecific. A persistently positive CEA postoperatively indicates the presence of metastatic disease.

Treatment Modalities

Simple resection to radical ileocolonic and perineal resections as well as en bloc dissection of involved intraperitoneal organs and lymph nodes may be performed. Therapeutic and palliative measures depend on the location of the tumor and the extent of the disease process. The following approaches may be used:

1. Surgery
   a. Anal carcinoma: Abdominal perineal resection (A&P and groin dissection with creation of a permanent colostomy).
   b. Rectosigmoid carcinoma: Abdominoperineal resection and creation of permament colostomy with or without groin dissection; anterior resection with primary anastomosis; and proctosigmoidectomy with "pull-through" and anastomosis and preservation of external sphincter muscle.
   c. Right colon carcinoma: Resection with end-to-end anastomosis of the colon.
   d. Metastatic tumor: Permanent colostomy or permanent ileostomy and abdominal-perineal resection and dissection of mesentery, lymph nodes, and organs (e.g. bladder, uterus, adnexae, ovaries) attached to the primary tumor. When such organs are removed, the term total pelvic exenteration is used and the patient will therefore have, in addition to either ileostomy or colostomy, a urinary diversion. (Urinary diversion procedures will be discussed in cancer of the genitourinary tract.)
2. Radiotherapy: Doses of 6000 rads given in six weeks may eradicate the primary lesion in 50 to 75% of cases since colorectal adenocarcinomas are only moderately sensitive. This mode of therapy is usually indicated in the treatment of local perineal recurrence to reduce pain and tumor size, inoperable lesions to relieve obstruction and hemorrhage, and poor surgical risk patients and who refuse surgery.
3. Heat coagulation or radon seed implantation: May be used for local palliation of symptoms and reduction of the size of the tumor.
4. Chemotherapy: Various chemotherapeutic agents have been tried as adjuvant therapy. Refer to Part III, Chapter 7 for the listing of these drugs and the nursing implications.
5. Combined therapy (chemotherapy, radiation, and surgery): Some centers have used preoperative irradiation. The Radiation Therapy Oncology Group (RTOG) and Central Oncology

Group (COG) are investigating the effectiveness of low dose (3000 rads) versus high dose (4500 rads) preoperatively on survival rate. Other groups are investigating the combination of chemotherapy (e.g., 5-fluorouracil and moderate dose (3500 to 4000 rads) for unresectable and recurrent cancers.

Nursing Implications

1. Preoperative care of the patient with ileocolonic and rectal malignancy: psychological preparation is of utmost importance, especially in patients who will have an ostomy.[23] Some institutions have enterostomal therapists who can play a major role in the care of the patient preoperatively and postoperatively. In the absence of such health care givers, the nurse assumes the primary responsibility in caring for the patient and family. Psychosocial principles related to the care of the ostomy patient have been discussed in Part 4, Chapter 11. Patient teaching is discreetly carried out and may include information regarding the presence of nasogastric tube, cecostomy tube, an ileocolostomy appliance, and a urinary collection bag for exteriorized ureters or ileal bladder. Physical preparations include "bowel prep" (low residue diet or liquid diet three days prior to surgery), cleansing enemas the night before surgery, and antibiotics to "sterilize" the bowel given either orally or per enema, or in some cases the patient may receive antibiotics parenterally.[24]

2. Postoperative care of the patient with ileocolonic and rectal surgery: The emotional care and rehabilitation of the enterostomate or ostomate (ostomy is coined from a suffix denoting a surgically created artificial opening into a hollow cavity),[8] are influenced by the patient's perception of his body image. Body image is defined as a mental picture of the body's appearance[31] which changes and is continuous in its process of development. It involves the individual's experiences, memory, past association, will power, attitude, and goals.[31] It is believed that people who have firm ego integrity and a clear, definitive body image are usually more independent with definite goals and have positive approaches to daily living. Other factors which influence the patient's rehabilitation are: the degree and length of the disease process, conditions after surgery, radical versus nonradical operations, and sexual functions before surgery. One sexual activity study indicated that only 15% of male ostomates have decreased sexual activity after surgery. It is well to note, however, that male patients who had wide

abdominal-perineal resections can become impotent. In order to be supportive to the patient and family, the nurse must have adequate patient-family assessment of their coping behaviors and support systems as well as accurate knowledge of specific nursing care related to the therapeutic or palliative treatments upon which she tailors her nursing care. For some helpful information on specific nursing care related to types of surgery, refer to Table 13 starting on page 321.

The related nursing care listed in Table 13 is by no means exhaustive and complete. Emphasis is placed on the prevention of complications such as skin irritation. An ileostomy and a urinary diversion procedure predisposes the patient to severe skin excoriation and infection. Enzymes in ileostomy drainage and urine drainage are irritating to the skin. Should fungal infection occur, antifungal and antiinflammatory drug preparations such as triamcinolone acetonide (Kenalog spray) may be applied. Protection of the skin may also be achieved by using karaya powder, coating peristomal skin with tincture of benzoin, and placing a karaya-ring seal or stomahesive around the stoma. Patients with concave abdomen, protruding abdomen, irregular sized or shaped stoma, excessive abdominal scar tissues or a stoma proximate to the waistline may require a custom-made appliance. As a rule, one-eighth inch clearance all around the stoma is provided.

Too frequent changing of the cemented appliance can also irritate the skin. Properly fitted and secure collecting bags may remain in place for as long as five to seven days. Permanent-type collecting bags should be washed thoroughly and allowed to dry in order to prevent retention of odor.

After the period of convalescence, the patient should be encouraged to resume his former lifestyle, resume his previous occupation and recreational activities as long as his constitutional makeup and strength allow. Follow-up care may be provided by the enterostomal therapist, the doctor, the VNA (Visiting Nurses Association) nurse or board of health nurses. The patient should be made aware of the services of local community organizations as well as the Ileostomy Association and its branches. Instruction should further include observation and consulting with the health care professionals for any problems such as change in ostomy drainage consistency, odor, amount, excessive weight loss or gain, protrusion or prolapse of the stoma, stricture, or retraction of stoma and periostomal skin infection.

Table 13: Nursing Care Related to Type of "Ostomy"

Cecostomy and A&P Resection	Colostomy	Ileostomy	Ileal Conduit or Percutaneous Ureterostomy
Tube connected to gravity collecting bag	Drainage is well formed	Drainage is more liquid and continuous. Permanent appliance is worn	Urine flow is continuous
Prevent tugging or dislodgement	Evacuation can be controlled or regulated by irritation and diet	Irrigation cannot regulate bowel evacuation	Ileal-conduit (ileal-bladder) is preferable to percutaneous ureterostomy unless ileum is cancerous
Cecostomy and drainage tubes or catheter post resection are temporary	Depending on condition of patient, use of permanent appliance can be replaced by single gauze dressing upon achievement of evacuation control	Prevention of impaction can be accomplished by chewing foods well and avoiding hard to digest foods such as corn kernels, peanuts, other kinds of nuts	Measure stoma size properly. Opening of collecting bags should fit snugly.
Note drainage for signs of infection, consistency, color, odor	Control of bowel evacuation also depends on site of colostomy. Ascending colostomy has liquid feces and may be difficult to control. It may require daily irrigation	To decrease watery drainage, fresh fruits and vegetables should be limited	Too large an opening can cause leakage into peristomal skin
Irrigation to declog tube as ordered			Too small an opening may impede drainage flow or blood circulation
			Unlike the colostomy or ileostomy the ureterostomy stoma is not markedly swollen after surgery. (The colo-ileostomy

Table 13 (Cont'd)

Cecostomy and A&P Resection	Colostomy	Ileostomy	Ileal Conduit or Percutaneous Ureterostomy
Cleanse skin with mild soap and water to prevent skin irritation around cecostomy tube	Irrigation may be started on the 4th day to the 5th postop day	Odor control may be achieved by avoiding or limiting intake of eggs, fish, onions, cabbage, asparagus and beans	stoma takes about 1-3 weeks for the edema to subside)
Perineal drains (mushroom catheters, penrose) may be connected to intermittent suction or left to drain. Change dressing frequently	It should be done at the same time daily and after meals. Food stimulates peristalsis and emptying of the colon.	Drugs to help decrease fecal odor include charcoal and chlorophyl tablets, bismuth subcarbonate or bismuth subgulate.	A good stoma protrude about half an inch above abdominal surface
	Irrigating solution is at body temperature. Initial amounts at 350 ml to 500 ml until 1,000 ml can be effectively instilled.		Abdominal distention or pregnancy can cause prolapse of an ileocolostomy and ileal-bladder but unlikely for a ureterostomy.
Culture drainage when infection is suspected	Observe for abdominal cramping which may be caused by too rapid flow of solution. If it occurs, lower the	Odor may also be diminished by putting in the collecting bag commercial products such as: banish, ostobon, mouthwash, sodium benzoate or two tablets of aspirin. Aspirin, however,	Reflux of urine can be prevented by emptying bag at regular intervals or as needed and by connecting a drainage tube into a collecting bottle or bag placed below the bed when the patient is in bed.
Warm sitz baths as ordered			

Avoid using rubber ring for patient to sit on post A&P resection. This may cause tension on suture lines which can cause disruption of wound and delay healing.

Patient teaching re: dressing changes, use of ointments and sitz baths (these may need to be continued post hospital discharge

irrigating can and resume irrigation

Lubricate tip of irrigating tube or bulb syringe before inserting into the stoma

Prevent injury to the stoma, remember the colon mucosa has no nerve endings, thus the patient cannot feel pain

should not be used if reflux of drainage unto the skin or stoma cannot be avoided. The acidity of the aspirin may cause skin or stoma irritation.

Collecting appliance (bags) should fit the stoma properly. In 1/8 inch clearance

Replace fluid losses

Electrolytes should be replaced

Adjust fluid intake as soon as ileostomy drainage becomes less watery. Gurgling sound from gas or flatulence can be muffled by gently pressing hand over the stoma

For continued ileostomy: a) continuous drainage is

Table 13 (Cont'd)

Cecostomy A&P Resection	Colostomy	Ileostomy	Ileal Conduit or Percutaneous Ureterostomy
		necessary initially since the reservoir holds only about 150-200 ml. b) maintain patency of catheter to prevent distention and possible rupture or leakage c) catheterization or emptying of the reservoir should be done at least 3-4 times/day within 5-6 months after successful surgery at which time it can hold up to one-half to one liter of fluid d) a silastic catheter (French 28) is best for catheterizing e) lubricate catheter and insert gently into	

stoma

f) a deep breath will fa-
cilitate catheter en-
trance

g) a severe resistance
may be due to anxiety,
patient should lie
down, take a deep
breath and then the
catheter is pushed
gently.

h) complete emptying
may be accomplished
in 10 minutes

i) very thick drainage
may require an irri-
gation

j) use 30-40 ml tap wa-
ter, or normal saline
and instill with an
asepto syringe or
Toomey syringe. Re-
peat as necessary

k) coughing, placing the
hand over abdomen
and exert gentle man-
ual pressure (valsalva
maneuver) can force

Table 13 (Cont'd)

Cecostomy and A&P Resection	Colostomy	Ileostomy	Ileal Conduit or Percutaneous Ureterostomy
		force the thick feces out	
		l) unplug any obstruction of catheter by rotating catheter gently and milking it or stripping it towards and away from the patient	
		m) wash catheter and syringe, cover peristomal area with soft-absorbent dressing after thorough cleansing and drying	
		Chewing food with mouth closed minimizes gas; also using a straw is helpful	

REVIEW QUESTIONS

1. What are some predisposing factors to the development of cancer of the esophagus?
2. Why is esophageal cancer associated with high mortality and morbidity?
3. Which portion of the esophagus most often develops a malignant neoplasm?
4. List at least six of the presenting signs and symptoms of esophageal carcinoma.
5. Discuss the rationale for the staging workup and pretreatment laparotomy for patients with esophageal cancer.
6. What are the local complications of radiation treatment?
7. Enumerate the principles of gastrostomy feeding.
8. List some predisposing factors to the development of gastric cancer.
9. Why is early detection of gastric neoplasms difficult?
10. Give 4 diagnostic tools which may be used in diagnosing cancer of the stomach.
11. Differentiate between Billroth I and Billroth II.
12. Why is gastric drainage necessary after a gastric resection?
13. Give at least 8 possible complications of gastric surgery for stomach cancer.
14. Differentiate afferent loop syndrome from dumping syndrome. What are some of the therapeutic measures which may be utilized to alleviate the symptoms of each condition.
15. Why do anemia and osteoporosis occur as complications of gastrectomy?
16. List six signs and symptoms of small bowel tumors.
17. In contrast to the longitudinal (contiguous) spread of esophageal tumor, describe the metastatic spread of ileocolonic and rectal cancers.
18. Why should proctoscopy be done?
19. What are some predisposing factors to colon and rectal cancers?
20. Differentiate right colon from left colon tumor signs and symptoms.
21. Describe five diagnostic tests which may be used for suspected cancer of the colon.
22. What are the indications for radiation therapy?
23. Define total pelvic exenteration.
24. Compare and contrast a colostomy from ileostomy and an ileal conduit or ureterostomy.
25. Discuss the related nursing care according to type of ostomy.

26. What is a continent ileostomy?
27. What factors influence the patient's rehabilitation?

REFERENCES

1. American Cancer Society. Current Concepts in Cancer, Multidisciplinary Views: Cancer of the Gastrointestinal Tract, Part One, New York (February, 1975).
2. Cancer Advisory Committee, Optimal Criteria for Cure of Patients with Cancer. JAMA, 227:57-63 (January, 1974).
3. Rubin, P. and Bakemeier, R. (eds.), Clinical Oncology for Medical Students and Physicians. The University of Rochester School of Medicine and Dentistry and American Cancer Society, New York (1974).
4. Gillespie, I., Carcinoma of the Esophagus. Nursing Times, pp. 1644-1647 (December 6, 1973).
5. Beatty, J.D., et al., Carcinoma of the Esophagus: Pretreatment Assessment, Correlation of Radiation Treatment Parameters with Survival and Identification and Management of Radiation Failure. Cancer, 43(6):2254-2267 (June, 1979).
6. Reid, H.A.S., Oat Cell Carcinoma of the Esophagus. Cancer, 45(9):2342-2347 (May, 1980).
7. Herrington, J.L., Antiperistaltic Jejunal Interposition for Control of Dumping. Hosp. Pract., 7: (January, 1972).
8. Rubin, P., Cancer of the Gastrointestinal Tract. D. Gastric Cancer. JAMA, 228:1283-1296 (June 3, 1974).
9. Lehane, C., Carcinoma of the Stomach Complicated by Metastasis. Nursing Mirror, pp. 38-40 (February, 1973).
10. Welch, C., Surgery of the Stomach and Duodenum. 5th ed., Yearbook Medical Publishers, Inc., Chicago (1973).
11. Wintrobe, M.M., et al., Harrison's Textbook of Medicine. 7th ed., McGraw Hill Book Co., New York (1974).
12. Kaneko, H., et al., Somatostatinoma of the Duodenum. Cancer, 44(6):2273-2274 (December, 1979).
13. Dent, D.M., Prospective Randomized Clinical Trial of Combined Oncological Therapy for Gastric Carcinoma. Cancer, 44(2):385-391 (August, 1979).
14. Shani, A., Schutt, A.J., and Weiland, L.H., Primary Gastric Malignant Lymphoma Followed by Gastric Adenocarcinoma: Report of 4 Cases and Review of the Literature. Cancer, 42(4):2039-2044 (October, 1978).
15. Olearchyk, A.S., Gastric Carcinoma. A Critical Review of 243 Cases. Am. J. Gastroenterol. 70(1):25-45 (July, 1978).
16. Morton, J., Alimentary Tract Cancer. In: Clinical Oncology for Medical Students and Physicians. Rubin, P. and Bakemeier, R. (eds.), The University of Rochester School

of Medicine and Dentistry and American Cancer Society, New York, pp. 164-197 (1974).

17. Beahrs, O.H. and Adson, M.A., Ileal-Pouch with Ileostomy Rather Than Ileostomy Alone. Am. J. Surg., pp. 154-158 (February, 1973).
18. Beahrs, O.H., Colorectal Malignancies: A Diagnostic Guide. Hosp. Med., 12(4):44-53 (April, 1976).
19. Cole, W.H., Cancer of the Colon and Rectum. Surg. Clin. North Am., pp. 871-882 (August, 1973).
20. Connors, M., Ostomy Care. Am. J. Nurs., pp. 1422-1425 (August, 1974).
21. Dericks, V. and Donovan, C., The Ostomy Patient Really Needs You. Nursing 76, pp. 30-33 (September, 1976).
22. Cosper, B., Physiological Colostomy. Am. J. Nurs., pp. 2014-2016 (November, 1975).
23. Grubb, R. and Blake, R., Emotional Trauma in Ostomy Patients. Am. Assoc. Operat. Room Nurses J., pp. 52-55 (January, 1976).
24. Gutosko, F., Ostomy Procedure: Nursing Care Before and After Am. J. Nurs., pp. 262-267 (February, 1972).
25. Hamilton, M.S. and Schalper, N.J., Pelvic Exenteration. Am. J. Nurs., pp. 266-272 (February, 1976).
26. Leffall, L.D., Early Diagnosis of Colorectal Cancer. CA, pp. 152-159 (May/June, 1974).
27. Schauder, M.R., Ostomy Care: Cone Irrigations. Am. J. Nurs., pp. 1424-1427 (August, 1974).
28. Lamanske, J., Helping the Ileostomy Patient to Help Himself. Nursing 77, pp. 34-39 (January, 1977).
29. Wentworth, A. and Cox, B., Nursing the Patient with a Continent Ileostomy. Am. J. Nurs., pp. 1424-1425 (September, 1976).
30. An Ileostomy a Swimmer Can Wear. Med. World News, p. 34 (February 18, 1974).
31. Plourde, M.C., Reflections on Urinary Diversion. AORNJ, 22(1):45-51, pp. 45-51 (January, 1976).
32. Herrman, R., et al., Gastrointestinal Involvement in Non-Hodgkin's Lymphoma. Cancer, 46(1):215-222 (July, 1980).
33. Cummings, J.H., Dietary Factors in the Etiology of Gastrointestinal Cancer. J. Human Nutr., 32(6):455-465 (December, 1978).
34. Enker, W.E., Carcinoma of the Colon and Rectum. Chicago Year Book Medical (1978).
35. Corman, M.L., The Sigmoidoscope: An Underused Tool. Consultant, 19(10):73-82 (October, 1979).
36. Davis, H.L. and Kisner, D.L., Analysis of Adjuvant Therapy in Large Bowel Cancer. Cancer Clin. Trials, 1(4):273-287 (Winter, 1978).

37. Horne, B.D. and McCulloch, C.F., Squamous Cell Carcinoma of the Cecum: A Case Report. Cancer, 42(4): 1879-1882 (October, 1978).

38. Valdivieso, M. and Mavligit, G.M., Chemotherapy and Chemoimmunotherapy of Colorectal Cancer: Role of the Carcinoembryonic Antigen. Surg. Clin. North Am., 58 (3):619-631 (June, 1978).

39. Stevens, K.R. Jr., Fletcher, W.S., et al., Anterior Resection and Primary Anastomosis Following High Dose Preoperative Irradiation for Adenocarcinoma of the Recto-Sigmoid. Cancer, 41(5):2065-2071 (May, 1978).

CHAPTER 32
Hodgkin's Disease

Hodgkin's disease is characterized by a painless progressive enlargement of lymphoid tissue. This disease constitutes 40% of malignant lymphomas and affects mostly those between the ages of 20 and 40 years (about 50% of cases). Less than 10% occur after age 60 and less than 10% before age 10. Males are predominantly affected (4:3 ratio) and generally have a worse prognosis.[1,2,6]

The first sites of involvement are usually the lymph nodes in the upper half of the body. Spread of the disease is usually contiguous, extending from the primary site to the adjacent lymph nodes.

ETIOLOGY

1. Infectious etiology has been implicated due to the chills, fever, and leukocytosis present during the course of the disease.
2. Recent investigations suggest that it is of tumoral origin as evidenced by the presence of atypical mitosis and invasion and destruction of surrounding tissue that are characteristic of malignant growth.
3. Abnormalities in cellular immunity have been demonstrated as evidenced by the increased susceptibility to a variety of bacterial, viral, fungal, and protozoal infections when the disease has become widespread.[4]
4. Heredity is not a significant factor in the development of the disease, even though some instances of familial Hodgkin's disease have been documented.[13,14,18]

CLINICAL MANIFESTATIONS

1. Unusual lump, mass, or swelling, usually in the cervical area.
2. The enlarged lymph nodes are painless and frequently become large before the patient notices them. Whereas 60 to

331

   80% of cervical lymph nodes are enlarged at the time of onset of the disease, only about 6 to 20% of mediastinal, axillary, and inguinal nodes are enlarged.
3. Pressure and obstructive symptoms occur, resulting from
   enlarged lymph nodes, such as pain and edema of involved
   extremity. Cough, dyspnea, stridor, and pleural effusion
   may be present if there is lymphadenopathy in the mediastinum. Inferior vena cava obstruction by the enlarged
   lymph nodes can cause ascites and edema.
4. Systemic symptoms include chills, sweating, fever, pruritus, weight loss, malaise, anorexia, fatigue and anemia.
   Characteristic of the fever in advanced Hodgkin's disease is
   the Pel-Ebstein fever pattern, i.e., a high fever for several days which alternates with normal and subnormal temperatures. This pattern occurs in just a few cases, however. Most patients with Hodgkin's disease suffer from a
   low-grade fever that they are not even aware of.
5. In a few instances, it has been found that pain may be experienced by the patient almost immediately after imbibing
   alcohol, and lasts from a few minutes to an hour.

DIAGNOSTIC TESTS AND DIAGNOSIS

1. Lymph node biopsy: The largest cervical lymph node is
   usually biopsied to avoid false positives from chronic inflammatory changes in the inguinal nodes or retroperitoneal
   nodes. Presence of Sternberg-Reed cells is essential for
   diagnosis.
2. History and physical examination with special emphasis on
   involvement of lymph nodes will aid in the detection of the
   extent of the disease.
3. Liver function tests and liver and spleen scans should be
   done.
4. Lymphangiography is still the most accurate and complete
   assessment of the extent of the disease.
5. Exploratory laparotomy with splenectomy is done to determine the extent of the disease.
6. Chest films to detect mediastinal involvement and skeletal
   films to detect bone involvement are done.
7. Bone marrow biopsy may also be done.
8. Laboratory findings of anemia may indicate bone marrow
   infiltration. Leukocytosis is present and elevated serum
   alkaline phosphatase indicates liver or bone involvement.
   A BSP (bromsulphalein excretion) test may be done to evaluate liver function.

CLINICAL STAGING OF THE DISEASE

A generally accepted classification of anatomic staging in Hodgkin's disease is that of the 1971 Ann Arbor Symposium on Staging in Hodgkin's disease as follows:1

Stage I: Involvement of one anatomical region or a localized extra lymphatic organ or site.

Stage II: Involvement of two or more anatomic regions on the same side of the diaphragm or extra involvement of extralymphatic organ or site of one or more lymph node regions on the same side of the diaphragm. Spleen may be involved if localization occurs below the diaphragm.

Stage III: Involvement of lymph node regions on both sides of the diaphragm, which may also be accompanied by localized involvement of extralymphatic organ or site or by involvement of the spleen.

Stage IV: Diffuse or disseminated involvement of one or more extralymphatic organs or tissues with or without associated lymph node enlargement.

TREATMENT MODALITIES

Treatment is designed according to the individual's needs based on the anatomic extent of the disease, the presence or absence of underlying medical problems not necessarily related to Hodgkin's disease, such as orthopedic problems. 2,5,11,14

Localized Hodgkin's disease responds very well to early and vigorous therapy with radiotherapy and chemotherapy. Advanced Hodgkin's disease does not usually respond as well to treatment.

Radiation is the primary form of treatment for localized Hodgkin's disease. Megavoltage radiotherapy delivers tumoricidal doses with little, if any, of the cutaneous reactions that can occur in a kilovoltage therapy. While radiotherapy is the treatment of choice in stage I and II Hodgkin's disease, chemotherapy is believed to be the primary treatment for disseminated cases.

In stage III Hodgkin's disease, radiotherapy is also used followed by chemotherapy when relapse occurs. Chemotherapy is also useful in stage IV. 9,16,17

The sequential protocol for chemotherapy of Hodgkin's disease may be as follows:4,6,8,18

1. Alkylating agent, such as cyclophosphamide, is initially given.
2. If relapse occurs, a plant alkaloid is used such as vinblastine and is followed by procarbazine (Matulane).
3. Bleomycin may also be given to provide still further remissions.
4. Procarbazine, a chemical relative to monoamine oxidase (MAO) inhibitors can be given if the patient is no longer responsive to the alkylating agents and alkaloids and will yield six months or more of remission.
5. Combined chemotherapy of mechlorethamine (Mustargen), vincristine (Oncovin), procarbazine, and prednisone has achieved more complete remissions than sequential chemotherapy. This MOPP protocol has proved superior to any single-drug therapy in long-term effects and has improved the survival rates of the disease.

NURSING IMPLICATIONS

The nursing care of the patient involves the psychosocial aspects of cancer nursing that have been discussed in Part IV. Some important considerations need to be emphasized in the specific care of the patient with Hodgkin's disease.

1. At the time of diagnosis, the nurse should make the patient and his family feel hopeful instead of grim about the illness by sharing the reality of the situation and by being supportive. Once the physician has established the diagnosis and has explained the implications of the illness from a medical viewpoint, the nurse can reinforce the physician's explanations. It may be useful to share with the patient that to date in carefully staged, optimally treated patients, the relapse-free survival rates at five years may be expected to be 85 to 90% in stage I and II, 70% in stage IIA and 40 to 50% in stage IIIB, with an overall survival rate of 65 to 70% considering all patients, all stages, and all cases. Since about 95% of all primary relapses occur during the first five years, relapse-free survival for more than five years has been considered almost equal to cure.[2]
2. Since the mainstay of therapy is usually chemotherapy for the early stages of the disease, the nurse should inform the patient of the possible side effects of the drugs and reassure the patient that something will be done to relieve these untoward effects.
3. The nursing care of the patient who suffers from side effects of chemotherapy and radiation therapy as discussed in Part Three should also be followed for the patient with Hodgkin's disease.

REVIEW QUESTIONS

1. What type of tissue is mainly affected by Hodgkin's disease?
2. What type of cell would establish confirmatory diagnosis of Hodgkin's disease?
3. List some of the etiologic factors implicated in Hodgkin's disease.
4. What is the initial clinical manifestation of Hodgkin's disease?
5. Enumerate some of the systemic and pressure symptoms of Hodgkin's disease.
6. What age group is mostly affected by the disease?
7. When a patient with Hodgkin's disease is considered to be in stage I or II, what is the treatment of choice?
8. In disseminated cases of Hodgkin's disease, what is the best treatment?
9. Describe the sequential chemotherapy for Hodgkin's disease.
10. What is the MOPP protocol for treating Hodgkin's disease.
11. What is the advantage of megavoltage radiation therapy over the kilovoltage therapy?
12. Describe the nursing care of the patient with Hodgkin's disease.

REFERENCES

1. Rubin, P. (ed.), Current Concepts in Cancer Multidisciplinary Views. Updated Hodgkin's Disease. American Cancer Society, New York (1973).
2. Bolin, R.H. and Auld, M.E., Hodgkin's Disease. Am. J. Nurs., pp. 1982-1986 (November, 1974).
3. Rodman, M.J., Drug Therapy Today. RN Magazine, pp. 30-34 (February, 1972).
4. Rubin, P. and Bakemeier, R. (eds.), Clinical Oncology for Medical Students and Physicians. The University of Rochester School of Medicine and Dentistry and American Cancer Society, New York (1974).
5. Houghton, A.N., Acute Hepatic Vein Thrombosis Occurring During Therapy for Hodgkin's Disease. A Case Report. Cancer, 44(6):2224-2229 (December, 1979).
6. Jenkin, D., et al., Hodgkin's Disease in Children: Treatment with Low Dose Radiation and MOPP without Staging Laparotomy. A Preliminary Report. Cancer, 44(1):80-81 (July, 1979).
7. Straus, D., et al., The Eight-Drug/Radiation Therapy Program (MOPP/ABOV/RT) for Advanced Hodgkin's Disease. Cancer, 46(2):233-240 (July, 1980).
8. Kaplan, H.S., Hodgkin's Disease: Unfolding Concepts Concerning Its Nature, Management and Prognosis. Cancer, 45(10):2439-2474 (May, 1980).

9. Wollner, N., et al., Improved Prognosis in Children with Intra-Abdominal Non-Hodgkin's Lymphoma Following LSA2L2 Protocol Chemotherapy. Cancer, 45(12):3034-3039 (June, 1980).

10. Gattiker, H., et al., Spontaneous Regression in Non-Hodgkin's Lymphoma. Cancer, 45(10:2627-2632 (May, 1980).

11. Long, J.C., et al., Terminal Deoxynucleotidyl Transferase Positive Lymphoblastic Lymphoma, A Study of 15 Cases. Cancer, 44(6):2127-2139 (December, 1979).

12. Smith, G.R., et al., Identification of Lymphoblastic Lymphoma Cells Using a Dual Assay for T-Cell Differentiation Markers. Cancer, 44(6):2059-2082 (December, 1979).

13. Bremer, K., Cellular Renewal Kinetics of Malignant Non-Hodgkin's Lymphomas. Rec. Results Cancer Res., 65:5-11 (1978).

14. Murphy, S.B., Childhood Non-Hodgkin's Lymphoma. N. Eng. J. Med., 299(22):1446-1448 (December, 1978).

15. Aisenberg, A.C., The Staging and Treatment of Hodgkin's Disease. N. Eng. J. Med., 299(22):1228-1232 (November, 1978).

16. Prosnitz, L.R. and Montalvo, R.L., The Therapy of Hodgkin's Disease - 1978: A Combined Modality Approach. Prog. Clin. Cancer, 7:97-112 (1978).

17. Devita, V.T. Jr., et al., The Chemotherapy of Hodgkin's Disease: Past Experiences and Future Directions. Cancer, 42(Suppl. 2):979-990 (August, 1978).

18. Ragab, A.H. and Lui, V.K., Hodgkin's Disease in Children. Pediat. Ann., 7(7):491-499 (July, 1978).

CHAPTER 33
Cancer of the Urogenital Tract

Primary kidney tumors are frequently asymptomatic, although in some cases the triad of a palpable mass, hematuria, and pain are the presenting symptoms. Unfortunately the symptoms appear only during the late stage of the disease. The most common malignant neoplasms are classified as:[2]

1. Adenocarcinoma: Arising from renal tubular epithelium or pre-existing renal adenoma.
2. Transitional cell carcinoma: From the epithelial lining of the pelvicalycine system.
3. Wilms' tumor or neuroblastoma: Arising from immature parenchymal tissue.
4. Other rare tumors which arise from the mesodermal elements of the kidney.

ADENOCARCINOMA OF RENAL PARENCHYMA AND TRANSITIONAL CELL OR SQUAMOUS CELL CARCINOMA[1]

Renal adenocarcinoma (adenocarcinoma of the renal parenchyma) is also called hypernephroma. Some authorities disagree in so far as the use of nomenclature because the tumor has variable patterns. Other terms which have been used to designate renal adenocarcinoma are Grawitz tumor, malignant nephroma, and metanephroma.

Adenocarcinomas comprise about 80% of all the primary renal tumors with a 2:1 male predominance, ages 50 to 60. Few families have been noted to become afflicted with the disease, although there is no consistent familial or hereditary tendency. Occasionally there is bilateral occurrence of the tumor in any part of the renal parenchyma.

Transitional or squamous cell carcinomas of the renal pelvis equally affects males and females. It is conjectured that they might be related to the presence of chronic irritation and

337

inflammation of the pelvicalycine system from renal calculous. In experimental animals, development of the renal tumors have been related to (1) hormones, e.g., diethylstilbestrol, (2) chemical carcinogens, e.g., various nitrosamines, and (3) viruses, polyoma and simian (SV40) viruses.

Signs and Symptoms

1. As previously stated, the presenting triad of a palpable mass, pain, and hematuria may be manifested when the disease process is at an advanced stage.
2. Occult bleeding or a palpable abdominal mass warrants further diagnostic methods.
3. Other symptoms which may accompany an advanced disease include: fever, polycythemia, gross hematuria with or without pain, or colicky pain with passage of blood clots, anemia, weakness, and weight loss.
4. In far-advanced metastatic disease, associated organ dysfunctions will accompany metastasis to the inferior vena cava (venous obstruction), lungs, bones, liver, and brain.

Diagnostic Tests

To differentiate a renal cyst from a neoplasm as well as to determine the extent of the disease, the following diagnostic procedures are advocated:

1. Selective renal arteriography: Shows the neoplastic vasculature and extent of the tumor.
2. IVP: Shows presence of a space-occupying mass, displacement or filling defect of the pelvicalyceal system.
3. Nephrotomography or ultrasound: Helpful in differentiating cystic versus solid tumors.
4. Venocavography: Helpful in determining the extent of the disease, e.g., obstruction or filling defect of the vena cava or renal vein from thrombus or nodal compression.
5. Needle aspiration or ureteral catheter irrigation: Used as adjunct in determining presence of malignant cells or for cytologic studies.
6. Urinary LDH: Elevation is associated with malignant lesions but not in renal cysts.

Therapeutic and Palliative Measures

1. Surgery: Anatomic staging of the disease (TNM classification is not widely used) is necessary in order to afford the best method of treatment. As a rule, surgical removal is the treatment of choice for all potentially curable cancers.

Therapeutic alternatives in renal cancers such as radiation, chemotherapy, cryosurgery, or use of the laser beam are not preferable to surgery. Surgical management should include removal of the tumor and its capsule or a radical nephrectomy with dissection of the perirenal fat and fascia, renal veins, periaortic and pericaval nodes, adjacent muscle, and viscera, such as removal of invaded portion of the bowel. (The large bowel rather than the small intestines is more often implicated in renal cancers.) This type of radical surgery is indicated for stages I through III. In far-advanced (stage IV) cases, palliative nephrectomy and resection of solitary metastasis to the bone, lung, brain, or other viscera may be done.

Operable carcinoma of the renal pelvis warrants a nephro-ureterectomy. The tendency of the transitional or squamous cell carcinoma of the renal pelvis to seed down the ureter and into the bladder requires removal of the ureter.

2. Radiation: Preoperative and postoperative irradiation have been tried. Preoperative radiation has the following advantages:
   a. Inoperable tumor may become operable.
   b. Dissemination of the cancer cells during nephrectomy is minimized.
   c. Tumor bulk is reduced and therefore facilitates an easier removal.

   Postoperative irradiation with 4500 to 5000 rads is used for recurrent or residual carcinomas. Definitive irradiation has also been utilized for nonresectable tumor.

3. Hormonal Therapy: Hormones from the anterior (adenohypophysis) and posterior (neurohypophysis) pituitary gland, the adrenal cortex, and parathyroid glands influence the functioning of the normal kidney. Whereas cortical adenomas and carcinomas are found more frequently in males than females, and spontaneous regression of renal cancers occurs predominantly in males, it is postulated that hormones may be involved in the development and metastatic processes of renal cancers. Various experiments have also shown a direct relationship between hormones and neoplastic renal diseases. Hormonal preparations which have been used for patients with progressive advanced diseases and in whom neither surgery nor irradiation seem feasible are: (1) medroxyprogesterone acetate, (2) testosterone propionate, (3) diethylstilbestrol, and (4) prednisone.

4. Immunologic Response: Spontaneous regression of carcinomas (hypernephromas) of the kidney as well as disappearance of distinct metastases, e.g., solitary pulmonary lesions, have been well documented. This phenomenon is attributed to immunologic response of the body or the presence of hormonal control, particularly in cases where regression of distant metastases has occurred after the removal of the primary renal cancer. In view of the above, it is presumptive that very soon immunotherapy will also be employed in treating renal cancers.

WILMS' TUMOR

Wilms' tumor of the kidney was first described in 1899 by Wilms as an embryonic renal neoplasm consisting of a variety of tissues. Other terms which have been used to describe this highly malignant, congenital mixed tumor include: embryoma, nephroblastoma, adenorhabdomyosarcoma, and mixed congenital tumor. The tumor may be present at birth but may not manifest itself until later in adult life. It affects both sexes equally, occurring mostly between four months and six years, with a peak incidence between two-and-a-half and three-and-a-half years. Bilateral renal involvement varies from 1 to 5% of cases. The tumor tends to be encapsulated for some time but may grow very rapidly. Metastases to the lymph nodes and hematogenous spread into lungs, liver, and bones can occur making a fatal prognosis. Children under two years and over nine years old have the best prognosis. When treated early, cure can be effected. [13,18,23]

Clinical Manifestations

1. The presence of solid, nontender, spherical mass in the flank may be the only presenting sign.
2. Low-grade fever which is intermittent, pain, malaise, and hematuria may accompany the disease process.
3. Hypertension is also commonly present (about 75% of cases).

Diagnostic Tests and Diagnosis

1. Presence of a palpable mass.
2. Occult blood in urine (gross hematuria indicates poor prognosis).
3. Flat plate film of the abdomen (may reveal presence of tumor).
4. Intravenous or excretory urogram (usually adequate for establishing diagnosis).

5. Retrograde pyelography if IVP is not diagnostic.
6. Aortogram and ultrasound may be useful.
7. X-ray of the chest to determine presence of metastases.
8. Exploratory laparotomy to determine primary tumor and nodal involvement.
9. Vena cavogram is done when renal function is altered to determine vascular invasion by the tumor.

It is important to differentiate Wilms' tumor from polycystic kidney disease, neuroblastoma, retroperitoneal mass, and hydronephrosis as requisite to establishing diagnosis, appropriate staging, and implementing an optimum course of therapy.

Treatment Modalities[44]

1. Surgical resection (simple nephrectomy) should be done as soon as possible. Radical nephrectomy is rarely done.
2. Preoperative radiation may be indicated in cases of large tumor mass.
3. Postoperative radiation therapy which is initiated as early as 24 hours postoperatively or earlier.
4. Combined radiotherapy and chemotherapy (e.g., dactinomycin and vincristine) administered preoperatively and postoperatively. It has been documented that the use of radiotherapy and chemotherapy have tumoricidal effects and are effective in preventing metastases. Dactinomycin also acts as a radiosensitizer and therefore augments the effects of radiation.
5. A solitary tumor metastasis (the lungs are first affected) should be removed surgically.
6. In case of a bilateral Wilms' tumor, an open biopsy and exploratory laparotomy are done to determine the extent of the disease. If indicated, a simple nephrectomy of the most involved kidney is carried out or this may be performed at a later time after a course of radiation treatment. Irradiation of both kidneys with 1200 rads (may vary according to child's age) and administration of chemotherapy are carried out. In some institutions, another exploratory laparotomy is done approximately one-and-a-half months later whereby the tumors may be "shelled out" or partial nephrectomy may be performed.[2]

Nursing Implications and Measures
To Prevent Metastatic Spread

1. The child should be cared for with extra caution to help prevent rupture of the tumor and subsequent spread of the cancer cells. No one should be allowed to indiscriminately

palpate the tumor mass. It is imperative that the active child should not be left on his affected side or be placed or allowed in the prone position.

2. Early ligation of the renal pedicle, renal artery, and vein is done during the surgery to minimize escape of cancer cells into the circulation.

3. Careful handling of the tumor during resection must be done since the tumor is highly fragile.

4. Monitor the child for radiation reactions such as skin irritations (burns), **debilitation** and dehydration, bone marrow depression, contralateral nephritis, and, rarely scoliosis.

CANCER OF THE URETER

Primary carcinoma of the ureter is relatively uncommon. It occurs predominantly in males (2:1) ages 60 to 70 and affects mostly the lower third of the ureter. The tumor cell type is transitional or squamous cell carcinoma, which is similar to that found in the bladder and renal pelvis. Some authorities claim there is a variety of ureteral tumors (22 types of epithelial cancers) including adenocarcinomas and sarcomas. Contiguous spread along the ureters and soft tissues as well as lymph nodes occurs more frequently than in bladder cancers.

Clinical Manifestations

1. Painless hematuria: This is the earliest sign.
2. Localized pain over the region of the kidney as the disease progresses.
3. The pain which begins as dull later becomes excruciating in nature. This is due to ureteral obstruction and pressure of the tumor over nerve roots. Severe pain may also accompany passage of blood clots.
4. Hydronephrosis and impaired renal function: This results from obstruction of the renal flow.

Diagnostic Tests and Diagnosis

1. Retrograde ureterography or pyelography
2. Cystoscopy and IVP
3. Cytology for abnormal cells
4. Urinalysis for presence of ureteral casts and blood cells.

Treatment Modalities

1. Nephroureterectomy for resectable tumors.
2. Local excision: Done for solitary kidney or if kidney function is impaired.

3. Radiation therapy and chemotherapy: Used for advanced stage and for residual or recurrent cancers.

CANCER OF THE BLADDER

Malignant tumor of the bladder which commonly affects elderly males (3:1) ages 50 to 70 is the most frequent malignancy of the urinary tract, although other authorities claim that cancer of the bladder is the second most common neoplasm of the genito-urinary tract. Most of the tumors are located in the posterior and lateral bladder wall with approximately 40% located at the trigone area. Most authorities claim that 95 to 97% of these neoplasms are epithelial tumors with predominantly transitional cell and squamous cell carcinomas and only a few adenocarcinomas. These tumors may be papillary with just a small stalk or they may have a tree-like appearance. They may also be flat, ulcerated, and hemorrhagic.

Etiological Factors

Factors which have been proven and suspected as causative agents to the development of carcinoma of the bladder are categorized as:[4]

1. Cigarette smoking (tobacco tar).
2. Industrial chemicals and dyes: aniline, beta naphthylamine, p-biphenylamine (xenylamine), 4-amino diphenyl and auramine.
3. Metabolites of foodstuffs, e.g., tryptophan, which is an essential amino acid. Excretion of excessive tryptophan metabolites in patients with bladder cancer has been documented.
4. Chronic mechanical irritation: chronic bladder infection, vesical schistosomiasis.
5. Chlornaphazine (for long-term treatment of Hodgkin's disease and polycythemia) have also been suspected.

Clinical Manifestations[14]

1. Unless proven otherwise, hematuria indicates cancer of the urogenital tract. Microscopic or gross hematuria which may be intermittent is the most common presenting sign (75% of cases) of bladder cancer.
2. Frequency, dysuria, burning, and urgency may be present.
3. Bladder-neck obstruction and prostatic enlargement may be diagnosed during performance of diagnostic workup.

Diagnostic Tests and Diagnosis

1. Urinalysis.
2. Cystoscopy or cystourethroscopy with deep muscle biopsy.
3. Excretory urography.
4. Bimanual examination under anesthesia (usually spinal).
5. Radiographic and radioisotopic survey for advanced cancer.
6. Pelvic arteriography combined with air contrast intravesically and perivesically (abnormal blood supply, tumor size, depth of penetration of bladder wall, as well as invasion of adjacent structures may be visualized).
7. Laparotomy may be done to assess the extent of the primary tumor, lymph nodes, and other visceral invasion. Placement of clips on identified positive nodes will be carried out for specific localization (seen on x-ray) for irradiation.

Treatment Modalities and
Palliative Measures

Prior to initiation of a treatment regimen, several factors must be taken into consideration, such as the anatomic and histologic classification of the tumor, the general health status of the patient, his ability to survive therapy, capability to care for any urinary diversion appliance which might be used postoperatively, and the skills of the surgeon and radiation therapist.[32,33,34]

Prognosis and treatment methods largely depend on the stage of the disease process.[35] Staging is a crucial determinant of optimum therapy. There is a variety of staging and classification of bladder carcinoma. The TNM system is not widely used in the United States. Anatomic, histologic, and combined staging are shown in Table 13.

Treatment Modalities

1. Surgery
   a. Simple transurethral resection (TUR) (endoscopic resection) with fulguration is usually used for superficial stage and for control of bleeding in advanced cases or poor operative risk patients.
   b. Segmental bladder resection is used for a large single tumor with well-defined margin located at the lateral wall or at the dome of the bladder. (If the tumor is near the ureteral orifice, a ureteral reimplantation is necessary.)
   c. Open diathermy excision with or without radioactive implantation is used as an alternative to segmental resection

Table 14: Staging of Bladder Carcinoma[31]

Anatomic	Histologic	Combined
(Based on depth of infiltration of bladder wall)	(Based on degree of cell differentiation or of anaplasia)	(Consider both anatomic extent and histologic feature)
Stage O: Carcinoma in situ, confined to superficial mucosa	Grade I: Least degree of anaplasia	Group I: Superficial stage (O, A, B); low-grade malignancy
Stage A: Invasion of submucosa	Grade IV: Highest degree of cancer	Group II: Deep muscle invasion (B_2, C); high-grade malignancy (III, IV, V)
Stage B_1: Invasion of superficial muscle	*UICC Staging:	Group III: Metastatic stage; high-grade malignancy (III, IV, V)
Stage B_2: Deep muscle	T_1: Carcinoma in situ	
Stage C: Perivesical fat infiltration	T_2: Submucosal infiltration	
Stage D_1: Spread outside the bladder wall (two nodes involved)	T_3: Deep muscle and fat infiltration	
Stage D_2: More than two nodes and adjacent organ involvement	T_4: Metastatic spread	

*Adapted from: UICC – Union Internationale Contre le Cancer (International Union Against Cancer)

when segmental resection necessitates sacrificing both ureteric orifices.
   d. Total cystectomy with urinary diversion.
   e. Total cystoprostatectomy with urinary diversion and removal of pelvic nodes, seminal vesicles, and as much of the urethra as indicated (cystoprostatourethrectomy).
   f. In females, total cystectomy and hysterectomy with removal of fallopian tubes, ovaries, and the anterior vaginal wall.
2. Radiation
   a. Preoperative dose range from 3000 to 5000 rads enhance beneficial effects of surgery and survival rate.
   b. Intracavitary balloon with central radium source or isotope is used.
   c. Cystostomy and interstitial implantation are used for thick tumors of the bladder wall.
   d. Supervoltage is used for deep lesions. Tumor dose of 6000 rads is given in five to six weeks with booster doses of 500 to 1000 rads.
3. Chemotherapy[25,26]
   a. Topically, thiotepa (using a urethral catheter) may be used for treating superficial, multiple, well-differentiated papillary tumors and as prophylaxis to minimize recurrences.
   b. Systemic treatment using 5-fluouracil has been tried with no evidence of enhancing therapeutic results of other treatment modalities nor any curative effects.

Nursing Implications

Patients afflicted with carcinoma of the bladder are elderly who therefore not only suffer from the sequelae of surgery or radiation therapy but also from the psychophysiologic stresses of aging. They are also vulnerable to radiation reactions (preoperative radiation and definitive treatment in unresected bladder) which include: nocturia, frequency, urgency, dysuria, and diarrhea. Other reactions that can occur 6 to 12 months after treatment include a contracted bladder, hemorrhage, cystitis, ulceration, colitis, and ileitis. Attendant marrow depression as well as other systemic effects of radiation treatment are inevitable. Emotional and physical needs are of changing priorities. Body image change and coping with the rigorous care of urinary diversion procedures are vital nursing considerations. The nurse should know the type of urinary diversion performed. Some of the common forms of diversions include:[20,37]

1. Ureterostomy (percutaneous) or ureterocutaneous: This may be performed with a single or double stoma. To create a

single stoma, one ureter is anastomosed to the other ureter or the ureters are delivered side by side and sutured together.

2. Bilateral ureteroenterocutaneous loops or conduits: These can be ileal loop or sigmoid loop. The ileal loop (ileal bladder) has been mostly used. In an ileal conduit (ileal bladder), a section of the ileum is resected with its blood supply and the remaining bowel segment anastomosed. One end of the resected ileum is sutured closed and the other end is brought to the skin as an ileostomy and the ureters are transplanted into it. Occasionally a segment of the jejunum is used if the ileum cannot be used. The proximal end of the loop is closed and the distal end is united to the skin surface, usually in the ileac fossa.

3. Ureterotransverse colostomy: The "rectal bladder" is also called ureterorectal with colostomy fecal diversion.

4. Colocystoplasty: A portion of the sigmoid colon is resected into the bladder. The urethra and ureters are anastomosed to it in an anatomic position that is as nearly normal as possible. After healing this will function as a bladder.

5. Ureterosigmoidostomy: The ureters are implanted into the sigmoid colon. In ureterosigmoidostomy, the following must be closely observed:

   a. Resorption of urinary electrolytes. Electrolyte imbalance may be indicated by nausea, diarrhea, and lethargy. Rectal tube drainage is used at night to prevent urinary electrolyte reabsorption.

   b. Obstructive uropathy at site of anastomosis between the bowel and the ureter (hydroureter and hydronephrosis with related complications can occur).

   c. Ascending kidney infection (acidifying the urine by supplemental vitamin C and drinking liberal amounts of cranberry juice can minimize infection).

   d. Hyperchloremic acidosis (alkalinization will be necessary to counteract the acidosis).

   e. Fluid intake of about 3000 ml/day and regular bowel emptying will minimize complications.

   f. Low-salt diet may also help prevent electrolyte imbalance. No other food restriction is indicated, although asparagus is known to cause a musty odor in the urine.

Isolated bowel loops for urinary diversion minimize the risks of ascending kidney infection and electrolyte imbalance. The bowel serves as a conduit rather than as a reservoir.[15]

Cutaneous ureterostomy conveys the urine directly from the kidney to the outside stoma. This can be used if the ureters are well dilated and can be made to extent 1.5 cm beyond the level of the skin surface. Complications to watch for include stenosis, stricture, and necrosis. Dilation of the stoma may be useful in some cases. This is done by using a well-lubricated catheter (rubber) or the little finger covered by a well lubricated finger cot. Inflammation, irritation, and bleeding (slight) of the stoma may be caused by a too-tight appliance, urine deposits forming a sandpaper-like crust (this may be dissolved by soaking appliance in a water solution of vinegar), or it may be due to allergic reaction to material in the appliance.

Protective skin and odor control have been discussed in the care of the patient with an ostomy in Chapter 31.

There is no activity restriction except for contact sports. The patient, like any other enterostomate, can swim, go horseback riding, ski, and play tennis as long as his condition permits.

Special apparel is not necessary. Very tight girdles are to be avoided. A professional model can resume modeling. I once met someone who, during her ill-prepared adjustment, revealed how an artificial eyelash cement had rescued her from an appliance leakage during one of her costume changes!

Since the most common method of urinary diversion is through an ileal bladder, a brief discussion of the nursing care of a patient with an ileal conduit is important.

1. Preoperative Nursing Care of the Patient for Ileal Conduit.
   a. Psychological preparation is very essential. An enterostomal therapist can assist the patient in the emotional adjustment needed to cope with the idea of having to have a different way of elimination after surgery. If there is no enterostomal therapist, the nurse can help the patient by being able to reinforce the advantages of having the procedure done, clarifying the patient's concerns, and by being accepting of the patient's reactions to surgical intervention.
   b. In addition to deep breathing, coughing, and leg exercises, the patient should be informed of the various equipment he might see after surgery so that there will be no cause for anxiety or alarm.
   c. Physical preparation is aimed at decreasing the bacterial content of the bowel by giving the patient a clear-liquid diet for three days prior to surgery, sulfonamides such as sulfathalidine or neomycin to "sterilize" the bowel, and giving enemas till clear the day before surgery.

2. Postoperative Care of the Patient with Ileal Conduit
   a. Immediately postoperation the patient will have a catheter inserted through the ileostomy opening for urinary drainage.
   b. Gentle irrigation of this catheter is necessary every two to four hours to remove any mucus secreted by the ileum.
   c. If no catheter is used, the patient will have an ileostomy bag (usually a plastic, disposable one) which is secured over the stoma to collect drainage from the ileal conduit.
   d. Observe for any complaints of lower abdominal pain or distention of the isolated segment of the ileum with urine. This may cause backpressure on the kidneys and rupture of the suture line.
   e. Empty the ileostomy bag frequently to prevent reflux of urine and ensure drainage.
   f. Sometimes a special ileal conduit bag can be used and attached to a drainage apparatus.
   g. Observe any swelling about the stoma which may prevent proper emptying of the conduit.
   h. Observe for any signs and symptoms of peritonitis such as fever and abdominal pain. Report immediately to the physician if any occur.
   i. Maintain the patency of the intestinal tube that will be in place for several days to prevent bowel distention which may impair the intestinal anastomosis.
   j. The dilatation of the stoma will be done daily by the physician for several days. Subsequently, it becomes a nursing responsibility. To dilate the stoma, the finger cot is used over the finger, lubricated (with water-soluble jelly), and is then inserted gently into the conduit. Proper aseptic technique should be observed in carrying out this procedure.

The ileal conduit bag is usually temporary until about six weeks, when the stoma has shrunk to its permanent size. After this, measurement of the stoma is done for a properly fitted permanent ileostomy bag. Two bags are ordered preferably so the patient can have one available when he needs to change the bag, cleanse it, and air it before reuse. The care of the appliance and the skin has been previously discussed in Chapter 31.

REVIEW QUESTIONS

1. Differentiate renal adenocarcinoma from a transitional cell carcinoma of the kidney.
2. What are the triad symptoms of a renal neoplasm?

3. List six signs and symptoms of a metastatic kidney tumor.
4. Give two diagnostic procedures used to differentiate a cystic versus a solid lesion of the kidney.
5. What is the purpose of venocavography?
6. What is the treatment of choice for a hypernephroma?
7. When is nephroureterectomy indicated?
8. List three advantages of preoperative radiation in treating malignancy of the kidney.
9. Discuss the rationale for hormonal therapy in renal neoplasms.
10. Discuss the pathology in Wilms' tumor.
11. Why are chemotherapy and radiotherapy used as adjunctive therapy in Wilms' tumor?
12. Discuss some preventive measures to metastatic spread of neoplastic cells in cases of Wilms' tumor. Why is it that Wilms' tumor lends itself to "mechanical" spread of the disease?
13. Discuss two treatment modalities for ureteral cancer.
14. List five etiologic factors associated with bladder carcinoma.
15. What is the main advantage of performing selective angiography, combined with intravesical and prevesical air contrast in assessing bladder carcinoma?
16. What are the indications for a TUR and segmental bladder resection?
17. Explain four procedures utilized in urinary diversion.
18. What are the advantages of chemotherapy as adjunct to surgical intervention in carcinoma of the bladder?
19. Give four complications of radiation treatment in carcinoma of the bladder.
20. List four disadvantages of a ureterosigmoidostomy.
21. How is dilation of the urinary stoma done?
22. Give four complications of a cutaneous ureterostomy.
23. Discuss preventive measures to the development of ascending kidney infection and electrolyte imbalance due to urinary diversion procedures.
24. Discuss the advantages of an isolated bowel loop used as a conduit for urinary diversion.

REFERENCES

1. American Cancer Society, Clinical Oncology for Medical Students and Physicians, A Multidisciplinary Approach, 4th ed., New York (1974).
2. American Cancer Society, Current Concepts in Cancer, Multidisciplinary Views: Cancer of the Urogenital Tract, Part I. New York (May, 1975).

3. Bearhs, O.H. and Adson, M.A., Ileal Pouch with Ileostomy Rather Than Ileostomy Alone. Am. J. Surg., pp. 154-158 (February, 1973).

4. Campbell, D., Primary Adenocarcinoma of the Bladder. Nursing Mirror, pp. 86-89 (August, 1973).

5. Cole, W.H., Cancer of the Colon and Rectum. Surg. Clin. North Am., pp. 871-882 (August, 1973).

6. Connors, M., Ostomy Care. Am. J. Nurs., pp. 1422-1425 (August, 1974).

7. Casper, B., Physiological Colostomy. Am. J. Nurs., pp. 2014-2016 (November, 1975).

8. Dowd, J., Methods of Urinary Diversion. Am. Assoc. Oper. Room Nurs. J., pp. 37-44 (January, 1976).

9. Grubb, R. and Blake, R., Emotional Trauma in Ostomy Patients. Am. Assoc. Oper. Room Nurs. J., pp. 52-55 (January, 1976).

10. Gutoski, F., Ostomy Procedure: Nursing Care Before and After. Am. J. Nurs., pp. 262-267 (February, 1972).

11. Hamilton, M.S. and Schlaper, N.J., Pelvic Exenteration. Am. J. Nurs., pp. 266-272 (February, 1976).

12. Jensen, W., Better Techniques for Bagging Stomas. Nursing 74, pp. 60-64 (July, 1974).

13. Marlow, D., Textbook of Pediatric Nursing. W.B. Saunders Company, Philadelphia (1975).

14. Paulson, D.F., Carcinoma of the Bladder and Urethra. Hosp. Med., p. 63 (November, 1975).

15. Plourde, M.G., Reflections on Urinary Diversion. Am. Assoc. Oper. Room Nurs. J., pp. 45-51 (January, 1976).

16. Ruiz, J.O. and Lillehi, R.C., Intestinal Transplantation. Surg. Clin. North Am., pp. 1075-1091 (August, 1972).

17. Schauder, M.R., Ostomy Care: Cone Irrigations. Am. J. Nurs., pp. 1424-1427 (August, 1974).

18. Scipien, G., et al., Comprehensive Pediatric Nursing, McGraw Hill Book Company, New York (1975).

19. Shapbell, N.S., et al., A Urinary Device for a Patient with Problem Stomas. Nurs. Clin. North Am., pp. 383-386 (June, 1974).

20. Watt, R.C., Urinary Diversion. Am. J. Nurs., pp. 1806-1811 (October, 1974).

21. Wood, R.Y., Catheterizing the Patient with an Ileal-Conduit Stoma. Am. J. Nurs., pp. 1592-1595 (October, 1976).

22. Zamcheck, N., Promising Approaches to Colonic Cancer. Consultant, pp. 149-150 (September, 1974).

23. Green, D.M. and Jaffe, N., Wilms' Tumor - Model of a Curable Pediatric Malignant Solid Tumor. Cancer Treatm. Rev., 5(3):143-172 (September, 1978).

24. Eidinger, D., Immunotherapy for Genitourinary Cancer.

In: Immunotherapy of Human Cancer. Raven Press, New York (1978).

25. Carter, S.K., Chemotherapy and Genitourinary Oncology. I. Bladder Cancer. Cancer Treatm. Rev., 5(2):85-93 (June, 1978).

26. Goldstein, G., Chemotherapy of Uroepithelial Tumors. Prog. Clin Biol. Res., 25:105-115 (1978).

27. Hoppmann, H.J. and Fraley, E.E., Squamous Cell Carcinoma of the Penis. J. Urol., 120(4):393-398 (October, 1978).

28. Stribling, J., Weitzner, S., and Smith, G.V., Kaposi's Sarcoma in Renal Allograft Recipients. Cancer, 42(2): 442-446 (August, 1978).

29. Limas, C., et al., A, B, H Antigen in Transitional Cell Tumor of the Urinary Bladder. Cancer, 44(6):2099-2107 (December, 1979).

30. Haid, M., et al., Urinary Bladder Metastases from Breast Carcinoma. Cancer, 46(1):229-232 (July, 1980).

31. Prout, G.R., Classification and Staging of Bladder Cancer. Cancer, 45(7):1832-1841 (April, 1980).

32. Utz, D.C., et al., Carcinoma in Situ of the Bladder. Cancer, 45(7):1842-1848 (April, 1980).

33. Cummings, K.B., Carcinoma of the Bladder: Predictors. Cancer, 45(7):1849-1856 (April, 1980).

34. Soloway, M.S., The Management of Superficial Bladder Cancer. Cancer, 45(7):1856-1865 (April, 1980).

35. Skinner, D.G., Current Perspectives in the Management of High-Grade Invasive Bladder Cancer. Cancer, 45(7): 1866-1874 (April, 1980).

36. Recht, K.A., Ureterosigmoidostomy Followed by Carcinoma of the Colon. Cancer, 44(5):1538-1542 (November, 1979).

37. Bricker, E.M., Current Status of Urinary Diversion. Cancer, 45(12)2986-2991 (June, 1980).

38. Levine, R.L., Urethral Cancer. Cancer, 45(7):1965-1972 (April, 1980).

39. Merrin, C.E., Cancer of the Penis. Cancer, 45(7):1973-1979 (April, 1980).

40. Haile, K. and Delclos, L., The Place of Radiation Therapy in the Treatment of Carcinoma of the Distal End of the Penis. Cancer, 45(7):1980-1984 (April, 1980).

41. Mount, B.M., Psychological Impact of Urologic Cancer. Cancer, 45(7):1985-1992 (April, 1980).

42. DeKernion, J.B. and Berry, D., The Diagnosis and Treatment of Renal Cell Carcinoma. Cancer, 45(7):1947-1956 (April, 1980).

43. Jaffe, N., Childhood Urologic Cancer Therapy Related Sequelae and Their Impact on Management. Cancer, 45(7): 1815-1823 (April, 1980).

44. D'Angio, G.J., et al., Wilms' Tumor: An Update. Cancer, 45(7):1791-1798 (April, 1980).
45. Jacobs, E. and Muggia, F.M., Testicular Cancer: Risk Factors and the Role of Adjuvant Chemotherapy. Cancer, 45(7):1782-1790 (April, 1980).

CHAPTER 34
Malignant Tumors of the Brain

Brain tumors in general are of insidious onset. These tumors are usually grouped according to the substance from which they originate, such as meninges, blood vessels, embryonal, cranium, or metastatic.[1] The course and prognosis of growth is usually slow except in medulloblastomas and some metastatic neoplasms.[2] In children, brain tumors are considered developmental; that is, they arise from abnormal growth of cells already present in the brain. Very few are from metastases of noncerebral neoplasms. Most tumors in children are located beneath the tentorium cerebri in contrast to adults which are above it.[10]

GENERAL CHARACTERISTICS OF BRAIN TUMORS

1. Local invasiveness.
2. High morbidity and mortality.
3. Cure rate very rare due to deep-seated invasion of areas of the brain.
4. All "gliomas" are malignant in that they are highly invasive locally.
5. Seeding of tumor cells in the subarachnoid space of the brain and spinal cord.
6. Complete surgical removal is almost impossible except in localized cerebellar tumors in children.[3]

CLINICAL MANIFESTATIONS

Clinical manifestations of brain tumors are variable and are directly related to tumor type and characteristics, specific anatomic location, and the extent of invasiveness. As a rule, an expanding neoplasm in the brain would cause:

1. Increased intracranial pressure (ICP)
2. Cerebral edema
3. Altered brain perfusion

4. Altered cerebrospinal fluid (CSF) circulation
5. Altered neural function
6. Destruction of brain tissues.

General assessment of the patient should elicit specific information on neurological status, such as appropriate affect and response; orientation and intactness of memory (past and immediate events); changes in vital signs and level of consciousness; changes in optic nerve (such as papilledema and atrophy); visual field defects; presence of nystagmus, aphasia, apraxia, abnormal reflexes, paralysis and/or paresis; and ataxia and other unpurposeful or incoordinated movements.[4]

Specific symptoms and signs according to tumor type, characteristics, treatment, and prognosis appears in Table 15.

DIAGNOSTIC TESTS AND DIAGNOSIS

Accuracy of diagnosis is based on the positive findings on neurological examination, history, and scientific diagnostic tools. Principles of diagnostic methods and associated nursing implications were already discussed. In summary, the most commonly used diagnostic tests are:

1. Roentgenogram (skull x-rays)
2. Electroencephalogram (EEG)
3. EMI x-ray scanner (Electronic Musical Instrumentation, Ltd.)
4. Cerebral angiography
5. Ventriculography
6. Pneumoencephalography
7. EMI and CAT (Computerized Axial Tomography), ACTA scanner (Automated Computerized Transverse Axial)[5]
8. LP (Lumbar Puncture) with CSF analysis.

A more detailed presentation of lumbar puncture and CSF analysis is presented below.

Lumbar puncture is contraindicated in the presence of increased intracranial pressure. The withdrawal of cerebrospinal fluid (CSF) can cause cerebellar herniation or shift of intracranial content, thereby compressing vital centers in the brain.

Positive findings include:

1. Pressure elevated above normal (normal: 70-180 mm of water in adults, 50-100 mm of water in children, and 30-80 mm of water in newborn).

Table 15: Brain Tumors

Tumor Type and Characteristics	Clinical Manifestations	Treatment and Prognosis
GLIOMAS - no known cause - affect 40-60 years old - seizure may be an early symptom but not very common Astrocytoma: - most common type of glioma - slow growth - frequently cystic - arise from the differentiation of adult cells rather than primitive cells Glioblastoma Multiforme: (Astrocytoma Stage III, IV) - treatment is palliative with 50% relief of symptoms - survival of 1-2 years or less	General signs associated with increased intracranial pressure and cerebral edema: - headache - usually diffuse. If unilateral, usually on same side as the tumor. - anorexia, nausea, vomiting (vomiting may not be projectile initially) - changes in vital signs: increasing systolic pressure and widening of pulse pressure - positive Macewen's sign associated with separation of sutures in children	Surgical removal (complete removal possible for Stage I, II) - surgery and postoperative irradiation - prognosis good with complete surgical extirpation otherwise survival is limited to 1-2 years for Stage III and IV. - poor prognosis - Treatment: palliative resection and/or decompression with corticosteroids plus intensive radiotherapy

Oligodendroglioma:

- 3rd most common type of glioma
- grows slowly
- often benign
- often mixed with glioblastoma multiforme
- radiosensitive
- 5-10 years survival

Localizing symptoms:

1) central region sensory-motor strip of opposite hemisphere: convulsive seizures confined to group of muscles or one side of body

2) temporal lobe: contralateral homonymous hemianopsia, psychomotor seizures, jerking, repetitive grand mal seizures, hallucinations: memory, visual, smell and taste

3) midbrain and third ventricle: behavioral and personality changes often early, positive signs of increased intracranial pressure and pyramidal tract symptoms (see 4)

4) brain stem and cerebellar signs: papilledema, nystagmus, flashing lights, dizziness, ataxia, hearing loss, paresthesias of face, cranial nerve palsies (V, VI, VII, IX, X, primarily sensory) suboccipital tenderness, hemiparesis, and

- prognosis good for the benign growths
- surgical removal with or without extensive x-ray therapy

Table 15 (Cont.)

Tumor Type and Characteristics	Clinical Manifestations	Treatment and Prognosis
	due to compression of supra-tentorial area can include the other symptoms (general and focal)	- partial surgical removal or decompression
MEDULLOBLASTOMA - frequent in children - greatest during school age - 30% of primary brain tumors - rapidly growing - infiltrative and metastatic - seeding in subarachnoid space in brain and spinal cord - radiosensitive in children but lesser tolerance	Cerebellar symptoms (see 4 above)	- intrathecal or perfusion of site with methotrexate or other an-tineoplastic drugs - 3-5-1/2 years survival (25%-30% 5 years survival with postoperative irradiation)
EPENDYMOMAS - 12% of all tumors - located mostly in 4th and lateral ventricles	Similar to gliomas affecting brain neural functioning due to pressure. Positive symptoms of increased intracranial pres-sure and obstructive hydroceph-alus depend on size of tumor	- surgical removal - surgery plus irradiation - 58%-87% 5-year survival with postoperative irradiation

MENINGIOMAS

- almost always benign
- seizures most common if located in cerebrum

- symptoms related to location and may be multifocal
- headaches, seizures, and hyperthermia may occur

- decompression with corticosteroids and diuretics such as Mannitol and Urevert
- irradiation (extensive x-ray therapy)
- 63% palliative relief of symptoms
- 1-2 years survival or lesser

2. Glucose is decreased in metastatic tumors and highly malignant tumors and highly malignant primary neoplasms (normal: 50-75 mg/100 ml or 20 mg/100 ml less than blood).
3. Tumor cells are occasionally found.
4. Increased levels of total protein are found in one-third of cases (normal: 15-45 mg/100 ml; albumin, 52%; alpha globulin, 5-14%; beta globulin, 10%; and gamma globulin, 19%).[9]

Normally globulin is low and there may not be positive reaction with Pandy reagent. As a rule the globulin is increased in relation to the total protein but it may be increased even if the total protein is within normal limits.

TREATMENT MODALITIES

The goals of therapy include removal of resectable tumor, reduction of bulk of unresectable tumor, decompression of cerebral edema and increased intracranial pressure, palliation of clinical symptoms, and alleviation and/or prevention of further complications such as neurological death, e.g., impaired mentation, sensory, and motor functions.

Treatment regimen is determined by histologic type of the tumor, its radiosensitivity, and anatomic location.

The various types of therapy that may be done are listed below.

1. Surgical removal: Complete removal is possible with localized cerebellar astrocytoma. Invasive tumors can be partially resected.
2. Nonsurgical decompression: This can be effected by drugs (corticosteroids, diuretics) and CSF shunting (ventriculo-atrial shunt, ventriculoperitoneal shunt).
3. Radiation: The dose and technique of administration depends on the type of tumor. Although most malignant tumors are radiosensitive, in general, radiotherapy is indicated in:[15]
   a. Medulloblastomas
   b. Multiple metastatic deposits
   c. Centrally located tumors
   d. Astrocytoma stage II-IV
   e. Sarcomas
   f. Tumors in midbrain and third ventricle
   g. Postoperatively if resection was incomplete.

There are certain problems associated with radiation:

1. Edema as an immediate response aggravates increased ICP and mimics progression of tumor growth.

2. Late recurrent symptoms occur in 6 to 12 months after radiation therapy.
3. Delayed effect on brain is necrosis, usually of the white matter of the brain stem. [4]
4. Systemic effects are as previously discussed.

CHEMOTHERAPY

Intrathecal or site perfusion with chemotherapeutic agents have been tried and are still under investigation. [12] Progress in research is limited due to neurotoxicity of the drugs as well as their effectiveness in crossing the blood-brain barrier. The drugs which have been used are:

1. Methotrexate
2. Nitrogen mustard
3. Cyclophosphamide (Cytoxan)
4. Hydroxyurea
5. Vincristine sulfate (Oncovin)
6. Thiotepa
7. Radioactive gold.

NURSING CARE OF THE PATIENT
UNDERGOING SURGICAL INTERVENTION

Preoperative Care

Patient management is focussed on safety, supportive measures, and alleviation of symptoms. Patient-family supports and positive coping behaviors should be maximized. Discreet discussion of changes in body appearance and possible neurologic deficits should be done. Physical preparation involves shaving the head. CNS depressant drugs should not be given as well as enemas and other maneuvers likely to cause or aggravate increased intracranial pressure.

Postoperative Care

Objectives of care are directed toward prevention of increased ICP, hemorrhage, loss of CSF, improve circulation of blood and CSF, maintenance of adequate respiration, regulation of temperature, seizure precautions, prevention of decubiti formation, and emotional support.

Table 16: Specific Nursing Measures According to Type of Surgical Approach

Infratentorial	Supratentorial
Position flat on either side, head aligned with spinal column, nose in line with breastbone. Use small pillow or folded towels for head support.	Position on unoperated side if large tumor was removed or if bone flap was removed to allow for brain expansion. Bone flap may be saved and replaced at a later date.
Log roll at least every two hours. Turning sheet should extend from buttocks to above head.	Keep on side lying with head elevated 45 degree angle. Do not place patient in Trendelenberg position (sudden increase in circulation and pressure may initiate bleeding).
Gradually elevate head.	
Activity and ambulation: (passive ROM) Active-resistive exercises and ambulation done as ordered.	
Dressing and Drains: check for bleeding and yellow-tinged drainage. Circle area to assess increase in drainage. • Reinforce dressing with sterile sponges. • Incision is just above nape of the head but dressing may cover entire head. Check downhill flow of drainage; • Clear, yellow rhinorrhea may indicate CSF leakage.	Dressing and drains: Dressing is applied over entire head and anchored around neck and back; • Maintain firm support to prevent neck flexion; • Check drainage for character and amount; • Rhinorrhea and otorrhea may be due to CSF leakage.

Fluids and feedings: Patient may take fluids post nausea (gag reflex present);
- No fluid restriction unless indicated;
- Evaluate ability to swallow;
- Prevent aspiration by immediate suctioning.

Note: Other aspects of care are similar and congruent with those listed under infratentorial approach.

Fluids and feedings may be NPO for 24 hours;
- Check for return of gag reflex and swallowing ability;
- Tube feeding is done as needed;
- Monitor output for possibility of diabetes insipidus.

Respiration suctioning should be done cautiously;
- Suction to prevent aspiration as gently as possible (vigorous coughing increases ICP);
- Deep breathing every hour (hypoxia increases ICP).

Temperature: Do not take orally in case of seizures;
- Check frequently, every 15 minutes in hyper- or hypothermic patients (hypothalamic and brain stem involvement, dehydration, thrombophlebitis, and infection may be the cause of hyperthermia);
- Control fever by hypothermia blanket or tepid water and alcohol sponges (massaging stimulates vasodilation, alcohol cools by evaporation).

Note: Prevent frostbite from skin moisture and hypothermia blanket.

Table 16 (Cont.)

Infratentorial	Supratentorial
Eye care: For periocular edema • Coat lightly with petrolatum jelly then apply light ice-cold compress; • Lubricate cornea with "artificial" tears or apply eye patch to prevent drying or irritation if corneal reflex is absent (gauze patch may irritate cornea if lid is not completely closed); • Tarsorrhaphy (suturing together of part or all of eyelids) may be done in the unconscious patient. Seizure precautions: Tongue blade should be at bedside, insert only if jaws are not clenched; • Pad side rails; • Assess presence of "aura" and/or precipitating events; • Do not apply restraint during convulsive seizures; • Administer anticonvulsant drugs.	

Prevention of decubiti formation: Use an
air mattress
flotation pads, or
alternating air pressure mattress

Emotional support and rehabilitation: Role
change and adaptation and speech and physical therapy should be implemented.

• Turn patient as indicated;
• Use cotton doughnuts under pressure areas.
Note: Other measures that may be undertaken to
prevent decubiti are:

• Massage pressure areas such as cheeks, ears,
ribs, acromial process, back of head, scapula, el-
bows, heel malleolus, sacrum, medial and lateral
condyles;
• Prevent drying of skin (do not use soap for washing skin of debilitated patient);
• Check for source of pressure, i.e., bed linen,
equipment.11

REVIEW QUESTIONS

1. List six characteristics of brain tumors.
2. What are the signs and symptoms of increased intracranial pressure?
3. Differentiate gliomas, medulloblastomas, ependymomas, meningiomas, and metastatic brain tumors.
4. Enumerate specific signs and symptoms of the various types of brain tumors in the above question.
5. Identify the treatment and prognosis for:
   a. Astrocytoma
   b. Glioblastoma
   c. Oligodendroglioma
   d. Medulloblastoma
   e. Ependymomas
   f. Meningiomas
   g. Metastatic brain tumors.
6. Name some of the diagnostic tests that may be done for diagnosis of brain tumor.
7. What are the positive findings in a lumbar puncture procedure that indicate the presence of brain tumor?
8. List some of the therapeutic treatments done for brain tumor.
9. What are some problems associated with radiotherapy as a form of treatment in brain tumors?
10. Describe the nursing care of the patient with surgery for brain tumor both preoperatively and postoperatively.
11. Differentiate the positioning of the patient in infratentorial surgery versus supratentorial surgery. What is the rationale for such positioning in either case?
12. Why is lumbar puncture contraindicated in a patient with increased intracranial pressure?

REFERENCES

1. Mazola, R. and Jacobs, J., Brain Tumors: Diagnosis and Treatment. RN Magazine, pp. 42-45 (March, 1975).
2. Luckman, J. and Sorensen, K., Medical-Surgical Nursing - A Psycho-Physiologic Approach. W.B. Saunders, Philadelphia, pp. 482, 530-541 (1974).
3. McDonald, J. and Lapham, L., Central Nervous System Tumors. In: Clinical Oncology for Medical Students and Physicians. Rubin, P. and Bakemeier, R., (eds.), The University of Rochester School of Medicine and Dentistry and American Cancer Society, New York (1974).
4. Peterson, B.H. and Kellog, C.J., Current Practice in Oncology Nursing. C.V. Mosby Co., St. Louis, pp. 118-131 (1976).

5. Pohutsky, L. and Pohutsky, K., Computerized Axial Tomography of the Brain: A New Diagnostic Tool. Am. J. Nurs., pp. 1341-1342 (August, 1975).
6. How to Color the Brain Tumor Blue. Med. World News., p. 41 (November 2, 1973).
7. New, P.F.S., Computerized Tomography: A Major Diagnostic Advance. Hospital Practice, 10(2):55-64 (February, 1973).
8. Mandrillo, M., Brain Scanning. Nurs. Clin. North Am., 9(4):653-669 (December, 1974).
9. Gillies, D.H. and Alyn, I., Patient Assessment and Management by the Nurse Practitioner. W.B. Saunders Co., Philadelphia, pp. 114-122; 224 (1976).
10. Marlow, D., Textbook of Pediatric Nursing, 4th ed., W.B. Saunders Co., Philadelphia, pp. 661-665 (1973).
11. Gruis, M. and Innes, B., Assessment: Essential to Prevent Pressure Sores. Am. J. Nurs., pp. 1762-1764 (November, 1975).
12. Avellanosa, A.M., et al., Chemotherapy of Nonirradiated Malignant Gliomas. Phase II: Study of the Combination of Methyl-CCNU, Vincristine, and Procarbazine. Cancer, 44(5):839-863 (November, 1979).
13. Littman, P., Pediatric Brain Stem Gliomas. Cancer, 45 (11):2787-2792 (May, 1980).
14. Bloom, H.J., Management of Some Intracranial Tumors in Children and Adults. Progr. Clin. Biol. Res., 25:55-84 (1978).
15. Scheithauer, B.W. and Rubinstein, L.J., Meningeal Mesenchymal Chondrosarcoma: Report of 8 Cases with Review of Literature. Cancer, 42(6):2744-2752 (December, 1978).

CHAPTER 35
Skin Cancer

Carcinoma of the skin is considered the most common type of all malignant diseases and an individual who has had a cancer will have a 50 to 60% chance of developing a second cancer, usually a skin cancer.[3] This disease frequently occurs after the fourth decade of life, although children are occasionally affected.

The areas of the body usually affected by skin carcinoma are those that are exposed, particularly the "T zone" areas of the face: lips, nose, cheeks, eyelids, and forehead. The three most frequent types of cutaneous cancer, accounting for the great majority of all malignant tumors of the skin, are basal cell carcinoma, squamous cell carcinoma, and malignant melanoma.[1] The cure rate for squamous cell carcinoma and basal cell carcinoma is between 75 and 95% with any adequate treatment modality whereas a malignant melanoma only affords a 70% five-year survival for a lesion confined to the epidermis that is less than 2 cm in diameter.

Melanocarcinoma (malignant melanoma) is considered the most malignant skin cancer. It is a neoplasm of the melanin-producing cells (melanocytes) which are primarily located in the basal layers of the skin epidermis. It occurs mainly in Caucasians and affects males more than females, occurring most often in the soles of the feet or near fingernails. Unlike basal cell carcinoma, which does not metastasize, squamous cell carcinoma and malignant melanoma metastasize by contiguous spread and by lymphatic and venous routes. Malignant melanoma also has a high rate of recurrence, with new primary lesions invading the cartilage and bone.

ETIOLOGY

Among the etiologic factors implicated in the development of skin cancer are:

1. Exposure to electromagnetic radiation (sunlight, x-rays).
2. Chemical carcinogens (arsenic).

Table 17: Clinical Manifestations of Skin Cancer[3]

Basal Cell Carcinoma	Squamous Cell Carcinoma	Malignant Melanoma
Nodular basal cell carcinoma: Elevated lesions with an umbilicated, ulcerated center; raised margin and waxy or "pearly border"; moderately firm.	Appearance varies from an elevated nodular mass to a punched-out, ulcerated lesion or a large fungating mass. Unlike basal cell carcinoma, these are opaque.	Usually pigmented (black, gray, blue, brown, red): often under 2.5 cm in size. The lesion may be flat or elevated, eroded or ulcerated.[2]
Superficial basal cell carcinoma: Plaque is present, usually with a crusted and erythematous center and a raised pearly border; often multiple.		

3. Genetic predisposition (nevoid basal cell carcinoma syndrome, xeroderma pigmentosa).
4. Thermal burns

CLINICAL MANIFESTATIONS

The clinical manifestations vary according to the types of skin cancer as shown in Table 17.

DIAGNOSTIC TESTS AND DIAGNOSIS

1. Persistent ulcer not explained by any other cause.
2. Ulcer in an old thermal burn scar or x-ray treated site.
3. Suspicious cutaneous lesion in a patient previously exposed to large amounts of ultraviolet irradiation, arsenicals or petroleum products.
4. Firm cutaneous or subcutaneous mass of unusual nature.
5. Pigmented or nonpigmented mole that is undergoing a growth pattern significantly different from its expected biologic behavior.

Table 18: Skin Cancer Treatment Modalities

Squamous Cell Carcinoma	Malignant Melanoma
Excisional removal of 2 cm of tumor	Wide and deep local excision with or without en block nodal dissection
Wide excision combined with skin graft	Radiotherapy used prophylactically postoperatively
Radical neck dissection for nodal metastases	Radioisotope therapy such as 198Au injected into the lymphatics
Radiation (used if extensive surgical excision is contraindicated)	Chemotherapy through regional perfusion using dimethyl triazeno aminoimidazocar (DTIC)
Chemosurgery using multiple biopsy and topical application of drugs containing zinc chloride	Immunotherapy using either BCG intralesionally applied or by melanoma cell vaccines, or use of a transfer factor or lymphocyte transfusion[5]
Chemotherapy by either topical application, local injection or intra-arterial infusion	
Immunotherapy using DNCB applied topically over lesion	

Careful examination of the patient's entire integument should be done to insure complete examination of any skin abnormality.

TREATMENT MODALITIES

The treatment of the disease again depends upon the type as shown in Table 18.

NURSING IMPLICATIONS

A unique nursing concern in caring for the patient with skin carcinoma is that of disruption of body image and self-concept by the disease process, particularly as it affects the face and other exposed areas of the body, the side effects of surgical, chemo-radiation, and immunotherapy. The nursing principles that can be utilized in meeting the needs of the patient with distorted body image and self-concept have been discussed earlier.

Careful postoperative care of full thickness or pedicle skin grafts to ensure optimum cosmetic effect is one of the nursing care goals. Avoid pressure on the graft side, do not position patient on affected areas, and inform the patient of the importance of avoiding pressure.[4]

It should be emphasized that the cure rate for skin cancer is excellent with adequate treatment except in malignant melanoma. The patient should be reassured of the good prognosis as determined by the physician.

REVIEW QUESTIONS

1. What areas of the body are predisposed to the development of skin cancer?
2. Differentiate basal cell carcinoma, squamous cell carcinoma, and malignant melanoma in terms of clinical manifestations and rate of cure.
3. Which type of skin cancer does not metastasize?
4. List chemotherapeutic modalities used in the treatment of squamous cell carcinoma.
5. Name four immunotherapeutic agents used as treatment of malignant melanoma of the skin.

REFERENCES

1. Gumport, S.L., Harris, M.N., and Kopf, A.W., Diagnosis and Management of Common Skin Cancers, Professional Education Publication, American Cancer Society, New York (1974).
2. Clark, Wilt, et al., The Histogenesis and Biologic Behavior of Primary Human Malignant Melanomas of the Skin. Cancer Res., 29:705-726 (1969).
3. Rubin, P. and Bakemeier, R. (eds.), Clinical Oncology for Medical Students and Physicians. The University of Rochester School of Medicine and Dentistry and American Cancer Society, New York (1974).
4. Cipollaro, A., Cancer of the Skin. Am. J. Nurs., 66(10) (October, 1966), (A Reprint by the American Cancer Society).
5. Gutterman, J.V., et al., Active Immunotherapy with BCG for Recurrent Malignant Melanoma. Lancet, pp. 1208-1212 (June 2, 1973).

CHAPTER 36
Retinoblastoma and Malignant Melanoma of the Eye

RETINOBLASTOMA

Retinoblastoma is the second most common cancer in childhood. About 30% of cases have bilateral occurrence of the disease. The tumor is believed to be present at birth but does not manifest itself until the age of three years. It is very seldom seen in children after the age of six. Retinoblastoma may occur as a solitary or multiple tumor with varying sizes. Some may involve over one-half of the retina. The tumor may outgrow its blood supply, thereby becoming calcified or necrotic, which has occasionally produced spontaneous regression. Local seeding into the vitreous tumor, into the iris and anterior eye chamber, and optic nerve involvement may serve as an avenue for metastases. Distant spread occur through the hematologic route.

Etiology

Retinoblastoma is a dominant autosomal gene, thereby one who survives the disease has a 50% chance of bearing a child who will develop the disease. The disease is also believed to be caused by genetic mutation. Some authorities contend that more than 90% occur sporadically without familial predisposition.[2]

Clinical Manifestations

The tumor in the retina may be seen by opthalmoscopy or retinoscopy. A large neoplasm may cause whitening of the pupil, strabismus, signs of inflammation, and increased intraocular pressure or glaucoma. There may also be nausea, vomiting, severe pain in and around the eye, halos or circles seen around bright lights, steamy cornea, blurred vision, and progressive blindness.

Diagnostic Tests

1. Retinoscopy
2. Radioactive uptake

3. Roentgenography
4. Echogram.

Treatment Modalities

1. Enucleation (complete removal of the eyeball) with resection of as much of the optic nerve as possible.
2. Radiation therapy to the cranium is done when there is involvement of the optic nerve.
3. Radiation and chemotherapy are used to treat the less affected eye in bilateral retinoblastoma.

MALIGNANT MELANOMA OF THE EYE

This neoplastic process involves the uveal tract. Malignant melanoma is the most common cancer of the eye affecting adults after the fifth decade of life. Like retinoblastoma, this type of cancer is primarily a disease affecting Caucasians. It differs from retinoblastoma in that this malignancy very rarely has a genetic predisposition. The tumor occurs independently from melanocarcinoma of the skin. Extraocular extension may involve the iris, ciliary body, orbital bones, and other distant tissues of the body.

Etiology

Factors associated with this type of carcinoma are pre-existing nevi, stromal melanocytes of the uvea, retinal pigmented epithelium, and severe inflammation or trauma.[2]

Clinical Manifestations

1. Tumor seen by ophthalmoscopy
2. Loss of peripheral vision as disease progresses
3. Presence of floaters before the eyes
4. Development of secondary glaucoma and/or cataract.

Diagnostic Tests

1. Ophthalmoscopy
2. X-ray of orbital bones to detect orbital involvement
3. Radioactive uptake.

Treatment Modalities

1. Excision for localized melanoma of the iris or ciliary body (most effective method).
2. Enucleation of the eyeball.

3. Exenteration of the eyeball, all contents of the orbital cavity, and perhaps the eyelids.
4. Radon seed implants.

Nursing Implications

The child who undergoes enucleation, exenteration, or radiation therapy suffers from the effects of separation and inability to comprehend the reasons for the treatment. The overall impact of the cancer is not fully grasped. However, for the parents, it is very distressing, as feelings of guilt may arise when the parents believe they have been instrumental in the development of their child's illness. The adult patient with malignant eye melanoma and the family members will invariably go through the grieving process associated with the loss of a body part and the threat of cancer as a killer disease. Holistic approach in caring for the patient should be maintained. Specific nursing care of the patient should include:[3,4]

1. Discussion of the possible complications of radiation regarding its effect on the facial bone. Radiation can arrest bone growth which may cause facial asymmetry.

2. Close observation of the possible complications of enucleation should be done. These complications include hemorrhage, thrombosis of blood vessels, and infection. Pressure dressings should be maintained for as long as five days to prevent possible hemorrhage.

3. Headache or pain in the operated side should be reported at once as it may indicate a complication of meningitis resulting from venous thrombosis of adjacent veins.

4. Ambulation may be allowed the day following surgery. The nurse should assist the patient in ambulating.

5. The patient should be informed that an artificial eye may be used as soon as complete tissue healing has occurred, which may be within six to eight weeks, although some patients may wear a prosthetic eyeball as early as three weeks.

6. The types of prostheses should be discussed so that the patient is afforded a choice of which to buy and wear. Prosthetic eyeballs can either be made of glass or plastic material. For longevity, glass eyes are better if not broken, although they are much heavier. Plastic prostheses are lighter, more expensive, and generally have to be replaced

every year or two because they get rough along the edges and may irritate the conjunctiva.[5]

7. It is important for the nurse to inform the patient who has an exenteration that it may not be feasible to use an artificial eye. In the case of the patient with enucleation, the artificial eye can either be shell-shaped or hollow, depending on what is needed as a result of the surgical procedure done. It is best to have the prosthetic eyeball match the color and size of the good eye for maximum cosmetic effect.

8. Care of the affected eye is important and is a nursing responsibility initially. This includes dressing changes and irrigation as ordered by the physician. The patient is gradually allowed to assume responsibility for his eye care after being taught how to do it by the nurse.

9. The patient should be taught how to insert and remove the artificial eye. To insert the eyeball, gently evert the lower lid, being certain that the narrower end of the eye is placed properly next to the inner angle of the orifice. Then grasp the upper eyelashes and gently raise the upper lid. With the finger of the other hand, gently slip the eyeball in place. To remove the eyeball, gently press upward on the lower lid, being certain that the cupped hand is held against the cheek so that the eye does not fall down and break or become lost.[1]

10. Care of the good eye is of utmost importance. The patient should be instructed to avoid strain on the good eye and protect it from injury by wearing protective eyeglasses.

11. Provide reassurance to the adult patient that in time he will get used to having only one eye to go about his daily activities. Driving a car may be a problem initially but with practice the patient may be able to drive with only one eye and with no particular difficulty.

REVIEW QUESTIONS

1. Differentiate retinoblastoma from malignant melanoma of the eye.
2. What is the most common type of intraocular malignancy?
3. List six signs and symptoms of retinoblastoma and of malignant eye melanoma.
4. Define enucleation and exenteration.

5. Explain the postoperative care of the patient with an exenteration of the orbit.
6. Give three complications of enucleation or exenteration.
7. Describe how to insert and remove a prosthetic eyeball.
8. How should the patient care for the prosthetic eyeball?

REFERENCES

1. Shafer, K., et al., Medical-Surgical Nursing. 5th ed., C.V. Mosby Co., St. Louis (1971).
2. Albert, C., et al., Tumors of the Eye. In: Clinical Oncology for Medical Students and Physicians. Rubin, P. and Bakemeier, R., (eds.), The University of Rochester School of Medicine and Dentistry and American Cancer Society, pp. 359-376 (1974).
3. Brunner, L. and Suddarth, D., Textbook of Medical-Surgical Nursing. J.B. Lippincott Co., New York (1975).
4. Smith, D. and Germain, C., Care of the Adult Patient: Medical Surgical Nursing. J.B. Lippincott Co., Philadelphia (1975).
5. Ruben, M., Contact Lenses, Shells, and Prosthesis. Nursing Times, 68:133 (February, 1972).

CHAPTER 37

Neuroblastoma (Sympathoblastoma)

Neuroblastoma is a highly malignant age-specific neoplasm which peaks during the first five years of life. It is considered the second or third most common solid tumor in infancy and early childhood. One third of all cases are believed to occur in infancy. The mode of spread is by local invasion which occurs early in the disease and by hematologic and lymphatic routes with distant metastases into the skin, lungs, liver, orbital bones, the skull, and rarely the brain. Mortality and cure rate are related to the age of occurrence. Five-year survivals of 70 to 90% have occurred in children under two years old and some cases of spontaneous regression of the tumors in this age group have been cited in various case reports.

ETIOLOGY

The neoplasm originates from neuroblasts that form the adrenal medulla or from any of the primitive or mature cells of the sympathetic ganglia. It is believed that mutational transformation of the normal cells occurs due to genetic predisposition or due to carcinogens. Some case reports also indicate that neuroblastoma is usually associated with other congenital conditions and that the child is also susceptible to the development of secondary tumors. The role of the immune system has also been cited in clinical studies which revealed the presence of specific immune complexes related to the disease.

CLINICAL MANIFESTATIONS

The presenting signs and symptoms of the disease are directly related to the involved part, its location, and the presence of metastases.

1. General manifestations
   a. Anorexia
   b. Nausea
   c. Vomiting

     d. Diarrhea
     e. Weight loss
     f. Failure to thrive
     g. Hypertension.
2. Local signs and symptoms
     a. Presence of a fixed, firm, solid mass in the neck (which may or may not be associated with Horner's syndrome)
     b. Referred pain down nerve roots
     c. Unilateral or bilateral and symmetrical abdominal mass
     d. Abdominal distension
     e. Cracked-pot sound on percussion of the skull
     f. Subcutaneous nodules.
3. Metastatic signs and symptoms
     a. Increased intracranial pressure
     b. Proptosis (exophthalmos) of the eyeball
     c. Periorbital ecchymosis
     d. Bone pain
     e. Delayed walking
     f. Paraplegia
     g. Hepatomegaly
     h. Dysphagia
     i. Tracheobronchitis.

DIAGNOSTIC TESTS

Besides the presenting signs and symptoms, the following tests may be done to confirm the diagnosis.

1. Chest x-rays: Thoracic tumors may be seen; rib involvement shows erosion or separation.
2. Bone x-ray: May reveal pathologic fractures or multiple lytic lesions with a moth-eaten appearance.
3. Intravenous urogram: Lateral and downward displacement of the kidney may be seen.
4. Arteriography: Shows outline of the tumor.
5. Bone marrow exam: Shows characteristic rosette cells or anaplastic neuroblasts.
6. Catecholamines: Elevated in functioning medullary tumors.

TREATMENT MODALITIES

Oncologists advocate total surgical removal of the tumor followed by deep megalovoltage radiation and use of folic acid antagonists, doxorubicin HCl (Adriamycin), vincristine, and cyclophosphamide. Other treatment protocols include:

1. Preoperative radiation.
2. Palliative radiation to orbital and other bone lesions.
3. Radiation therapy which has been used successfully as a primary mode of treatment. Neuroblastomas are highly radiosensitive, therefore cure may be effected by radiation.

NURSING IMPLICATIONS

The care of the child includes concern for the significant others in his immediate environment. The nurse acts as a liaison between the patient and his family, grandparents, and other members of the treatment team. The operative care of the child has been discussed in other chapters. General principles of care during infancy and early childhood should include the following approaches.

Sensory Stimulation

The infant needs appropriate stimuli in order to elicit a desirable response. The infant's responses to aversive stimuli should be assessed. Over the crib or overbed hanging, colorful objects or mobile and musical objects should be provided.[3]

Establishment of Trust and Reduction of Separation Anxiety

The most significant person to the infant is his mother. Adequate mothering should be maintained so that the infant achieves the sense of trust. Touch and cuddling, identifying the meaning of his cry and meeting his needs for comfort lead to the development of security and trust. The child who goes in and out of the hospital for palliative treatments of exacerbations of the disease should be given continuity of care. As much as possible a primary nurse for the child should be designated from the very beginning of his hospitalization. The primary nurse assesses his unique needs and establishes a rapport with him. She develops a trusting and therapeutic relationship with him and his family. This type of relationship is one of the priorities of care. In dealing with the child, the nurse and the other health care givers should pay close attention to the child's reaction to his illness. The child's reaction depends on his particular type of illness and its treatment, his personality, his developmental tasks or struggles, his previous experiences with illness and dying, and the reactions of his family and the significant persons in his environment.[5]

Specific Reaction to Acute And Chronic Illness

Those caring for the child with sudden, acute illness should be aware that the preschool child may show reactions to changes in body image, may become confused and frightened by the disease and hospitalization, may manifest regressive behavior and withdrawal, and may not understand why he is ill. Chronic illness carries with it the process of grieving which the child can experience and/or perceive from his family and those caring for him. The nurse should be alert to the development of mother/child symbiosis whereby the husband/father relationship becomes ignored or neglected The nurse should recognize the other extreme reaction of total neglect of the child by a parent, which usually stems from persistent denial of the child's condition and situation. Adequate and honest explanation of the disease process, treatment, and prognosis should be given and periodically reinforced by the nurse.

REVIEW QUESTIONS

1. Differentiate neuroblastoma from pheochromocytoma and Wilms' tumor.
2. List some signs and symptoms of neuroblastoma:
   a. General manifestations
   b. Local signs and symptoms
   c. Metastatic signs and symptoms.
3. Discuss possible x-ray findings in neuroblastoma with or without metastases.
4. Discuss general principles of care for the hospitalized infant and preschooler.

REFERENCES

1. Clark, C., The 1975 Year Book of Cancer. Year Book Medical Publishers, Chicago, p. 250 (1975).
2. Chung, H., et al., Abnormalities of the Immune System in Children with Neuroblastoma Related to the Neoplasm and Chemotherapy. J. Pediat., pp. 548-554 (February, 1977).
3. Hutchinson, J., Practical Pediatric Problems. Lloyd-Luke Medical Publications, London, pp. 177-179 (1967).
4. Knudson, A. and Meadows, A., Developmental Genetics of Neuroblastoma. J. Nat. Cancer Inst., pp. 675-682 (September, 1976).
5. Scipien, C., et al., Comprehensive Pediatric Nursing. McGraw Hill Book Company, New York (1975).
6. Silver, H., et al., Handbook of Pediatrics. Lange Medical Publishers, Palo Alto, CA (1975).

7. Kramer, S., et al., Bilateral Adrenal Neuroblastoma. Cancer, 45(8):2208-2212 (April, 1980).
8. Evans, A.E., A Review of 17 IV-S Neuroblastoma Patients at the Children's Hospital of Philadelphia. Cancer, 45(5): 833-839 (March, 1980).
9. Lopez, R., et al., Treatment of Adult Neuroblastoma. Cancer, 45(5):840-844 (March, 1980).

CHAPTER 38
Nutrition and Cancer

Dietary consumption, preparation, and storage of food are linked to the occurrence, treatment, and prevention of cancer. Replicated research provides ample evidence of a definite association of food, food additives and contaminants, vitamins, chemicals, and food coloring with specific cancers and treatments. Although some of the findings are conflicting and controversial due to uncontrolled rival causative factors and nonrandomized samples, there are specific forms of cancer which have been linked to nutritional elements such as gastric carcinoma; oropharyngeal and esophageal cancers; carcinomas of the breast, lung, and liver; lymphosarcomas, and osteogenic sarcomas.[1-10]

The foods and vitamins which have shown direct or indirect causal relationships with the above-mentioned cancers include: refined carbohydrates; sugar; sodium cyclamate; benzypyrene in coffee beans, bread and smoked foods; certain nuts; talc-treated rice; animal proteins; fats and reheated fats used in cooking; peas; fruits; stored or cured foods from which aflatoxin B_1 is formed, and a multiple list of vitamins.[1,3,9,10]

In light of the confirmed relationships between nutritional elements and cancer occurrence, the progression or rate of growth of cancerous tissue, and treatment effects and survival rate of patients, the significance of nutritional adjunctive therapy has had a tremendous impact in the holistic multidisciplinary care of cancer patients. There is growing evidence that maintaining, restoring, and forced enhancing of the patient's nutritional status improve the overall response of the patient to his illness and therapy. Moreover, lifespan has increased and the quality of life for the patient has become more meaningful and less pain-laden. Nonetheless, there is a persistent controversy among researchers relative to the cause-effect relationships between food and cancer.

One example of this is the effect of forced feeding or hyperalimentation in increasing or decreasing tumor growth rate. In a similar vein, studies concerning vitamins and other minerals and chemicals are still inexact and have bipolar effects. Thus, research findings cannot be conclusive in all situations.

Despite the controversial findings, it is important to recognize the value of data gathered in planning the therapeutic intervention. Some of the relevant data from the most recent research follow.

CAUSAL RELATIONSHIP BETWEEN NUTRITION AND CANCER

Vitamin C

Megadoses of vitamin C (orthomolecular therapy) of up to 10 gm daily have been claimed by some researchers to have effected prolongation of life, reduction of urinary hydroxyproline, tumor regression, pain relief from skeletal muscle metastasis, and reduced need for high opiate dosage. The interactional relationships between vitamin C and vitamin B_{12} in carcinogenesis has also been documented. The need for vitamin C therapy has become controversial in light of research findings that indicate increased tumor growth rate in guinea pigs and in providing protection of lung cells against abnormal growth and malignant transformations induced by marijuana and tobacco smoking. Some findings also indicate that normal amounts of dietary intake of ascorbic acid alleviate certain effects of some other forms of cancer. It should be noted that megadoses of vitamin C or prolonged daily intake of 1 gm may cause changes in the bone marrow by suppression of normal levels of vitamin B_{12}. Moreover, it is speculated that vitamin C may provide cell protection from radiotherapy due to hypoxia resulting from increased oxygen consumption produced by the interaction of ascorbate and radiation-induced chemicals.[8]

Vitamin A

Vitamin A and its synthetic analogues (retinoids) are considered as "chemopreventive" by blocking critical metabolic pathways to tumor genesis. This claim is supported by a study of 8000 Norwegian male smokers whose low vitamin A intake was associated with the incidence of lung cancer. There are also laboratory experiments that indicate that retinoids control cell differentiation and growth in tissue cultures from the bladder, kidney, bronchi, trachea, pancreas, skin, uterus, testis, and prostate.

Vitamin E

Vitamin E, which is an antioxidant, is believed to afford lipo-protein structural protection and/or oxidation of liquid components. Administration of supplemental vitamin E to patients during the course of doxorubicin HCl (Adriamycin) therapy have reduced cardiotoxicity of the drug.[5]

Vitamin K

Vitamin K and its antagonist have been investigated in relation to cancer metastasis. There is some conclusive evidence that vitamin K and its antagonist have a role in carcinogenesis. Addition of phenprocoumon in the drinking water in mice produced spontaneous reduction of lung metastasis from Lewis lung carcinoma.

Vitamin B6

Vitamin B6, which is essential in antibody formation and cell-mediated immunity, has been studied specifically in relation to decrease in serum levels in advanced carcinoma and drug therapy. Prevention of recurrence of stage I bladder cancer and the toxic effects of 5-fluorouracil (5-FU) and mitomycin-C used in the treatment of primary and metastatic liver carcinoma have been achieved with pyridoxine administration.

Vitamin B12

Vitamin B12 still has an unclear relationship with carcinogenesis. In certain conditions, this vitamin may increase lifespan; in others it may accelerate disease progression or tumor growth. It has also been documented that high vitamin B12 serum levels in liver cancer usually indicate poor prognosis.

Other Vitamins and Compounds

1. Vitamin B2 (riboflavin), niacin, and thiamine have been considerably researched but results are also inconclusive and conflicting. Riboflavin deficiencies have inhibited tumor growth in man and animals as well as stimulated carcinogenic effects of some chemicals.
2. Interferon as a treatment for cancer was accorded the largest treatment research grant of $2 million by the American Cancer Society in 1978.[5] The effectiveness of interferon against herpes zoster, viral hepatitis, and chicken pox have been proven. Unexpected prevention of recurrence of certain cancers such as non-Hodgkin's lymphoma, slow-growing

lymphatic cancer, and osteogenic sarcoma have also occurred. International meetings on the uses of interferon were held in 1979. Some research has been conducted on its topical use in skin and cervical cancers, analysis of the 180 amino acids that comprise interferon, mixing two forms of crude interferon which potentiates its effectiveness by a factor of 100, and isolating human gene(s) that produce interferon.[4,6,8] The development of synthetic analogues or interferon potentiators are likely within the next four to five years. It is hoped that such compounds would help alleviate the high cost of cancer treatment. Thus far, it costs $20.00 to $25.00 per million units of interferon. This is astronomically expensive, since one unit is required to treat a single cancer cell and multi-million units would be necessary to treat an advanced metastatic cancer.

The effects of interferon are currently being tested at 10 medical centers across the United States. Some 70 patients who have not responded to conventional treatment to their advanced carcinoma are being given tiny quantities of the drug. In March, 1980 the first data from these tests were revealed with very good results. Of 11 patients with multiple myeloma, a cancer of the bone marrow, three had their tumors shrink substantially. In the case of those with metastatic breast carcinoma, seven out of 16 patients showed noticeable improvement, five of them enough to be considered as partial remissions (Time, March 31, 1980, p. 61). Due to these promising results, various drug companies have taken interest in the development of new mass production techniques of interferon. To date, scientists estimate that a pound of interferon would cost between $10 and $20 billion. This is attributed to the painstaking effort involved in its production, such that only 400 mg (0.014 oz) were obtained from 45,000 liters (90,000 pints) of blood in 1979.

In summary, there is sufficient evidence provided by clinical research data on the association of nutritional factors with cancer and its treatment to indicate the following advantages:

1. Reduction in tumor growth.
2. Increased survival rates and prolongation of quality of life.
3. Decreased side effects of chemotherapy and radiation therapy.
4. Increased tolerance to combined treatment modalities or combination chemotherapy.
5. Increased or restoration of immunocompetence.

Thus, many cancer centers and oncologists are implementing nutritional therapy as adjunctive therapy to either surgery, chemotherapy, or radiation therapy. Specific research findings, however, need not be generalized as apropos to all situations and conditions. A thorough assessment of the individual patient, his needs and active participation in the treatment process, the availability of resources and facilities for care, and the prognosis of the disease should constitute the parameters for the implementation of nutritional therapy. Moreover, each institution may develop certain protocols to follow in the implementation of adjunctive nutritional therapy. An example of such protocol is the use of intravenous hyperalimentation (IVH) 7 to 10 days prior to surgery. In some instances, IVH may also be required for a certain length of time prior to and in conjunction with chemotherapy or radiotherapy. A suggested guideline in assessing the need for supplemental or forced enhancement of nutrients is shown in Table 19.

Nutritional derangement may be caused by chemical effects produced by the cancer, tumor-host competition for nutrients, sequelae of surgery, and toxicity of chemotherapy and/or radiotherapy. Specifically, altered nutrition-enzyme systems may be grouped under:[1,2,9,12-15]

1. Inadequate food ingestion
   a. Nausea, vomiting, anorexia (which may be due to intermediary metabolites produced by the cancer and mobilized lipids which depress the appetite-regulatory center in the hypothalamus).[3]
   b. Psychoemotional causes, such as depression.
   c. Abnormal taste and food smell.
   d. Difficulty in masticating, swallowing due to decreased saliva, xerostemia, gum shrinkage, stomatitis, dental deterioration, and radical surgery of the head, neck, and/or upper GI tract.
2. Altered digestion and absorption
   a. Postgastrectomy disturbances, such as dumping syndrome.
   b. Villous atrophy of the GI tract.
   c. Alimentary diversion and massive GI resections.
   d. Protein-losing enteropathy caused by some intestinal cancers and lymphomas.
   e. Pancreatic enzyme disturbances.
   f. Gastrointestinal fistulas.
   g. Local effects of radiotherapy.
   h. Systemic effects of chemotherapy and radiotherapy.
   i. Carcinoid syndrome
   j. Complete bowel obstruction.

Table 19: Assessment Parameters for Nutrition Therapy

Specific Indicators	Individual Patient Needs
Weight loss (10% or more) Anergic reaction to recall antigen skin test Decreased immunoglobulins Serum albumin below 3.4 gm% Protein losing enteropathy Postgastrectomy syndrome Ileus or intestinal obstruction Gastrocolic and enterocolic fistula Extended chemotherapy Head and neck and GI surgery Cachexia	Physical: Negative nitrogen balance, concurrent disabilities, one or more of the indicators Psychoemotional: Receptivity of patient and family, risk-benefit factors in terms of possible complications and cost, home care services and other support systems, cultural and religious constraints Nutritional history: Dietary habits, including preparation, temperature of foods and liquids, meal schedule (if on elemental feedings), special foods that symbolize nurturing, feeding assistance and assistive devices (e.g., dentures, appliances), use of drug appetizers, antiemetics, and pain relief prior to meals (analgesics given routinely rather than as necessary), socialization during meal time

Nutritional enhancers or repleters may be administered in the form of elemental feedings (commercially prepared complete nutrient foods such as Vivonex) via tube feedings through a nasopharyngeal tube, gastrostomy tube, esophagostomy tube, jejunostomy or pharyngoesophagostomy tubes. In considering this method of feeding, it should be noted that the patient's ability to metabolize the nutrients and the risk of aspiration must be carefully assessed and monitored closely. Elemental feedings also have other side effects such as diarrhea which may be due to rapid administration, volume, and consistency of the feeding. Thus, the rate of flow, consistency, and specific nutrients to be given (e.g., lactose and milk) as well as the amount per feeding must be tailored to the patient's individual needs. The rationale for the use of elemental feedings, such as stimulation of biliary and pancreatic secretions, augmentation of intestinal luminal mass by direct epithelial cell contact with food, and stimulation of other enzyme-systems in the gastro-intestinal tract, must outweigh the side effects.

Intravenous hyperalimentation (IVH) is a method of choice in most instances. IVH can now be administered in home-care settings and hospices. For the nursing care of the patient receiving IVH, see Part VI, Chapter 39.

HOLISTIC CARE OF THE PATIENT

Central to the nutritional concerns of the cancer patient is the role of the nutritionist. This is specifically needed in the use of elemental feedings, although the nurse still assumes a key role in the nutritional assessment and monitoring of the patient. The cancer care team have distinct yet interrelated and mutually goal-directed roles.

REVIEW QUESTIONS

1. Discuss the indications for nutritional adjunctive therapy.
2. List 10 specific indicators for nutrition therapy.
3. Cite some research findings related to the use of interferon and vitamins in cancer treatment.
4. List four therapeutic results of forced-nutrient feedings.
5. Explain why the nutritional assessment of the cancer patient is necessary in his holistic care.

REFERENCES

1. Nutrition and Cancer. American Cancer Society, New York (1972).
2. Bjelke, E., Dietary Vitamin A and Human Lung Cancer. Int. J. Cancer, 15:561-565 (1975).
3. Burkhalter, P. and Donley, D., Dynamics of Oncology Nursing, McGraw-Hill Book Co., New York (1978).
4. Cameron, E., et al., Ascorbic Acid and Cancer: A Review. Cancer Res., 39:663-681 (1979).
5. Cancer News, The American Cancer Society, New York (Winter, 1980).
6. Copeland, E.M., et al., Effect of Intravenous Hyperalimentation on Established Delayed Hypersensitivity in the Cancer Patient. Ann. Surg., 184:60-64 (1976).
7. Copeland, E.M., Intravenous Hyperalimentation as an Adjunct to Cancer Patient Management. CA, 6:322-330 (October, 1979).
8. DiPalma, J.R. and McMichael, R., The Interaction of Vitamins with Cancer Chemotherapy. CA, 5:280-286 (September/October, 1979).

9. Kellog, C.J. and Sullivan, B.P., Current Perspectives in Oncologic Nursing, Vol. 2, C.V. Mosby Co., St. Louis (1978).

10. Lipkin, M., Dietary, Environmental and Hereditary Factors in the Development of Colorectal Cancer. CA, 6:322-330 (November/December, 1978).

11. Potera, C., et al., Vitamin B_6 Deficiency in Cancer Patients. Am. J. Clin. Nutr., 30:1677-1679 (1977).

12. Shils, M.E., Enteral Nutrition by Tube. Cancer Res., 37:2432-2439 (1977).

13. Shils, M.E., Enteral Nutritional Management of the Cancer Patient. CA, 2:78-83 (March/April, 1979).

14. Theologides, A., Pathogenesis of Cachexia in Cancer. A Review and a Hypothesis. Cancer, 29:484-488 (1972).

15. Theologides, A., Anorexia-Producing Intermediary Metabolites. Am. J. Clin. Nutr., 29:552-558 (1976).

16. Time Magazine. March 31, 1980, p. 61.

PART VI
Cancer Metastases and Management

CHAPTER 39
Metastatic Cancer and Related Management

It is common knowledge that a malignant neoplastic growth manifests itself mostly by pressure upon adjacent organs, obstruction, and distortion of organs and tissues resulting in interference with functions and body processes. Major, nonspecific manifestations of cancer include bleeding, cachexia, pleural and peritoneal effusions, infections (of the tumor and of the host due to decreased immune response) and anemia.

Metastatic cancer, regardless of its primary site, will invariably present any or all of the major, nonspecific symptoms listed in the preceding paragraph. Approximately 60 to 80% of patients with cancer will have disseminated cancer during their lifespan that will necessitate medical and nursing (interdisciplinary) interventions. The problems of cancer metastases can be broadly categorized as follows:

1. Target organ effects which comprise the signs and symptoms of local organ involvement.
2. Systemic effects which refer to those clinical manifestations that occur as remote effects of the malignant neoplasm.

TARGET ORGAN EFFECTS
AND MANAGEMENT

Lung

The most common metastatic site which may involve solitary or multiple lesions is the lung. Management comprises the following:

1. Surgical excision for solitary or few nodular lesions after extirpation of the primary neoplasm.
2. Radiation therapy if primary neoplasm is radiosensitive, i.e., Wilms' tumor and lymphomas.
3. Chemotherapy in combination with radiotherapy.

4. Thoracentesis for small pleural effusion and chest tube drainage for large effusions followed by instillation of chemotherapeutic drugs, which may include antibiotics such as tetracycline and antineoplastic drugs such as nitrogen mustard.[1]

It is important to note that if the lung lesions (tumors) are responsive to the treatment, tumor necrosis can occur causing complications which include hemoptysis and/or pneumothorax. Large pneumothorax can lead to heart and major vessel compression as well as opposite lung compression due to mediastinal shift resulting in cardiopulmonary embarrassment. Check for the presence of: tachypnea, dyspnea, chest pain, tachycardia, restlessness and anxiety, and lack of fremitus (vibration) when the patient speaks. (To check for fremitus, place hands on thorax and let patient speak. Normally, vibration is felt. Decreased or absence of vibration may indicate large accumulation of air and tracheal displacement into the contralateral side of the pneumothorax.) A substantial atelectasis or obstruction of the bronchus will cause an ipsilateral displacement of the trachea.

Emergency management can be effectively instituted by inserting a 16 to 18 gauge needle (connected to a three-way stopcock) into the anterior and intercostal space below the clavicle at the midline. Air escaping from the needle will produce a hissing sound. When indicated, a chest tube connected to a water-seal drainage may be used.

Bone

Metastases of bone are very rarely solitary. Severe pain and pathological fractures can occur. Management comprises the following:[2]

1. Radiation is the treatment of choice for bone pain when occurrence of pathological fracture is not likely.
2. Chemotherapy using alkylating agents (bone metastases are more responsive to these agents).
3. Hormonal manipulation is used more effectively if primary cancer is from the breast or prostate.
4. Internal fixation of long-bone fractures, bed rest and corsets for spine and pelvic fractures, and casts may be used for distal-end fractures of the extremities.

Spinal Cord

Direct involvement of the spinal cord does not usually occur but compression may result from tumors of the spine, most commonly associated with lymphomas and Hodgkin's disease. When infarction of the cord itself has developed, there is no effective management, since regeneration does not occur. Depending on the location of spinal cord arrest, death, quadriplegia, or paraplegia will ensue. Therefore, suspicion of spinal cord compression manifested by leg weakness, paresthesias, and sometimes bowel and bladder symptoms should be confirmed by myelography to localize cord involvement. Depending on the level of compression, the following procedures may be utilized:

1. Surgical decompression via a laminectomy.
2. Radiotherapy, which is particularly effective in slow-developing paresis and primary cancers such as oat cell, neuroblastoma, Wilms' and lymphomas.
3. Corticosteroids, though controversial in their use, may be given for palliation of edema.

Liver

Metastases in the liver are also rarely solitary. Depending on the degree of involvement, metabolic and enzyme systems are altered and ascites becomes a problem. Management comprises the following:[1]

1. Chemotherapy is employed. Drug of choice depends on the tissue origin of the tumor and drug administration may be either systemically or by hepatic artery infusion.
2. Radiation therapy may be used for pain palliation, although caution is exercised due to the adverse effects of the treatment such as worsening of the hepatic function which can lead to hepatic coma and death.

Malignant Effusions

The accumulation of fluids in the lung, pericardial space, and peritoneal cavity may result from lung and liver involvement as well as irritations of serous membranes from solid tumor implants or by obstruction of lymphatics and small vessels. Management comprises the following:[1]

1. Peritoneal effusion (ascites) may be treated by using intracavitary instillation of chemotherapeutic drugs or by placing radioactive isotope in cases where the ascitic has a cell count greater than 4000 cells/ml.

2. Diuretics are used for indirect control of fluid accumulation.
3. Pericardial effusion may be treated by needle aspiration. For long-term control or prevention of pericardial effussion, a pericardiectomy or pericardial window is created.

Gastrointestinal

Any portion of the GI tract may be involved by contiguous extension or by metastasis giving rise to obstruction. Management comprises the following:[1]

1. Radiation therapy is best used for obstruction of the esophagus or rectum.
2. Surgical decompression for small and large intestines.
3. Adjuvant use of tube decompression proximal to the obstruction.
4. Enteroenterostomy to bypass the obstruction when surgical resection is contraindicated or when the mesentery or several loops of the bowel are involved.

Brain

Personality and behavioral changes will give clues to brain involvement. Brain scan will establish the diagnosis. Management comprises the following:[1]

1. Radiation therapy and corticosteroids, either alone or in combination, work best for the majority of patients.
2. Steroids alone are preferred by most authorities when the lifespan is somewhere between one and two months.

The above management thus far has shown no evidence of increasing length of survival, but the quality of survival has improved. Health care givers should understand and condone the unpredictable behavior of the patient. A colleague who was helping take care of her hospitalized friend undergoing radiation therapy for brain metastases once said, "I understand . . . but what can I do? Shall I reason it out with her? Be firm in explaining why she is angry with me?" Previous rapport or therapeutic relationship may not guarantee a solution to the barrage of emotional or behavioral displays at the particular moment. One eventually tailors his specific approach after a careful and thorough assessment of the situation, although in most instances the unpredictable behavior does not follow a specific pattern. Rational explanations may work or you may just simply remain attentively with the patient during his emotional outburst or crisis.

SYSTEMIC EFFECTS
AND MANAGEMENT

Anemia

This may be due to multiple etiology and mechanisms, including:

1. Hemolysis and nonhemolytic shortening of RBC survival from either effects of chemotherapy, radiation therapy, or other toxic metabolites.
2. Blood loss due to bleeding from the tumor or as sequela of therapy.
3. Autoimmune hemolysis which is most often associated with chronic lymphocytic leukemia or lymphomas.
4. Decreased red cell production due to bone marrow depression and/or decreased erythropoietin production by the kidneys.
5. Insufficient iron and folic acid intake.

Management of the anemia includes blood transfusion (packed red cells as needed), specific tumor therapy, folic acid, multivitamin and iron supplements, as well as minerals. Decreasing oxygen consumption and mental activity readjustments are imperative in the overall patient management.

Fever and Infection

Fever is most common with hematologic malignancies, especially leukemia. The presence of fever heralds a fatal disease. Infection is associated with the depression of the host defense mechanisms induced by the malignancy or by chemotherapy and radiation therapy. Depression of the humoral immune response from chemotherapy, lymphosarcoma, multiple myeloma, or lymphatic leukemias makes the patient susceptible to the pathogens pneumococci, streptococci, hemophilus influenza, and Pseudomonas aeruginosa. Depression of the cellular immune response caused by chemotherapy or radiation therapy, corticosteroids, Hodgkin's disease, or advanced cancer causes the individual to be more susceptible to fungus infection (e.g., candidiasis), viral infection (e.g., herpes), tuberculosis, and Pneumocystis carini.[1]

Management of the patient with fever includes use of hyperthermia blanket and antipyretics, most commonly acetaminophen (Tylenol). Aspirin should be avoided as it can cause abrupt lysis of fever, which may be accompanied by hypotension.[1] Antibiotic therapy is based on results of culture and sensitivity.

Antiviral chemotherapy is still limited in its clinical application due to its toxic effects on the cells. The signs and symptoms of the viral infection only become apparent after the peak replication of the virus in the body and the course of the disease has been established. Some drugs which have been used are:

1. Amantadine hydrochloride (Symmetrel), which has prophylactic effects on certain myxoviruses such as some tumor viruses, rubella, and influenza A.
2. Idoxuridine (Dendrid, Herplex, Stoxil) which inhibits replication of some viruses and is primarily used in the treatment of herpes simplex keratitis.[3]

Antifungal chemotherapy is not as well developed as antibacterial therapy. The most commonly used drugs are:

1. Amphotericin B (Fungizone) is an antibiotic agent but is both fungistic and fungicidal and has no direct effect on bacteria or viruses but is the only effective drug for treating very deep fungal disease. Very little absorption of the drug occurs in oral, subcutaneous, or intramuscular administration. Therefore, intravenous administration is the method of choice. Monitor the patient for the concomitant drug-induced fever, chills, headache, and vomiting as well as renal and hepatic dysfunction resulting in anemia, shocklike syndrome, electrolyte imbalance, and various neurologic symptoms. These side effects may be minimized by temporarily reducing the dosage and administering corticosteroids, slowly increasing the dosage, and administering the drugs on alternate days. Another important thing to remember is to refrain from mixing amphotericin with any other drug.[3]

2. Griseofulvin (Fulvicin, Arifulin), which has toxic effects that are relatively low. Leukopenia, headache, photosensitivity, and mild hepatic dysfunction can occur. It is important to know and remember that concurrent use of phenobarbital reduces the effectiveness of the drug while milk and other fatty foods enhance the absorption of the orally administered drug.[3]

3. Nystatin (Mycostatin) is an antibiotic obtained from Streptomyces noursei. It is primarily used for Candida Albicans. It may be given by suppository or topically as cream, powder, or ointment, or it may be given orally for suppression of candidiasis of the bowel. Although side effects

are uncommon, mild gastrointestinal discomfort from oral administration may occur.

Hypercoaguability

The mechanism for the hypercoaguability in the cancer patient is not well delineated. However, considerable evidence show that tumor cells release thromboplastic substances into the blood stream. Deep venous thrombophlebitis and thromboembolic problems in extreme form are known as disseminated intravascular clotting (DIC).[1] Management of the patient includes:[1]

1. Ambulation as much as feasible.
2. Heparin administered intravenously. The dose requirement is higher for cancer patients.
3. Oral anticoagulants are useful for chronic treatment for thromboembolic problems other than DIC.

Hypercalcemia

This can develop in 10% of all cancer patients resulting from either bone metastases or ectopic production of parathormone with squamous cell carcinoma of the lung and hypernephroma. Management of the patient includes:[1]

1. Restriction of calcium intake in the diet.
2. Hydration and steroids.
3. Other drugs
   a. Mithramycin (blocks osteoclastic activities): Side effects include nausea and liver and bone marrow dysfunction.
   b. Thyrocalcitonin (inhibits osteoclasts): Side effects include nausea and flushing.
   c. Phosphate (helps increase calcium deposition in bones): Side effects include ectopic calcification in kidneys.[1] Furosemide (Lasix) or Ethocrynic acid (edecrin) to induce forced calciuresis: Side effects include severe diarrhea, vertigo, tinnitus, permanent or temporary deafness, and electrolyte imbalance.

Pain

This is very real in the cancer patient. Long-term management is tailored to the individual patient. In general, a program of mild to potent analgesics, sedatives, and narcotics are used with the usual fashion of starting from aspirin (acetaminophen (Tylenol), oxycodone (Percodan), hydromorphone (Dilaudid),

morphine or meperidine (Demerol). The important thing to remember is that tolerance, on the average, occurs only after
two to three months of continued 3 to 4 hour usage. Incremen-
tal increase in the dosage may be necessary. Addiction should
not be of prime concern; rather, relief of the pain should be.
If localized pain cannot be adequately controlled, intrathecal
injection of cold saline may help. For severe, excruciating intractable pain, a cordotomy or a rhizotomy may be performed.

Anorexia, Nausea and Vomiting

These may be due to an unexplained mechanism produced by the
malignancy or it may be due to:

1. Effects of chemotherapy and/or radiation therapy.
2. Pressure or reflex stimulation of the sensory receptors of
   visceral organs (such as the kidneys and uterus), the gastrointestinal tract, the heart, and semicircular canals of
   the ears.
3. Pain, some narcotics, e.g., morphine sulphate and meperidine (Demerol), unpleasant odor, tastes, sight, and thoughts
   can initiate the vomiting reflex.
4. Anorexia is attributed to abnormalities in taste. Studies
   have shown that patients have an elevated threshold of sweet
   taste and a lowered threshold for bitter taste.

Management of the patient includes sweetening the foods, and
serving cheese and other high-protein foods, since with the increased intolerance to bitter taste patients complain that meat
taste bad. Avoid or minimize unpleasant odors, tastes, and
other initiators of vomiting reflex. Antiemetics administered
by rectal suppository would help decrease the episodes of anorexia and vomiting. (Oral forms may only be included in the
vomitus if the patient vomits, and injections can cause bleeding
due to the thrombocytopenia.) Other measures include deep
breathing and swallowing, drinking appropriate fluids, and avoiding hot or acidic fluids in the presence of buccal ulcerations.

Cachexia

This is usually characterized by wasting of body tissues and
hypermetabolic state attributed to the increased metabolic demands of the neoplasm and the effects of the tumor by-products.

Management of the patient is directed to optimum tumor treatment modality and induction of remission of signs and symptoms of cancer. Overall many terminally ill and cachetic patients who are unable to maintain nutrition to sustain life may

receive total body nutrition by administering parenteral hyper-alimentation (HA) fluids. The fluids consist of a balanced appropriate mixture of glucose, water, protein hydrolysates or amino acids, vitamins, electrolytes, and minerals in order to supply the body with the required calories and nitrogen. Specific nursing care should include:

1. Maintain flow rate as ordered. Full strength hyperal fluids have 20% glucose. The rate of infusion is gradually increased to allow the patient to increase his insulin production as his glucose intake increases.

2. Check for blood and urine glucose levels. Fractionals are usually done every four hours for the first three to four days (may vary with institution's protocol) followed by an eight-hour interval. A 4-plus glycosuria and elevated serum glucose may necessitate insulin administration. In the absence of a standing order for insulin coverage, the doctor should be notified.

3. Monitor vital signs. Increased temperature may indicate sepsis while an increased central venous pressure (CVP) can indicate fluid overload and heart failure. (The hyperalimentation line should not be used for measuring CVP. The hyperosmolar fluid may not accurately reflect the reading and any interruption of flow rate may cause backflow of blood which can clog the catheter.)

4. Observe for signs of pulmonary edema or circulatory overload: distended neck veins, cough, moist rales, copious frothy sputum, dyspnea, gurgling respirations, and cyanosis.

5. Accurate intake and output, daily weight, and periodic assessment of electrolytes including calcium, magnesium, and phosphorus should be performed and compared with previous parameters to evaluate the effectiveness of therapy.

6. Check and prevent allergic reactions and drug incompatibilities by knowing appropriate admixture of drugs. Antibiotics are never given (mixed) with hyperalimentation fluid. Calcium and bicarbonate cause precipitates. It is always best to use the hyperalimentation line solely for the administration of HA fluids. "Piggybacks" therefore should be connected to other peripheral IV lines.

7. Observe for skin rash which may be indicative of fatty acid deficiency. Topical application of fat-base ointment may be

used and prevention of the deficiency may be achieved by including folic acid in the HA mixture as well as fat-soluble vitamins and parenteral lipid administration.

8. Prevent contamination and sepsis. Almost all hyperalimentation fluids are prepared in the pharmacy under laminar airflow. Heat carmelizes the HA fluid. Refrigeration until 30 minutes prior to administration helps preserve potency. The solution should be prepared shortly before administration and the HA fluid once hung should be given within eight hours. Large volume, e.g., 1 to 2 liter bottles, should be avoided. Interline microfilters are used to filter precipitates, bacteria and microorganisms. A 0.22 μm filter is very effective but it requires the use of IV pumps. Intravascular pumps are readily available, such as IVAC, IMED, VIP, etc. The use of alarm systems to alert the nurse for changes in flow rate and complete infusion of the solution do not preclude close monitoring of the patient and his therapy. Malfunctioning of the pump can occur.

9. Dressing changes and catheter-site skin care varies. Some doctors prefer to use sterile strips to hold the catheter in place and maybe a spray dressing which can be left undisturbed for a number of days as long as there is no sign of infection or leakage. If a 4 x 4 dressing is used, routine changing are prescribed. Aseptic techniques, which include wearing of mask, cap and gloves, are used. The site may be cleaned with hydrogen peroxide or acetone, allowed to dry then providone-iodine (Betadine) solution or ointment is applied before placing the gauze dressing. Some studies have documented that antibiotics, e.g., polymixin B-Bacitracin neomycin (Neosporin) bacitracin routinely used do not prevent infection. The Betadine is effective in preventing bacterial and fungal infections.

10. Do not allow the HA solution to be abruptly discontinued. The patient can go into rebound insulin shock.

11. Observe for signs of air embolism such as cyanosis, hypotension, weak and rapid pulse, fainting and coma. Listen for air being sucked in the HA line. If air embolism occurs, place the patient on his left side in Trendelenberg position or place in prone position.

12. Observe for presence of precipitates in the solution and check expiration date and time of infusion on label. The HA fluid is normally clear yellow.

13. Ensure x-ray visualization to confirm placement of the catheter on superior vena cava. The catheter is most commonly threaded through the following approaches.

   a. The supraclavicular subclavian vein. This is the most convenient readily accessible approach and most dependable for prevention of pneumothorax. Arterial puncture is a possible complication.

   b. The modified infraclavicular approach: The two major complications of this approach are pneumothorax, particularly in patients with apical blebs in the lungs, and detouring of the catheter into the internal jugular vein.

   c. Basilic or arm veins: It is important to have the catheter exited from the skin at least 2 cm away from the point of entrance into the vein. The length of the catheter, preferably silicone which is less likely to cause thrombophlebitis after a prolonged use, can vary from 12 to 24 inches. This is the technique of choice for patients with large veins since it is the safest approach.

   d. Inferior vena cava: This is used when insertion into the superior vena cava is not possible. However, this technique should not be used in the presence of abdominal obstruction and in pelvic and lower extremity infection. The catheter may be inserted percutaneously or by a cutdown into the greater saphenous vein or femoral vein. The tip of the catheter may be placed in either the abdominal portion or supradiaphragmatic portion of the inferior vena cava. The catheter is exited further away on the thigh to minimize occurrence of infection.

   e. Internal jugular vein: This approach is most feasible on those patients who must remain in a prone position. Disadvantages and complications include position changes such as flexion and extension of the neck which can dislodge the catheter, pneumothorax, and arterial puncture of the common carotid.

14. Observe for infiltration of the HA fluid into the soft tissue which may be manifested by edema and swelling over the puncture site, pain in the shoulder and arm, and edema of the neck and face. Refer to Table 19 Chapter 38 for the management of the patient receiving parenteral nutrition.

REVIEW QUESTIONS

1. What is the most common target organ for metastatic cancer?

2. Discuss the management of metastatic lung lesions.
3. Explain why pneumothorax can occur as sequale of treatment.
4. List four signs and symptoms of mediastinal shift.
5. How is spinal cord involvement treated?
6. When is pericardiectomy indicated?
7. Give two palliative measures for peritoneal effusion.
8. When is it necessary to perform enteroenterostomy in cases of gastrointestinal obstructions?
9. Give eight systemic effects of disseminated cancer. Discuss at least two management principles for each systemic effect.
10. List at least eight nursing principles related to the care of the patient receiving intravenous hyperalimentation.

REFERENCES

1. American Cancer Society, Clinical Oncology for Medical Students and Physicians: A Multidisciplinary Approach, 4th ed., New York (1974).
2. Beland, L., Clinical Nursing: Pathophysiological and Psychosocial Approaches, Macmillan Company, New York (1974).
3. Bergensen, B., Pharmacology in Nursing, C.V. Mosby Company, St. Louis (1976).
4. Bilezikian, J., Hypercalcemia: The Changing Clinical Profile. Medical Times, pp. 153-163 (November, 1976).
5. Brunner, L. and Suddarth, D., The Lippincott Manual of Nursing Practice, W.B. Saunders Co., Philadelphia (1974).
6. Cowan, G. and Scheetz, W., Intravenous Hyperalimentation, Lea and Febiger, Philadelphia (1972).
7. Luckman, J. and Sorensen, K.C., Medical-Surgical Nursing: A Psychophysiologic Approach, W.B. Saunders Co., (1974).
8. Montana, G.S., et al., Brain Irradiation for Metastatic Disease of Lung Origin. Cancer, 49:1477-1480 (1972).
9. Peck, S.D. and Reiquan, G.W., Disseminated Intravascular Coagulation in Cancer Patients: The Supportive Evidence. Cancer, 31:1114-1119 (1973).
10. Theologides, A., A Pathogenesis of Cachexia in Cancer. Cancer, 29:484-488 (1972).
11. West, T.E.T., et al., Treatment of Hypercalcemia with Calcitonin. Lancet, pp. 675-678 (April 3, 1971).
12. White, W.A., et al., Role of Surgery in the Treatment of Spinal Cord Compression by Metastatic Neoplasm. Cancer, 27:558-561 (1971).

PART VII

Application of a Multidisciplinary Approach to
Care of the Cancer Patient

CHAPTER 40
Case Studies

CASE STUDY 1

This is a case study demonstrating the multidisciplinary approach to holistic care of the cancer patient.

Situation

Janet Lewis, a 41-year-old woman married to a business executive of a national sales corporation, a devoted Catholic, who lived with her husband and two children in a northern suburb of Chicago, was admitted to the hospital for a breast biopsy, and possible radical mastectomy in June 1979.

Mrs. Lewis' husband traveled frequently to other states for business meetings and conferences, although he tried to be home during weekends. Their two children were both in their early twenties and currently university students.

Upon admission, Mrs. Lewis was accompanied by her husband and her daughter. She was noticeably anxious about her condition and expressed concern that it might be cancerous. Breast biopsy was done, which revealed cancer of the right breast and a modified radical mastectomy was performed.

Postoperatively, Mrs. Lewis had a Hemovac suction for hemoserous drainage of the operative site and returned to her room in satisfactory condition. When her husband saw her for the first time after her recovery from anesthesia, the nurse noticed that Mrs. Lewis could not relate to her husband very well. This was in sharp contrast to the observed closeness preoperatively. As Mrs. Lewis progressed in her recovery, she exhibited signs of depression and anxiety. She was not motivated to participate in her rehabilitation exercises. At times, she was observed not talking to her husband during visiting hours.

Case Analysis	Multidisciplinary Intervention

Preoperative Phase

Mrs. Lewis' anxiety was probably due to fear of death, fear of anesthesia, fear of pain, fear of bodily disfigurement, fear of becoming less of a woman, and fear of the effects of the surgery upon her husband and her family.

Use of the nursing process to unveil the sources of fear (see Postoperative Intervention).

Preoperative visit by the anesthesiologist to explain type of anesthesia and course of anesthetic effects during and after surgery.

Physician's initiative to have a recovered mastectomy patient visit Mrs. Lewis.

Social service and/or psychologist involvement in eliciting adaptive responses to stress and Mrs. Lewis' self-concept.

Being a devoted Catholic, the possibility of cancer was perhaps more than a shock, thereby causing ambivalent feelings about God's justice

Visit by a priest to discuss Mrs. Lewis' feelings and attempt to restrengthen her religious belief.

The frequent travels of her husband could be a source of anxiety for Mrs. Lewis. Perhaps if something goes wrong after her surgery, her husband may not be present. Perhaps, if she ends up with a mastectomy, her husband may not view her as a woman any more and may cause him to look for another in other states (fear of infidelity of partner)

Nurse should initiate an open communication with both Mrs. Lewis and her husband

Assessment of marital relationship and Mrs. Lewis' concept of sexuality by the professional nurse

Involve psychiatric clinical specialist for psychosocial support

Case Analysis	Multidisciplinary Intervention
Postoperative Phase	
Inability of Mrs. Lewis to relate to her husband is a confirmation of her fear of bodily disfigurement, fear of being rejected by her husband, fear of being less than a woman	Identification by the nurse/clinical specialist of Mrs. Lewis' ego strengths, coping mechanisms she can effectively or ineffectively use in a healthy or unhealthy manner, the primary or secondary gains she can derive from the situation, and the adaptation response to her fears.
	Involvement of the psychologist in attempt to reintegrate Mrs. Lewis' self-concept and ego identity.
	Physician's reassurance of the positive prognosis in early cancer detection and surgical intervention.
	Visit by the priest to afford peace of mind and regain confidence and trust in the sanctity of marriage.
Lack of motivation in rehabilitation exercises	Encouragement by the nurse to do her exercises in order to strengthen her affected arm.
	Visit by a recovered mastectomy patient to discuss prosthetic appliances, thereby enhancing Mrs. Lewis' self-concept.
	Involvement of a physical therapist in the rehabilitation process.

CASE STUDY 2

The emphasis of this case study is on the identification of key concepts integrated in the holistic care of the cancer patient and the presentation of one example of interdisciplinary roles and functions from the prediagnostic phase to the bereavement phase of patient-family care.

Situation

Mr. Roy James, a 61-year-old white male business executive, a known cigarette smoker for over 30 years, a devoted Catholic, who lived with his wife upon whom he was very dependent, was scheduled for hip pinning surgery in October 1979. A preoperative chest x-ray revealed a small area of consolidation in the upper lobe. Bronchoscopy and biopsy confirmed the presence of an oat cell carcinoma of the right-upper lobe and right hilar involvement. A scalene node biopsy also was positive.

Mr. James' social history included having children, a son and a daughter. The son was married and had two boys, and the daughter was also married, living in the northern suburb with her self-employed husband and two sons. All of Mr. James' grandchildren were between the ages of 10 and 14. Mr. James' son-in-law had a sister who had died of breast cancer less than a year earlier.

Following diagnosis, Mr. James was placed on a six-week course of chemotherapy consisting of cyclophosphamide, methotrexate, and CCNU (Lomustine).

Followup diagnostic tests and results included: bronchoscopy, which revealed an endobronchial tumor; chest x-ray, which showed middle lobe collapse of the right lung with pleural effusion; bone scan, indicating posterior ribs, right shoulder, and lumbar spine metastases; and antigenic skin tests which were all negative.

Radiation therapy services were not available in the area where Mr. James lived. He and his wife moved in with their daughter for the two courses of radiation treatments, each given for 15 days. The first course of radiation was given following the chemotherapy and the second course was administered for the bone metastases early in January 1980.

Mr. James experienced pain during his illness. Asperin-phenacetin (Emprin) was given initially for pain control and oxycodone HCl (Percodan) was used during the latter part of his terminal illness. Two weeks prior to Mr. James' death, home-care services were made available to him. The daughter was told this care was part of a hospice care program. Mr. James' daughter was with him during the last three days of his life, which he spent in the hospital in his home town while his wife was beside him.

Key Concepts	Sample Interdisciplinary Roles and Functions
Nursing process	Nursing history utilizing the nursing process helped obtain data of long-standing cigarette smoking, germane to importance of preoperative chest x-ray.
Fear of the unknown	Physician's explanation of the need for bronchoscopy and biopsy and what the procedure entails.
	Nurse's open communication with the patient and family to allow expression of feelings and provide emotional support.
Fear of effects of chemotherapy	Explanation and sharing of information regarding the drugs used and side effects by both the nurse and physician
	Nursing interventions specific to side effects experienced by the patient.
Knowledge of radiation	Physician's explanation of the purpose of therapy, number of treatments, as well as expected side effects and potential side effects to patient and family.
	Nurse's reinforcement and clarification of physician's explanation, including procedure and expected outcomes.
	Nurse's attempt to reassure patient and family that he is not radioactive to himself and others so that family can visit.

Key Concepts	Sample Interdisciplinary Roles and Functions
Psychosocial and economic concerns (patient having to move to daughter's home)	Social service representative to discuss the possibility of financial assistance as needed and desired by the patient and family. Psychologist, psychiatric clinical specialist, or psychiatrist's availability as resources for crisis intervention on aspects beyond the nurse's ability to handle
Pain	Nurse's assessment of pain utilizing parameters and measurements as described in Chapter 14. Physician's prescription for medication for pain depends to a great extent upon the nurse's assessment shared with the physician.
Reactions to death and dying	Nurse's identification of the level of awareness of the patient and family of the impending death. Nurse's ability to cope with her own feelings about death influences her ability to meet the needs of the dying patient and his family. Physician has the moral obligation to tell the patient and his family that he is dying. Nurse, social worker, minister, psychiatric clinical specialist, and psychologist providing emotional support can promote a peaceful death.
Death with dignity	Family is informed of availability of hospice care by the physician and nurse. Patient and family are allowed to decide whether to have patient die at home, in a hospice facility, or in the hospital by the multidisciplinary team.